Edwards' Treatr of Drinking Problems

A Guide for the Helping Professions

Edwards' Treatment of Drinking Problems

A Guide for the Helping Professions

Sixth Edition

Keith Humphreys
Anne Lingford-Hughes

With contributions from

Griffith Edwards
Sole author of the first and second editions
Lead author of the third and fourth editions

and

David M. Ball
Co-author of the fifth edition

Christopher Cook
Co-author of the third and fourth editions
Chapter author in the fifth edition

E. Jane Marshall
Co-author of the third, fourth, and fifth editions

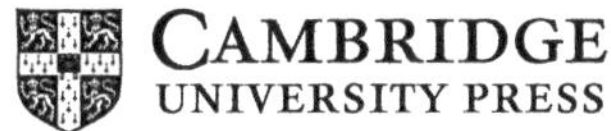

CAMBRIDGE
UNIVERSITY PRESS

University Printing House, Cambridge CB2 8BS, United Kingdom

Cambridge University Press is part of the University of Cambridge.

It furthers the University's mission by disseminating knowledge in the pursuit of education, learning and research at the highest international levels of excellence.

www.cambridge.org
Information on this title: www.cambridge.org/9781107519527

First published in 1982 by Wiley Blackwell
Second edition published in 1985 by McGraw Hill Higher Education
Third edition published in 1997 by Cambridge University Press
Fourth edition published in 2003 by Cambridge University Press
Fifth edition published in 2010 by Cambridge University Press

Printed in the United Kingdom by Clays, St Ives plc

A catalogue record for this publication is available from the British Library

Library of Congress Cataloging-in-Publication data
Humphreys, Keith, author. | Lingford-Hughes, Anne, author. | Edwards, Griffith, author. | Ball, David M., author. | Cook, Chris (Christopher C.H.), author. | Marshall, E. Jane, author.
Edwards' treatment of drinking problems : a guide for the helping professions / Keith Humphreys, Anne Lingford-Hughes; with contributions from Griffith Edwards and David M. Ball, Christopher Cook, E. Jane Marshall.
Treatment of drinking problems.
Sixth edition. | Cambridge, United Kingdom ; New York : Cambridge University Press, [2016] | Preceded by The treatment of drinking problems / E. Jane Marshall, Keith Humphreys, David M. Ball ; with contributions from Griffith Edwards and Christopher Cook. 5th ed. 2010. | Includes bibliographical references and index.
LCCN 2015041410 | ISBN 9781107519527 (pbk.)
| MESH: Alcoholism – therapy. | Alcohol Drinking – adverse effects. | Alcohol Drinking – psychology. | Alcoholics – psychology.
LCC RC565 | NLM WM 274 | DDC 616.86/106–dc23
LC record available at http://lccn.loc.gov/2015041410

ISBN 978-1-107-51952-7 Paperback

This book is dedicated to anyone struggling with a drinking problem

Contents

Acknowledgements and disclosures

The authors are very grateful to Remy Flachais and John Kelly for reviewing drafts of chapters. We also appreciate Janet Blodgett's assiduous work locating and updating scientific references. In addition, we are indebted to both the patients we have cared for and our colleagues in the treatment field for teaching us so much about the subject of this book.

Quite appropriately, it is now expected that authors will disclose their sources of financial support. During the writing of this book, Keith Humphreys was supported by grants from the U.S. Veterans Health Administration, the U.S. National Institute on Alcohol Abuse and Alcoholism, the Michael and Arlene Rosen Foundation, and the Greenwall Foundation. He has never accepted grants or honoraria from the drinks industry or from any manufacturer of medications used to treat drinking problems. Anne Lingford-Hughes received research grants from the UK Medical Research Council and the UK National Institutes of Health Research. She also received research funding from Lundbeck, as well as honoraria for speaking, presentations, and chairing events.

A note on the sixth edition

The Treatment of Drinking Problems: A Guide for the Helping Professions was first published in 1982 as a single-author text by Griffith Edwards, who wrote that he had drawn freely from the "two major resources which must be the foundations of any treatment text – the worlds of clinical experience and of scientific research." Edwards acknowledged the many clinical colleagues with whom he had worked for more than 20 years at the Maudsley and Bethlem Royal Hospitals. The 1982 edition was translated into German, Spanish, Portuguese, Japanese, and Swedish. The second edition appeared in 1987, again as a single-author work. For the third (1997) and fourth (2003) editions, Edwards was joined by Jane Marshall and Christopher Cook as equal partners in the writing team. In 2010, Edwards stepped back from direct authorial involvement and turned the fifth edition over to Marshall and two new authors: David Ball and Keith Humphreys. Humphreys continues as co-author of this sixth edition with a new writing partner, Anne Lingford-Hughes. After a long career as one of the world's foremost authorities on addiction and its treatment, Griffith Edwards passed away in 2012. Because the book he created has been repeatedly revised and updated by different authorial teams, it is not clear whether any of his original sentences remain in the text of this, the sixth edition. But because his spirit and intellect animate every page, the present authors and publisher were happy to rename the book *Edwards' Treatment of Drinking Problems: A Guide to the Helping Professions.*

Introduction

This book's primary intended audience is helping professionals whose responsibilities bring them into contact with people who have drinking problems. We hope that generalists will find it a helpful introduction to the field and that generalists and specialists from all backgrounds will use it to enhance their diagnostic and therapeutic skills. Some individuals who themselves have drinking problems or love someone who does may also find the book valuable as an aid to understanding and coping with their situation.

Drinking problems occur across all social structures and cannot be neatly confined to the specialist addiction treatment sector. The text therefore considers the treatment of drinking problems across a range of approaches from informal, through nonspecialist, to specialist treatment. Because varied helping professionals will encounter drinking problems in their work, we have employed the generic word "clinician" to describe the person doing the helping and hope that the text is equally relevant to the needs of general medical practitioners, psychiatrists, and other medical specialists, nurses, psychotherapists, pastoral counselors, psychologists, social workers, and occupational therapists, among others.

The generic terms "drinking problems" and its close cousin "problem drinking" are employed throughout the book to encompass a diverse range of difficulties that range from what is popularly described as "alcoholism" to far less severe cases that nonetheless would benefit from intervention. Indeed, a key message of the book is that there is no one sort of drinking problem and that interventions should be tailored to the realities of the patient's situation rather than being applied in a one-size-fits-all fashion.

The book is divided into two sections. The first provides essential context for understanding drinking problems and their effects, whereas the second digs into the specifics of treatment. The content of each chapter is synopsized here.

Part I: Background to understanding (Chapters 1–7)

Definitions of drinking problems (Chapter 1)

This chapter opens with a number of vignettes describing the many faces of drinking problems, and this is followed by an account of "sensible" drinking guidelines. Three categories of alcohol misuse are defined: hazardous drinking, harmful drinking, and alcohol dependence. The clinical genesis of the concept of the alcohol dependence syndrome is outlined, the individual elements of the syndrome are discussed, and the relevance of an understanding of dependence to the specifics of treatment is considered.

Alcohol as a drug (Chapter 2)

Alcohol is a drug that has important pharmacological and toxic effects on most systems in the human body. Knowledge of these pharmacological effects is basic to understanding the problems that arise from its use as well as the treatment adopted. The language in this chapter is necessarily technical, but we have tried to write the text in a way that is accessible to the nonmedical reader.

Causes of drinking problems (Chapter 3)

This chapter endeavors to explain why some people and not others develop drinking problems. Environmental factors, such as alcohol availability and cultural norms, are addressed, as well as economic factors, biological predisposition, and psychological mechanisms.

Alcohol-related problems (Chapters 4–7)

Chapter 4 through 7 deal with the complications of alcohol problems, which encompass a number of domains: social (Chapter 4), physical (Chapter 5), psychiatric (Chapter 6), and other drug problems (Chapter 7).

Part II: Treatment: Context and content (Chapters 8–17)

Introduction, settings, and roles (Chapter 8)

Only a small minority of people with drinking problems actually make contact with specialist services. This chapter thus takes a broader view of where problem drinkers may find help, exploring help-seeking trajectories that include informal, nonspecialist, and specialist treatment paths.

Case-finding and intervention in nonspecialty settings (Chapter 9)

Nonspecialist settings offer the opportunity to intervene earlier in the life course/drinking career, before problems become severe. Even a small intervention made early enough can have significant long-term impact. A number of nonspecialist settings are described, ranging from primary care to the workplace. We include general psychiatry services, where drinking problems are all too often overlooked despite the capacity to treat them. Case finding and detection are considered, and this is followed by a review of biological markers and screening questionnaires. Intervention within the nonspecialist setting is described, and a more detailed account of brief motivational interviewing and medical management is given.

Assessment (Chapter 10)

This chapter covers practical issues related to the art and technique of history-taking. Assessment of drinking as well as of other domains of a patient's life are addressed, as are ways to shorten assessment times when necessary. The role of assessment in guiding case formulation and treatment goal-setting is also discussed.

Withdrawal states and their clinical management (Chapter 11)

Detoxification is an important prelude to the further treatment of the dependent drinker. This chapter covers the medical and clinical basics of alcohol withdrawal, but also guides the nonmedical reader through the underlying principles. The diversity of withdrawal states, the choice between community and in-patient settings, and the correct use of medication are all addressed.

The therapeutic relationship (Chapter 12)

This chapter emphasizes that the relationship between the clinician and problem drinker is as important as the treatment techniques or therapeutic tactics used. Likewise, changing behaviour is impossible without significant motivation on the part of the patient, and the nurturing of this motivation is core work for the clinician. Some guiding principles for working with the patient are given, and the question of when treatment ends is also reviewed.

Specialist treatment (Chapter 13)

This chapter reviews the evidence base for specialist treatments, with a particular focus on motivational interviewing and motivational enhancement therapy, cognitive behavioural therapy, and pharmacotherapy. The chapter places particular emphasis on the view that treatment should be research-based.

Alcoholics Anonymous and other mutual-help organizations (Chapter 14)

Alcoholics Anonymous (AA) is an international self-help organization that has helped countless millions of people with drinking problems since it was founded in 1935. This chapter provides an introduction to how AA operates and to its beliefs and practices. The importance of effective cooperation between treatment professionals and AA is emphasized. Alternative mutual-help organizations are also discussed.

Religion, spirituality, and values in treatment (Chapter 15)

Values, whether religiously derived or not, shape how people understand their drinking problem, their treatment, and their goals in life. Spiritual and religious issues are also commonly addressed in the treatment of drinking problems. This chapter explores the meaning of spirituality and religious belief, considers the spiritual "fallout" that occurs as a result of addiction, and tries to make sense of what all of this means when working with someone who has an alcohol problem.

Pursuing treatment outcomes other than abstinence (Chapter 16)

Not all people with drinking problems need to abstain in order to live healthy and productive lives. This chapter explains when a goal of moderate drinking may be more appropriate in treatment. It also discusses situations in which clinicians may decide that drinking-related treatment goals must be subordinated to other urgent clinical concerns.

Managing setbacks and challenges in treatment (Chapter 17)

This is a practical chapter that deals with common clinical situations in which treatment comes up against difficulties. It considers how such problems arise and how to reconfigure the therapeutic strategy in such situations in order to get on course again.

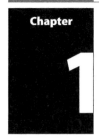

Definitions of drinking problems

The many faces of drinking problems

To many workers in the field, including readers of prior editions of this volume, the phrase "drinking problem" conjures up thoughts of cases like this one:

> Robert is a 45-year-old unemployed white man who was admitted to the in-patient alcohol unit for medically assisted withdrawal from alcohol for the second time in a year. He began drinking heavily in his teens. Since then, he has had only a few transitory periods of abstinence, all of them stimulated by short-term contacts with treatment professionals and mutual help groups. His wife became fed up with his drinking 5 years ago and kicked him out of the house. He has lived since in shelters, halfway houses, single-room occupancy hotels, and other marginal housing arrangements, including periods when he slept under a bridge with his "bottle gang." In morning group on the ward, his hands shake as he holds his cup of tea and tells his doctor and fellow patients in a trembling voice that "this time, I'm really going to make a go of it."

Individuals with severe alcohol dependence seen in specialist care settings, such as Robert, are familiar to anyone who works in the alcohol field and remain one focus of this edition of this book. Yet drinking problems occur and present across all social structures and health resources and are not neatly confined within the specialist addiction sector. This text, professing to address the treatment of all sorts of drinking problems, considers the whole range of approaches from informal through nonspecialist to specialist services. As such, it does not merely comment on the treatment of established alcohol dependence but also examines preventive factors that reduce the population prevalence of drinking problems and the clinical interventions that can benefit individuals with less severe alcohol problems. Cases as diverse as the following are thus within the ambit of this volume:

> Michael is a 50-year-old successful salesman of Indian descent. He is slightly overweight and is being monitored regularly by his primary care physician for elevated blood pressure. His doctor is mystified by the difficulty they experience in bringing Michael's blood pressure under control; the medications and diet recommendations do not seem to be working. During an early afternoon appointment, the doctor notices that Michael seems slightly tipsy and asks if he has been drinking. Michael smiles and says: "A three martini lunch with clients is standard practice in the sales game. But it's not like I'm an alcoholic or anything: I've got a house, a great family and I'm a star performer at my firm. So, on the blood pressure, are you going to switch my medication or what?"

> Emily is a 22-year-old honours college student whose roommate brings her to the Emergency Room[1] at midnight on a Saturday for treatment of facial bruising and a cracked

tooth. Emily had been assaulted by her boyfriend who was convinced that she had been flirting with the barman. Emily's boyfriend goes on pub crawls many times during the week; she accompanies him only on weekends. Her boyfriend is under arrest and Emily is sobbing hysterically that she doesn't want him in jail. With slurred words, she protests: "He's not really like that – it's the drink that makes him act that way. I've been after him to cut back." Emily attempts to leave as soon as her injuries are treated, but the doctor asks her to wait a moment so that the alcohol liaison nurse can have a word with her. "About my boyfriend's drinking?" Emily asks. "No," says the doctor kindly, "about yours."

George was a "workaholic," well-respected judge until the age of 65. During his retirement, he began for the first time in his life to experience long periods of boredom, which led him to spend inordinate amounts of time practising his hobby of wine tasting. After a particularly indulgent weekend, he experienced an episode of loss of consciousness, bit his tongue, and was incontinent of urine. Believing that George had suffered a stroke, his wife telephoned an ambulance that took him to hospital. He was admitted to the clinical decision unit overnight, and, the next day, transferred to a neurology ward for further investigation. Two days later, he started to become confused and suspicious, and, during an MRI scan, leaped off the trolley, pulling out his intravenous line. "That machine is trying to read my mind!" he yelled, maintaining that the stolen personal information would be used by the criminal fraternity to destroy his family in a final act of revenge. He was restrained by the hospital security team, and, following a short period of sedation with benzodiazepines, he recovered but still finds it difficult to understand this frightening period in his life.

A population perspective on drinking

Drinking within a population can be envisaged as a continuous spectrum ranging from nondrinkers, through "moderate" or "low-risk" drinkers, to individuals like those described in the preceding examples who have drinking problems of varying severities. Across populations, the proportion of people who fall into these categories ranges widely, for reasons explored in Chapter 3.

Defining drinks and low-risk drinking

A precondition for defining how much drinking is unhealthy is standardizing the term "drink." Standard drinks vary across different countries, and this must be taken into account when reading the literature or using instruments that quantify drinking behaviour (see Table 1.1). Many countries use the World Health Organization (WHO) standard of 10 g of pure alcohol, roughly equal to that found in a 100 mL glass of wine. In contrast, in the UK, a "unit of alcohol" is 8 g, roughly the amount contained in an Imperial Measure of a half-pint (284 mL). In the United States, product sizes are typically set in ounces, and a standard drink is 14 g, which is roughly equal to the alcohol contained in a 12-ounce can of beer.

In the UK, the drinking guidelines formulated by the Royal Colleges of Physicians, Psychiatrists and General Practitioners converged in the mid-1980s to define low-risk drinking as being less than 21 units of alcohol per week for men and less than 14 units per week for women (British Medical Association, 1995). Consumption of 22–50 units per week for men and 15–35 units per week for women was considered as hazardous and the consumption of more than 50 units per week for men and 35 units per week for women as harmful. In 1995, the Department of Health moved from weekly to daily limits and advised that "regular consumption of between 3 and 4 units a day by men of all ages will not accrue

Table 1.1. Example of standard drink sizes in different countries

Country	Standard drink (grams of ethanol)
Australia	10
Bulgaria	13
Canada	13.6
France	10
Ireland	10
Luxembourg	12.8
Mexico	14
UK	8
USA	14

Source: Kalinowski & Humphreys, in press

Table 1.2. Examples of recommended daily drinking limits in different countries (grams of ethanol)

Country	Men	Women
Australia	20	20
Canada	40.7	27
Japan	40	20
The Philippines	28	14
USA	28/56	14/42

Source: Kalinowski & Humphreys, in press

significant health risk" (Department of Health, 1995, p. 32). Likewise, women were advised that "regular consumption of between 2 and 3 units a day by women of all ages will not accrue any significant health risk" (Department of Health, 1995, p. 32). These guidelines, based on epidemiological data of alcohol-related morbidity and mortality, were similar to those available in many other countries (see Table 1.2). However in 2016, the UK Chief Medical Officers amended their advice based on the latest evidence about the impact of alcohol consumption on health, notably cancer (Dept of Health, 2016). They recommended to *both* men *and* women that "you are safest not to drink regularly more than 14 units of alcohol per week," "to spread this evenly over 3 days or more," and "adopting alcohol free days."

U.S. guidelines are based on 14 g units and somewhat confusingly define "moderate" and "low-risk" drinking differently. The former is up to one drink per day for women and two for men, whereas the latter is up to three standard drinks a day for women and four for men

(Kalinkowski & Humphreys, in press). Interestingly, not all guidelines around the world recommend lower drinking limits for women than men, despite evidence that women experience more health harm per unit of alcohol consumed than do men. For example, the Australian National Health and Research Council (2009) recommend for both men and women a limit of 20 g/d (two standard Australian drinks).

How much influence low-risk drinking guidelines have on alcohol consumption patterns is open to debate. Drinking above recommended levels is commonplace. Using data from the U.S. National Longitudinal Alcohol Epidemiologic Survey, Dawson and colleagues (Dawson, Archer, & Grant, 1996) calculated that a third of drinkers never exceed moderate alcohol consumption, a third do so occasionally, and for the rest it was their usual behaviour. Furthermore, 88 percent of the alcohol was consumed in a risky fashion. Similarly, in England, the General Lifestyle Survey reported that 39 percent of men and 28 percent of women had exceeded daily recommended limits on the days they drank the most alcohol (Lifestyle Statistics, Health and Social Care Information Centre, 2013). Notably, this was most common in the over-65 age group. In Australia, 24 percent of males and 17 percent of females reported drinking more than the recommended guidelines for acute harm on at least one occasion a month (Australian Institute of Health and Welfare, 2008), and 62 percent of the alcohol consumed was at a risky/high-risk level for acute harm (Chikritzhs et al., 2003). This percentage rose to more than 80 percent among the 14- to 17-year-old and 18- to 24-year-old age groups (Chikritzhs et al., 2003). Globally, alcohol contributes to about 4 percent of the burden of disease, with greater burden in higher income countries and in men (Rehm et al., 2009; World Health Organization, 2009).

Categories of high-risk drinking

Three categories of drinking outside of recommended limits make up the top three tiers of the pyramid in Figure 1.1: namely, hazardous drinking, harmful drinking, and alcohol dependence (Edwards, Arif, & Hodgson, 1981). *Hazardous drinking* refers to drinking that

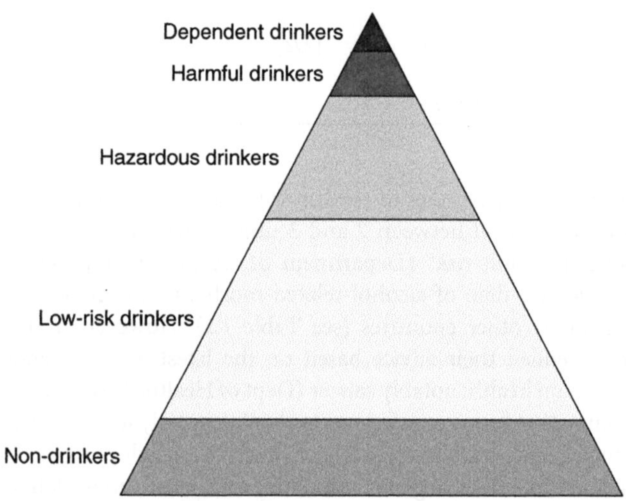

Figure 1.1: Drinking within the population. The areas are not accurate representations of the relative proportions of those exhibiting differing drinking behaviours because this varies among populations.

has not yet accrued any harm but exceeds safe limits. *Harmful drinking* describes drinking behaviour that has incurred damage. The division between these two is somewhat arbitrary because harms from drinking may go undetected (e.g., liver damage). The third category of high-risk drinking clusters with other problems (e.g., craving, blackouts) that together are suggestive of alcohol dependence.

Hazardous drinking

Hazardous drinking refers to drinking more than a certain limit that places the individual at risk of incurring harm (Edwards, Arif, & Hodgson, 1981). The WHO (1994) *Lexicon of Alcohol and Drug Terms* described hazardous use of a substance as:

> A pattern of substance use that increases the risk of harmful consequences for the user. Some would limit the consequences to physical and mental health (as in harmful use); some would also include social consequences. In contrast to harmful use, hazardous use refers to patterns of use that are of public health significance despite the absence of any current disorder in the individual user.

Hazardous drinking usually applies to anyone drinking more than the recommended levels. One common pattern of hazardous use is "binge drinking," a term and its synonyms (e.g., bout, bender, spree) used to describe drinking "a lot" in everyday speech. Clinical and scientific definitions vary nationally.

The U.S. National Institute on Alcohol Abuse and Alcoholism (NIAAA) defines binge drinking as a pattern of drinking that brings blood alcohol concentration levels to 0.8 mg/dL, which typically occurs after four drinks for a woman or five drinks for a man, consumed over 2 hours or less. Binge drinking is not represented in Figure 1.1 or in the diagnostic criteria because it is not specific to any level of consumption: hazardous, harmful, and dependent drinkers may all engage in drinking binges.

Hazardous drinkers do not usually seek help for an alcohol problem. They are typically identified opportunistically in the primary care, general hospital, and other nonspecialty care settings (see Chapter 9).

Harmful drinking

Unlike hazardous drinking, harmful drinking is known to have damaged the drinker (Edwards, Arif, & Hodgson 1981). *Harmful psychoactive substance use* (in this case, alcohol) is a diagnostic term within the International Classification of Diseases (ICD-10):

> A pattern of psychoactive substance use that is causing damage to health. The damage may be physical (as in cases of hepatitis from the self-administration of injected drugs) or mental (e.g. depressive episodes secondary to heavy consumption of alcohol). (World Health Organization, 1992, pp. 74–75)

Although harmful use often has adverse social consequences, social consequences in themselves are not sufficient to justify a diagnosis of harmful use. The parallel diagnosis in the fourth iteration of the *Diagnostic and Statistical Manual of Mental Disorders* (DSM-IV) was alcohol abuse: a "maladaptive pattern of alcohol use in the absence of a diagnosis of alcohol dependence" (American Psychiatric Association, 2000).

However, DSM-5 has replaced the diagnoses of alcohol abuse and alcohol dependence with alcohol use disorder (AUD). AUDs exist on a continuum, with mild, moderate, and severe subclassifications. Although many criteria remain the same in DSM-5, legal consequences have been removed and the term "craving" added (American Psychiatric Association, 2013). Of the 11 criteria, 2–3 are required for a diagnosis of mild AUD, 4–5 of moderate, and 6 or more for a diagnosis of severe disorder (see Table 1.3). As a consequence of these changes in DSM-5, an individual could now meet criteria for having an AUD with a level of drinking that would not have met DSM-IV alcohol abuse criteria. ICD-11 is in development and appears likely to maintaining the ICD-10 categories of harmful use and dependence.

Alcohol dependence (syndrome)

The top of the pyramid in Figure 1.1 represents the dependent drinker. These individuals typically have a history of alcohol-related problems and constitute most of the caseload in specialty alcohol treatment services (although they also present elsewhere). Moderately dependent drinkers will show evidence of tolerance, alcohol withdrawal, and impaired control over drinking. Severely dependent drinkers typically have long-standing problems and a history of repeated treatment episodes.

Based somewhat on the traditions imposed by different diagnostic systems, some scientific and clinical work on this population of drinkers has been organized under the concept of "alcohol dependence" (e.g., studies using the DSM-IV), whereas other work has been informed by the concept of the "alcohol dependence syndrome" (e.g., studies using the ICD-10). Etymologically, the English word "syndrome" derives from the Greek *syn* meaning "together" and *dromos* meaning "running." Thus, the "alcohol dependence syndrome" as operationally defined by the ICD-10 is a collection of symptoms that "run together," including a compulsion to take alcohol, difficulty with control, withdrawal symptoms and relief drinking, tolerance, predominance, and persisting use despite evidence of harm (see Table 1.4). Nonetheless, the ICD-10 requires only three of the criteria to be present, and so perhaps the strict definition of syndrome as "consistently occurring together" should not apply to the ICD-10. Many people diagnosed as alcohol dependent under ICD-10 will meet the DSM-5 criteria for severe AUD, which are similar and include tolerance, withdrawal symptoms, taking of alcohol in greater amounts than intended, desire or unsuccessful attempts to cut down, spending extensive time in activities to obtain alcohol or recover from consuming it, giving up of activities, and persistent use despite associated problems (see Table 1.3).

Making the diagnosis of dependence should not be a mechanistic tick-box exercise. Dependence cannot be conceived as "not present" or "present," with the diagnostic task then completed. Clinicians must recognize the subtleties of symptomatology, which will reveal not only whether this condition is there at all but, if it exists, the degree of its development. What has also to be learnt is how the syndrome's manifestations are molded by personality, environmental influence, or cultural forces. The ability to comprehend variations on the theme constitutes the real art of clinical diagnosis. For instance, craving may have a different meaning to the clinician and the patient, and alcohol-related consequences may depend on context. If clinicians cannot recognize *degrees* of dependence (or severity of AUD), they will be unable to adapt their approach to the particular individual, and they may retreat into seeing "alcoholism" as a fixed entity from which all individuals with drinking problems are presumed to suffer, for whom the universal goal must be total abstinence, and with the treatment offered being universally intensive.

Table 1.3. The DSM-5 criteria for alcohol use disorder

	DSM-IV	DSM-5	
Alcohol Abuse: Any 1 of these criteria	Recurrent alcohol use resulting in a failure to fulfil major role obligations at work, school, or home	Alcohol is often taken in larger amounts or over a longer period than was intended.	Alcohol use disorder
	Recurrent alcohol use in situations in which it is physically hazardous	There is a persistent desire or unsuccessful efforts to cut down or control alcohol use.	Mild: The presence of 2 to 3 symptoms
	Recurrent alcohol-related legal problems	A great deal of time is spent in activities necessary to obtain alcohol, use alcohol, or recover from its effects.	
	Continued alcohol use despite having persistent or recurrent social or interpersonal problems caused or exacerbated by the effects of the alcohol.	Craving, or a strong desire or urge to use alcohol.	
Alcohol dependence: Any 3 of these criteria	Tolerance, as defined by either of the following: a) A need for markedly increased amounts of alcohol to achieve intoxication or desired effect b) Markedly diminished effect with continued use of the same amount of alcohol	Recurrent alcohol use resulting in a failure to fulfil major role obligations at work, school, or home.	Moderate: The presence of 4 to 5 symptoms
	Withdrawal, as manifested by either of the following: a) The characteristic withdrawal syndrome for alcohol b) Alcohol is taken to relieve or avoid withdrawal symptoms	Continued alcohol use despite having persistent or recurrent social or interpersonal problems caused or exacerbated by the effects of alcohol.	Severe: The presence of 6 or more symptoms

Table 1.3. *(cont.)*

DSM-IV	DSM-5
Alcohol is often taken in larger amounts or over a longer period than was intended.	Important social, occupational, or recreational activities are given up or reduced because of alcohol use.
There is a persistent desire or unsuccessful efforts to cut down or control alcohol use.	Recurrent alcohol use in situations in which it is physically hazardous.
A great deal of time is spent in activities necessary to obtain alcohol.	Alcohol use is continued despite knowledge of having a persistent or recurrent physical or psychological problem that is likely to have been caused or exacerbated by alcohol.
Important social, occupational, or recreational activities are given up or reduced because of alcohol use.	Tolerance, as defined by either of the following: a) A need for markedly increased amounts of alcohol to achieve intoxication or desired effect b) A markedly diminished effect with continued use of the same amount of alcohol
Alcohol use is continued despite knowledge of having a persistent or recurrent physical or psychological problem that is likely to have been caused or exacerbated by the substance (e.g., continued drinking despite recognition that an ulcer was made worse by alcohol consumption).	Withdrawal, as manifested by either of the following: a) The characteristic withdrawal syndrome for alcohol (refer to criteria A and B of the criteria set for alcohol withdrawal) b) Alcohol (or a closely related substance, such as a benzodiazepine) is taken to relieve or avoid withdrawal symptoms.

(Adapted from National Institute on Alcohol Abuse and Alcoholism [NIAAA] [use square brackets not parentheses] 2015.)

Clinical genesis of the concept

A syndrome is a descriptive clinical formulation that is, at least initially, likely to be agnostic as to causation or pathology. The existence of alcohol dependence has been evident to acute observers for many years (see Box 1.1), but, in the 1970s, a detailed clinical description was enunciated within a syndrome model by Edwards and Gross (1976). These scholars' clinical observations revealed a repeated clustering of signs and symptoms in certain heavy drinkers. They postulated that the syndrome existed in degrees of severity rather than as a categorical absolute, that its presentation could be shaped by pathoplastic influences rather than its being concrete and invariable, and that alcohol dependence should be conceptually distinguished from alcohol-related problems. This clinically derived formulation was at that stage designated as only provisional, and, within the general research tradition of psychiatric taxonomy, the *validity* of the syndrome had then to be determined.

Elements of the alcohol dependence syndrome

Following the original description, extensive research has documented that the alcohol dependence syndrome is a reality rather than a chimera of the clinical eye. That is not to say that all elements are in psychometric terms equally well tied into the syndrome. Within a psychometric perspective, some elements may be redundant, and difficulties have been encountered in operationalizing elements, such as narrowing of repertoire, subjective change, and reinstatement.

The elements of the syndrome as originally formulated by Edwards and Gross will now be discussed sequentially, rather than the more restrictive formulations described in ICD-10 (Edwards & Gross, 1976). The alcohol dependence syndrome is a hypothetical construct that formal diagnostic criteria index to some extent. However, it is important to appreciate that the symptoms of this hypothetical construct are not, strictly speaking, equivalent to a diagnostic symptom list.

Narrowing of repertoire

The ordinary drinker's consumption and choice of drink will vary from day to day and from week to week; they may have a beer at lunch on one day, nothing to drink on another, share a bottle of wine at dinner one night and then go to a party on a Saturday and have several drinks. Their drinking is patterned by varying internal cues and external circumstances.

At first, a person becoming caught up in heavy drinking may widen their repertoire and the range of cues that signal drinking. As dependence advances, the cues are increasingly related to relief or avoidance of alcohol withdrawal, and the drinker's personal drinking repertoire becomes increasingly narrowed. The dependent person begins to drink the same amount of alcohol whether it is a workday, weekend, or holiday; the nature of the company or their own mood makes less and less difference. Clinical questioning may distinguish earlier and later stages of dependence by the degree to which the repertoire is narrowed. With advanced dependence, the drinking may become scheduled to a strict daily time table that maintains a high blood alcohol level. More careful questioning will, however, show that even when dependence is well established, some capacity for variation remains. The syndrome must be pictured as subtle and plastic

Table 1.4. The ICD-10 criteria for alcohol dependence syndrome

A cluster of physiological, behavioural, and cognitive phenomena in which the use of alcohol takes a much higher priority for a given individual than other behaviours that once had greater value. A central descriptive characteristic of the dependence syndrome is the desire (often strong, sometimes overpowering) to take alcohol. There may be evidence that the return to alcohol use after a period of abstinence leads to a more rapid reappearance of other features of the syndrome than occurs with nondependent individuals.
Three or more of the following have been experienced or exhibited at some time in the previous year.
(a) Strong desire or sense of compulsion to take alcohol.
(b) Difficulties in controlling alcohol-taking behaviour in terms of its onset, termination, or level of use.
(c) A physiological withdrawal state when alcohol use has ceased or has been reduced, as evidenced by: the characteristic withdrawal syndrome for alcohol or use of the same (or a closely related substance) with the intention of relieving or avoiding withdrawal symptoms.
(d) Evidence of tolerance, such that increased dosages are required in order to achieve effects originally produced by lower dosages.
(e) Progressive neglect of alternative pleasures or interests because of alcohol use, increased amount of time necessary to obtain or take alcohol or recover from its effects.
(f) Persisting with alcohol use despite clear evidence of overtly harmful consequences, such as harm to the liver through excessive drinking, depressive mood states consequent to heavy substance misuse, or alcohol-related impairment of cognitive functioning. Efforts should be made to determine if the user was actually, or could be expected to be, aware of the nature and extent of the harm.

Source: World Health Organization (1992).

rather than as something concretely set, but, as dependence advances, the patterns tend to become increasingly fixed.

Salience of drinking

The stereotyping of the drinking pattern as dependence advances leads to the individual giving priority to maintaining their alcohol intake. A partner's[2] distressed scolding – once effective – is later neutralized by the drinker as evidence of a lack of understanding. To avoid irksome advice to drink less, the drinker drifts into a social group composed entirely of those with equally heavy alcohol consumption. Income, which previously had to serve many needs, now supports the drinking habit as the first demand. Gratification of the need for drink may become more important for the individual with liver damage than considerations of survival. Diagnostically, the progressive change in the salience given to alcohol is important, rather than the drinker's behaviour at any one time. The individual may relate that they used to be proud of their house but now the paint is peeling; used always to take the children to football matches but now spend no time with the family; and used to have rather conventional moral standards but will now beg, borrow, or steal to obtain money for alcohol.

BOX 1.1 From the pages of history: Thomas Trotter's pioneering essay on drunkenness

> The habit of drunkenness is a disease of the mind – Thomas Trotter (1804)

Beginning in the late seventeenth century, the growing availability of inexpensive strong spirits triggered an epidemic of drinking problems across England. Reformers responded with efforts to limit the supply of alcohol (e.g., The Gin Act of 1751) and calls for religious and moral renewal of the drinking population. Not until the turn of the nineteenth century did a book-length discussion adopt an explicitly medical perspective on heavy drinking. *An Essay, Medical, Philosophical and Chemical, on Drunkenness and Its Effects on the Human Body* was penned by Dr. Thomas Trotter (1804) who had recently retired from a distinguished career as Physician to the Royal Navy (Vale & Edwards, 2011).

Trotter detailed the possible medical sequelae of chronic drunkenness, including ulcers, jaundice, and melancholy (i.e., depression), illustrating his points with vivid accounts of individual cases. In unpacking the etiology of problem drinking, Trotter blamed neither

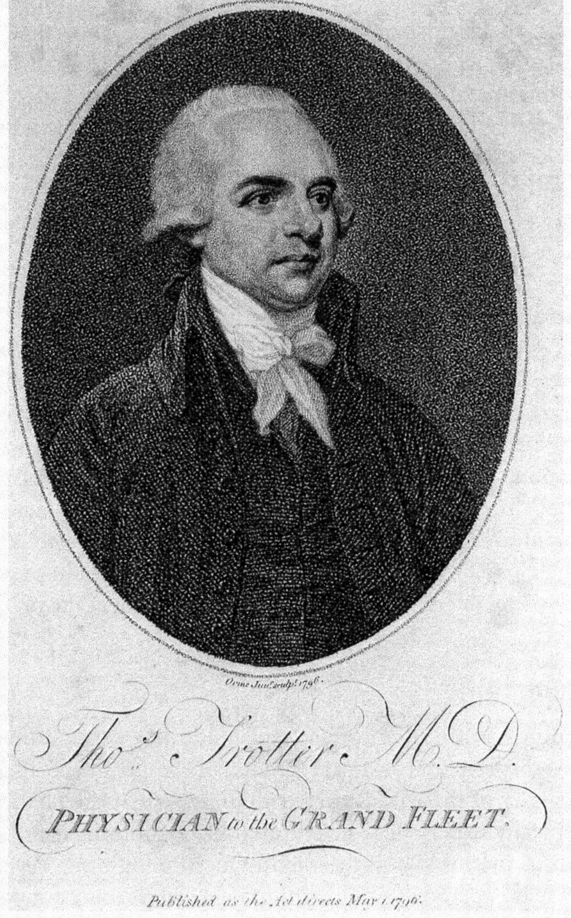

Figure 1.2: Portrait of Thomas Trotter used with permission of the Wellcome library.

spirits nor the drinker's bad character. Rather, he understood problem drinking as a learned habit made more tenacious by psychological forces. His concept of "disease" was not therefore strictly biological, but referred instead to psychological discomfort (Vale & Edwards, 2011).

Trotter was clearly wrong in some particulars (e.g., like Charles Dickens, he believed that heavy drinking could eventually make the human body combustible), and his essay never garnered as broad a hearing as it deserved. But reading it today provides a remarkable window into the historical emergence of a compassionate, medically oriented perspective on drinking problems that would eventually compete with religious understandings that had prevailed for centuries.

Increased tolerance to alcohol

Alcohol is a drug to which the central nervous system (CNS) develops tolerance (see Chapter 2). Individuals themselves report on tolerance in terms of "having a good head for alcohol." Acute tolerance may develop in regular nondependent alcohol drinkers, but this should be distinguished from the chronic tolerance that is a feature of the dependence syndrome. In dependence, tolerance is shown by the individual being able to sustain an alcohol intake and go about their business at blood alcohol levels that would incapacitate the nontolerant drinker. This does not mean that these drinkers' functioning is unimpaired – they will be a dangerous driver, but because of their tolerance they will (unfortunately) still be able to drive. Furthermore, an individual may present with very high blood alcohol concentrations that would be fatal for the nontolerant, yet not appear intoxicated, engage in a constructive interview, and even remember it afterwards! Being able to "breathalyze" an individual during assessment is therefore key in determining his or her degree of tolerance.

Cross-tolerance will extend to certain other drugs, notably the sedative-hypnotics such as benzodiazepines, which means that the person who has become tolerant to alcohol will also have a tolerance to these drugs and vice versa. Indeed, this cross-tolerance can be exploited by using benzodiazepines to prevent and manage alcohol withdrawal symptoms during detoxification. The rate of development of tolerance is variable, but the heavy drinker who is not dependent can manifest tolerance. In later stages of dependence, for reasons that are unclear, many individuals begin to lose their previously acquired tolerance and become incapacitated by quantities of alcohol that they could previously handle. After what was once a typical, tolerable evening of heavy drinking at the pub, they may fall down drunk in the street.

Withdrawal symptoms

At first, these symptoms are intermittent and mild; they cause little incapacity, and one symptom may be experienced without others. As dependence increases, so does the frequency and severity of the withdrawal symptoms. When the picture is fully developed, the individual typically experiences severe multiple symptoms every morning on waking and perhaps even in the middle of the night. Questioning often reveals that the severely dependent individual experiences mild withdrawal symptoms at any time during the day when their alcohol level falls. Complete withdrawal is therefore not necessary to precipitate disturbance. Although many individuals do associate their symptoms with alcohol withdrawal, some may not and instead describe themselves as suffering from anxiety or stress.

The individual often remembers rather exactly the dating of the period when he or she first began to experience withdrawal symptoms, and there is no necessary association with a sudden increase in alcohol intake. The spectrum of symptoms is wide and includes tremor, nausea, sweating, sensitivity to sound (hyperacusis), ringing in the ears (tinnitus), itching, muscle cramps, mood disturbance, sleep disturbance, hallucinations, generalized (*grand mal*) seizures, and the fully developed picture of delirium tremens. There are four key symptoms, outlined in the following sections.

Tremor

Tremor nicely illustrates that it is the *degree* of symptom experience that is essential to the clinical observation, rather than a recording in the case notes simply that the individual does or does not experience withdrawal tremor. Shakiness may have been experienced only once or twice, or intermittently and mildly – for example, after a heavy binge – or it may be experienced every morning and to a degree that is incapacitating, or it may appear with many intervening intensities and frequencies. As well as the hands shaking, there may be facial tremor or the whole body shaking. The therapist has to cultivate an awareness of something equivalent to the Richter scale used to categorize the strength of earthquakes and look out for the individual saying that they rattle their morning teacup against the saucer. In the extreme case, a drinker may rely on the kindness of a bartender or drinking companion to lift the day's first pint to their lips.

Nausea

The individual who is asked only whether they vomit may well deny it. Their experience, however, may be that if they attempt to clean their teeth in the morning, they will retch; or they may never eat breakfast because they know it would be too risky. A common story is that most of the first drink of the day is vomited back.

Sweating

This may be dramatic; the individual wakes regularly in the early hours of the morning with soaking sweats. At the earlier stages of dependence, the drinker may report no more than feeling clammy.

Mood disturbance

In the earlier stages, individuals may phrase the experience in terms of "I'm a bit on edge" or "my nerves are not too good," but when dependence is fully developed they may use vivid descriptions to indicate a state of appalling agitation and depression. Often, the anxiety seems to be characterized by a frightened reaction to loud noises or traffic (sometimes with a phobia of crossing the road), fear of someone approaching from behind, and fright at "the twigs on the trees rubbing together." A co-occurring mood disorder may at times exacerbate withdrawal symptoms.

Relief or avoidance of withdrawal symptoms by further drinking

In the earliest stages, the individual may be aware that a drink at lunchtime "helps to straighten me up a bit." At the other extreme, an individual may require a drink every morning before they get out of bed, as a matter of desperate need. As with withdrawal symptoms, relief drinking must not be conceived as only a morning event; the individual may wake in the middle of the night for the drink that will abort incipient withdrawal. They may be aware that if they go 3 or 4 hours without a drink during the day, the next drink is valued especially for its relief effect. Relief drinking is cued not only by frank withdrawal but also by minimal symptoms of subacute withdrawal, which signal worse distress if a drink is not taken. The dependent individual may try to maintain a steady alcohol level that they have learnt to recognize as comfortably above the danger level for withdrawal, and, to this extent their drinking is cued by withdrawal avoidance as well as by withdrawal relief.

Clues to the severity of an individual's dependence are often given by the small details they provide of the circumstances and timing of the first drink of the day and their attitude toward it. If they get up, have a bath, dress, and read the paper before that drink, then dependence is not very advanced. The person who runs some errands or finishes household chores before having a first drink is likewise at a different stage of dependence than the one pours whisky into the day's first cup of tea or coffee. Someone engaged in relief drinking may have ritualized the procedure. A man may go to the early morning pub and go straight up to the bar, where the barman will know immediately to give him a pint of lager, which the man will grab at clumsily with both hands and drink down fast. He may go to the lavatory and vomit some of this pint back, but he can then drink the next pint at greater leisure, and he will know that within 20 or 30 minutes of walking into that pub "the drink will have cured me." Drinkers may relate that they know the exact quantity of alcohol required for this "cure" and the exact time interval for the alcohol to take effect, and they report also that the "cure" is repeatedly so complete as to be almost miraculous. Sometimes, drinkers describe what is, presumably, a conditioned response; the mere fact of having a glass in their hands gives relief.

That the dependence syndrome is a plastic condition rather than something immutable is brought out again by the way this particular element is shaped by social and personal factors. For some, the idea of keeping drink in the house may be so against subcultural expectations that they will always wait for the pubs to open rather than "keep a drink indoors." The person of rigid personality may endure considerable withdrawal for some hours rather than take a drink before lunch. A dependent individual with a short-term competing activity (e.g., doing well on a job interview, attending a religious service, spending a weekend caring for an aging parent) may abstain throughout. To understand fully what the individual reports always requires that these shaping factors are taken into account.

Subjective awareness of compulsion to drink

The conventional phrases used to describe the dependent person's subjective experience are not altogether satisfactory. For instance, awareness of "loss of control" is said to be crucial to understanding abnormal drinking; sometimes a drinker may say, "If I have one or two, I'll go on," or "If I go into the pub, promises don't mean anything," or "Good resolutions dissolve in alcohol," or "Once I've really got the taste of it, I'm away." Control is probably best seen as variably or intermittently impaired rather than "lost." Although "loss of control" has in some of the classic texts been pictured as the touchstone for diagnosis of alcohol dependence, many so-called social drinkers at times drink too much and are sorry and embarrassed afterward. However, unlike a nondependent drinker, a dependent person will generally reply "alcohol" when asked "who is usually in control – you or alcohol?"

The experience of "craving" is often wrapped up in conventional phrasing. The patient may describe it in unambiguous terms – they are "gasping for a drink" or reports that "a drink will hit the spot." Characterizing an individual's experience of craving is essential for appropriate treatment. For example, is alcohol craved to relieve withdrawal (negative reinforcement) or to give a buzz (positive reinforcement)? Craving is dynamic and much influenced by environment, with the person who is withdrawing on a hospital ward not experiencing any craving compared to at home. Cues for craving may include the feeling of intoxication as well as incipient or developed withdrawal, mood (anger, depression, or elation), or situational cues (being in a pub or with a drinking friend).

The individual who is in a withdrawal state (or partial withdrawal) may report that they are compulsively ruminating on alcohol and that they have hit on the strategy of blocking these ruminations by bringing in other lines of thought.

Reinstatement after abstinence

When alcohol dependent patients begin to drink again (a lapse) following a period of abstinence, they generally, sooner or later, start to drink in a dependent fashion again (relapse). The time course is extremely variable. Typically, the person who had only a moderate degree of dependence may take weeks or months to reinstate dependence, perhaps pulling back once or twice on the way. A severely dependent individual typically reports that they are again "hooked" within a few days of starting to drink, although even here there are exceptions: on the first day, they may become abnormally drunk and be surprised to find that they have lost their tolerance. Within a few days they are, however, experiencing severe withdrawal symptoms and drinking for relief, the subjective experience of compulsion is reinstated, and their drinking is back in the old stereotyped pattern. A syndrome that had taken years to develop can be fully reinstated within 72 hours of drinking or sooner, and this is one of the most puzzling features of the condition.

Should dependence be diagnosed in the absence of withdrawal symptoms?

As noted earlier, the term "syndrome" suggests that certain symptoms and signs consistently run together. In contrast, the "pick and mix" nature of diagnostic criteria permit the diagnosis of alcohol dependence (in ICD-10) or severe AUD (in DSM-5) in the absence of withdrawal symptoms. As such, this approach will probably catch in the net many people who are drinking heavily but who are not experiencing any features of physical dependence on alcohol. The question is important and not merely semantic. In a large U.S. household survey, Schuckit and colleagues found that people with diagnosed alcohol dependence varied markedly according to whether physiological symptoms (withdrawal or tolerance) were or were not present. Those with physiological symptoms drank more heavily than the others and experienced more adverse consequences from their drinking (Schuckit et al., 1998). In another population study, the experience of tremors was predictive of poorer 1-year outcome and chronicity (Hasin, Paykin, Meydan, & Grant, 2000). A syndrome, by its nature, is a state difficult to differentiate absolutely from non-syndrome, and whilst some may understand the presence of withdrawal symptoms as merely a measure of severity, others recommend that the diagnosis of alcohol dependence be reserved for those who have experienced withdrawal symptoms to at least some degree. Our own view is that clinicians should weigh withdrawal symptoms more heavily than the other diagnostic criteria when judging how severe a case may be, particularly given its potential serious sequelae if not recognized and treated appropriately (see Chapters 4 and 5).

The time element

To discuss the severity of dependence inevitably introduces consideration of the time element. The longer someone has been putting themselves through repeated cycles of withdrawal and relief, the more severe the dependence they will have contracted. However, note also has to be taken of the rapidity or gradualness of the transition between heavy drinking and dependence, and of the age at which dependence developed. Why dependence should have become manifest at a certain phase in the life of a drinker is unexplained. For some with a strong family history of alcoholism, transition to dependence is likely to be more rapid. Some evidence suggests that women, on average, experience a more "telescoped" onset of dependence symptoms, whereas in men, symptoms of dependence develop over about 12 months from a long-standing heavy alcohol intake. As drinking patterns become more similar in men and women, such gender differences may not be evident in all societies and subcultures. With other cultures, personalities, and patterns of drinking, dependence may arise earlier or later in life, after longer or shorter alcohol exposure, and may advance with greater or lesser rapidity.

In summary, to understand fully the individual's dependence, the present picture has to be related to its evolution over time, and the determinants of that evolution must be identified.

Why an understanding of dependence matters

Having outlined the diagnosis of dependence, the manner in which degrees of the syndrome's development are to be identified, and the way in which personality and environment may shape the presentations, the question then arises: "What is the practical purpose of such diagnostic work, the gain from developing this kind of diagnostic skill?" The answers are both general and specific.

The dependence concept and the brokerage of understanding

The realization that such a condition as alcohol dependence exists and an understanding of the personal implications of this diagnosis may often assist in the relief of the person's sense of muddle and bafflement. It can contribute to a helpful framework for personal understanding and enable them to come to terms with a condition that they had previously only reacted to with confusion. The fact that alcohol is a drug that can produce dependence – "a drug of addiction" – often comes as a surprise to a person's family as much as to the individual themselves. The diagnosis, if sensitively explained, can – for the family, too – offer a way of restructuring a reaction to a situation that previously engendered confusion, fear, or anger. The spouse begins to realize that there is more than "weakness of the will" that has to be understood; that expecting their partner "to drink like other people" is not possible.

For the treating clinician, what flows from understanding the nature of dependence lies partly in accurate empathy for that person's experience. To impart baldly no more than the diagnostic label – a sort of magisterial sentencing – is not what is meant by building up understanding.

Furthermore, it would be useful health education if the public in general were aware that alcohol has dependence potential. The public needs to know more of the dangers and the danger signals and what dependence can mean for themselves, for someone in their family, for someone at work, or for someone they meet in the pub. An understanding of alcohol dependence should become part of ordinary social awareness, but it is equally important that society understands that alcohol problems also commonly occur without dependence.

The relevance of an understanding of dependence to the specifics of treatment

The ability to diagnose dependence and recognize its degrees is vital to setting the treatment goal (see Chapters 10 and 12). A severely dependent drinker is unlikely to be able to return to normal drinking, and the clinician's ability accurately to recognize the degree of dependence is vital to this important aspect of care (Edwards, 1986). Assessment of the person's degree of dependence is also relevant to the choice of withdrawal regime and a forewarning of the risk of delirium tremens or withdrawal fits (see Chapter 11). Understanding of the severity of relapse requires an ability to recognize whether dependence has been reinstated. Monitoring the progress of regression of dependence intensity over time is relevant to understanding the drinking career and drinking within the life course.

The range of drinking problems

It is essential to appreciate the full range of drinking problems that occur and manifest themselves in a rich variety of situations and settings. Many problem-drinking individuals who could benefit from treatment are not alcohol dependent, and such individuals are diverse in their difficulties, needs, and strengths. Even the more restricted population of drinkers who experience the cluster of symptoms that constitute the alcohol dependence syndrome vary in terms of severity and are subject to moulding factors including personal, environmental, and cultural forces. Rather than mentally categorizing all people with drinking problems into a single pigeon hole (e.g., alcoholics who should become abstinent), clinicians should be aware of the extraordinary diversity of drinking problems and the ever-present individuality and humanity of each patient they see.

Notes

1. In recent years, the term "emergency room" has spread from the United States to the UK, which historically had preferred the terms Accident & Emergency Department (A&E) or Casualty Department. For stylistic ease, this edition of the book uses "emergency room" as a catch-all term for all such settings.
2. In this book, we use the term "partner" as a catch-all term for a significant romantic attachment in the drinker's life, which may or may not involve legal marriage.

References

American Psychiatric Association (APA). (2000). *Diagnostic and statistical manual of mental disorders* (4th edition, text revision). Washington DC: American Psychiatric Association.

American Psychiatric Association (APA). (2013). *Diagnostic and statistical manual of mental disorders* (5th edition). Washington DC: American Psychiatric Association.

Australian Institute of Health and Welfare. (2008). *2007 national drug strategy household survey: Detailed findings.* Drug statistics series no. 20. Cat. no. PHE 98. Canberra, Australia: Australian Institute of Health and Welfare.

British Medical Association. (1995). *Alcohol: Guidelines on sensible drinking.* London: British Medical Association.

Chikritzhs, T., Catalano, P., Stockwell, T., Donath, S., Ngo, H. T., Young, D. J., & Matthews, S. (2003). *Australian alcohol indicators 1990–2001: Patterns of alcohol use and related harms for Australian states and territories.* Perth, Australia: National Drug Research Institute.

Dawson D. A., Archer L. D., & Grant B. F. (1996). Reducing alcohol-use disorders via decreased consumption: A comparison of population and high-risk strategies. *Drug and Alcohol Dependence*, **42**(1), 39–47.

Department of Health. (1995). *Sensible drinking: The report of an inter-departmental working group.* London: Department of Health.

Department of Health. (2016). *Alcohol Guidelines Review – Report from the Guidelines development group to the UK Chief Medical Officers.* London: Department of Health.

Edwards, G. (1986). The alcohol dependence syndrome: A concept as stimulus to enquiry. *British Journal of Addiction*, **81**(2), 171–183.

Edwards, G., Arif, A., & Hodgson, R. (1981). Nomenclature and classification of drug- and alcohol-related problems: A WHO memorandum. *Bulletin of the World Health Organization*, **59**(2), 225–242.

Edwards, G., & Gross, M. M. (1976). Alcohol dependence: Provisional description of a clinical syndrome. *British Medical Journal*, **1**(6017), 1058–1061.

Hasin, D., Paykin, A., Meydan, J., & Grant, B. (2000). Withdrawal and tolerance: prognostic significance in DSM-IV alcohol dependence. *Journal of Studies on Alcohol*, **61**(3), 431–438.

Kalinowski, A., & Humphreys, K. (in press). Governmental standard drink definitions and low-risk alcohol consumption guidelines in 37 countries. *Addiction.*

Lifestyle Statistics, Health and Social Care Information Centre. (2013). *Statistics on alcohol: England, 2013.* London: Health and Social Care Information Centre.

National Health and Medical Research Council. (2009). *Australian guidelines to reduce health risks from drinking alcohol.* Canberra, Australia: National Health and Medical Research Council.

National Institute on Alcohol Abuse and Alcoholism (NIAAA). (2015). *Alcohol use disorder: A comparison of DSM-IV and DSM-5.* NIH Publication 13–7999. Bethesda, MD: National Institutes of Health.

Rehm, J., Mathers, C., Popova, S., Thavorncharoensap, M., Teerawattananon, Y., & Patra, J. (2009). Global burden of disease and injury and economic cost attributable to alcohol use and alcohol-use disorders. *Lancet*, **373**(9682), 2223–2233.

Schuckit, M. A., Smith, T. L., Daeppen, J. B., Daeppen, J. B., Eng, M., Li, T. K., … Bucholz, K. K. (1998). Clinical relevance of the distinction between alcohol dependence with and without a physiological component. *American Journal of Psychiatry* **155**(6), 733–740.

Trotter, T. (1804). *An essay, medical, philosophical, and chemical, on drunkenness, and its effects on the human body.* London: T. N. Longman and O. Rees.

Vale, B., & Edwards, G. (2011). *Physician to the fleet: The life and times of Thomas Trotter, 1760–1832.* Woodbridge, UK: Boydell Press.

World Health Organization (WHO). (1992). *The ICD-10 classification of mental and behavioural disorders clinical descriptions and diagnostic guidelines.* Geneva: World Health Organization.

World Health Organization (WHO). (1994). *Lexicon of alcohol and drug terms.* Geneva: World Health Organization.

World Health Organization (WHO). (2009). *Global health risks: Mortality and burden of disease attributable to selected major risks.* Geneva: World Health Organization.

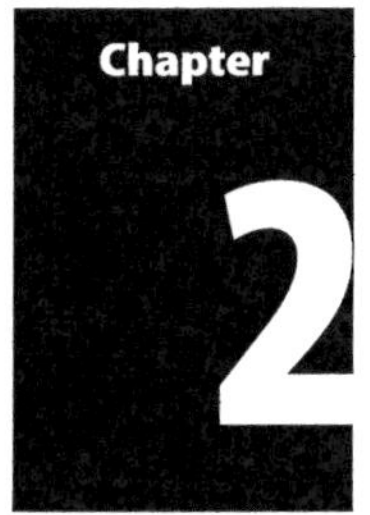

Alcohol as a drug

The purpose of this chapter

Humankind has long "enjoyed" a relationship with alcohol. Alcohol's properties have been familiar to – and greatly valued by – countless peoples around the world for thousands of years. Alcoholic drinks are imbued with symbolic significance when used within social, cultural, and religious custom and ritual. Yet alcohol is also a drug that has important pharmacological and toxic effects upon most systems in the human body. Knowledge of these pharmacological effects is basic to understanding both the problems that arise from its use as well as the treatment approaches adopted.

What's in an alcoholic drink?

The English word *alcohol* is derived from an Arabic word for the black powder of purified antimony (*al-koh'l*) that was used as an early form of eyeliner. The word was subsequently generalized to mean *purification* and later adopted into the English language to describe the distillate of wine as "alcohol of wine." Pharmacologically, alcohol describes organic compounds characterized by a hydroxyl group attached to a saturated carbon molecule.

There are many alcohols, including methyl alcohol (methanol, which is highly toxic – ingestion of 30 mL is potentially fatal), isopropyl alcohol (isopropanol – also highly toxic, with symptoms being reported at doses as low as 20 mL), and ethyl alcohol (ethanol – the primary active ingredient in alcoholic drinks; see Figure 2.1). Alcohol-containing drinks consist mostly of water (H_2O), ethanol (CH_3CH_2OH), and flavouring/colouring. Ethanol has been called a "stupid molecule" due to its simple structure, whereas the flavour, colours, and congeners (related chemicals produced during fermentation) are sometimes called the "dirt in the drink." Ethanol is the subject of this chapter; however, the inaccurate term "alcohol" is used in its place in deference to the common usage of this term while recognizing this inherent inaccuracy.

Pharmacology

Alcohol is a colourless liquid at room temperature. Relative to water, it has a lower density, freezing point, and boiling point (Table 2.1).

The complexity of scientific notation

Various ways of expressing alcohol concentrations are employed in different texts. Usually, concentration is expressed as a weight in a given volume of blood, breath, or urine. In this

Table 2.1. Properties of alcohol compared with water

	Alcohol (ethanol)	Water
Formula	CH_3CH_2OH	H_2O
Appearance	Colourless clear liquid	Colourless clear liquid with a hint of blue
Molecular weight	46 g/mol	18 g/mol
Density	0.79 g/cm^3 (liquid)	1 g/cm^3 (liquid)
Melting point	−114°C	0°C
Boiling point	78.4°C	100°C

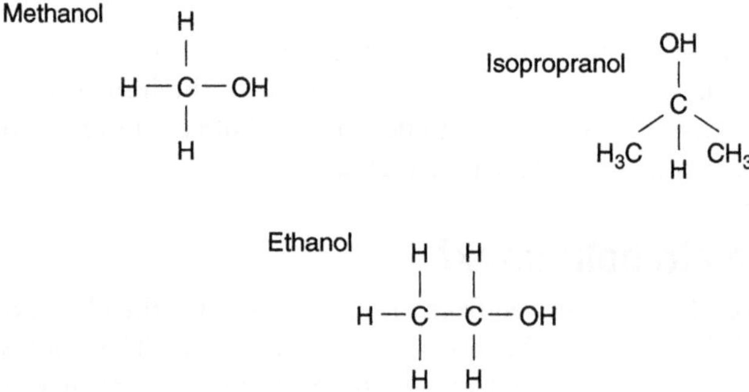

Figure 2.1: Chemical structure of some alcohols.

chapter, blood alcohol concentrations (BACs) are expressed as milligrams per 100 millilitres of blood (mg/100 mL). It should be noted, however, that the following reported BACs are all the same (see also Brick, 2004):

100 mg/100 mL
100 mg/decilitre (100 mg/dL)
100 mg/100 cc
100 mg percent (100 mg%)
0.1 g/100 mL
0.1 g/decilitre
0.1 grams percent (0.1 g%)
0.1 percent (0.1%)

Laboratory studies may report a millimolar concentration, and this can be converted to mg/100 mL by using the molecular weight. Thus, the millimolar concentration (mmol) of alcohol is multiplied by the molecular weight 46 g/mol and divided by 10 to achieve the same concentration in mg/100 mL. Clinical laboratories usually measure alcohol concentrations in serum rather than in blood. An approximate conversion between serum and blood concentration can be obtained by multiplying the value in serum by 0.85.

The term "proof" adds another layer of complexity, particularly across "two nations separated by a common language." *Proof* was used as a measure of the concentration of alcohol, and 100 percent proof represents the lowest dilution able to sustain combustion of equal amounts of gunpowder and the spirit under test and produce a clear blue flame. This represents a concentration of approximately 57 percent alcohol by volume (ABV) under the UK system, with pure alcohol being 175 percent proof. In the United States, *proof* is double the concentration expressed by volume; therefore, 100 percent proof is equivalent to 50 percent ABV. Thus, in the old UK system, 70 percent proof spirit is 40 percent ABV or 80 percent proof in the USA! (See Chapter 1 for more information about how much alcohol is present in a "unit" or "drink.")

Absorption and distribution

Absorption of alcohol is relatively slow from the stomach but occurs rapidly in the small intestine, and the time to maximum concentration in the blood ranges from 30 to 90 minutes after consumption (Brick, 2004). The presence of food in the stomach slows absorption by delaying gastric emptying into the small intestine, which is highly efficient at absorbing such substances due to the presence of villae. Villae are little projections into the gut that dramatically increase the surface area available for absorption. Furthermore, the prandial state can alter the efficiency with which drinks of differing alcohol concentrations are absorbed. The presence of carbon dioxide bubbles in fizzy drinks (e.g., champagne) increases absorption, whereas physical exercise reduces absorption. In addition, sugar-free mixers increase gastric emptying and absorption when compared with sugar-containing regular versions. Furthermore, peak blood levels are higher if the same quantity of alcohol is ingested in a single dose rather than in several small doses (Agarwal & Goedde, 1990).

Following absorption, alcohol is distributed throughout the body. It is hydrophilic (water-loving) and therefore is distributed with water. It can cross the placenta into the fetal circulation and is also found in breast milk in lactating mothers.

BAC is very similar to tissue levels in most of the body except fat. The usually smaller stature and relatively higher proportion of body fat (or lower proportion of water) in women often leads to a higher BAC than would occur in men after an equivalent dose of alcohol. This may explain, in part, the increased vulnerability of women to certain types of tissue damage.

Excretion and metabolism

Between 90 percent and 98 percent of ingested alcohol is eliminated from the body by oxidation to carbon dioxide and water. Most of the alcohol that escapes oxidation is excreted unchanged in expired air, urine, and sweat. Elimination by these routes may increase after a heavy drinking bout or at elevated temperatures. Indeed, the presence of alcohol in expired air can be used to estimate the BAC using a breathalyser. The breath alcohol concentration can be used to calculate a presumed BAC level using a conversion factor, which varies between countries (some breathalyzers do this automatically). Breathalyzers provide a more objective measure of alcohol levels than clinical examination alone, and they are widely employed to test motorists suspected of drink-driving offences (known as drunk-driving in the United States). Countries set differing legal limits for driving; for example, this ranges widely across Europe from 0 to 80 mg/100 mL in blood.

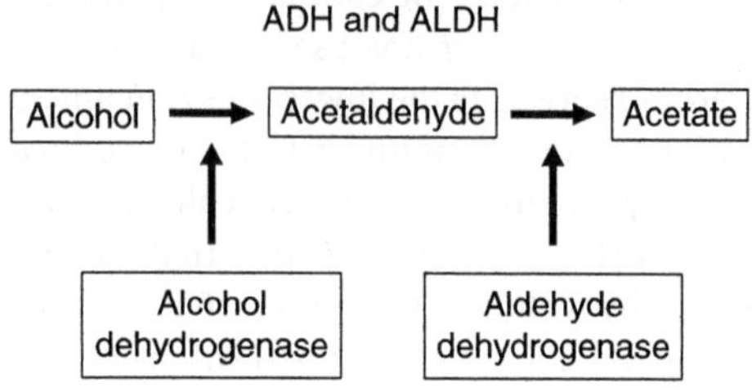

Figure 2.2: Metabolism of alcohol.

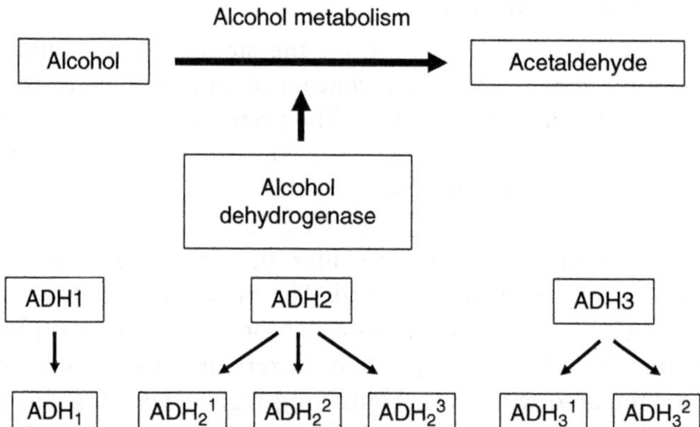

Figure 2.3: Genetic variation I alcohol dehydrogenase (ADH). There are three genetic variants in ADH2 and two in ADH3 that affect the speed of the enzyme.

Hepatic alcohol metabolism

The amount of alcohol oxidized per unit time depends on body weight. In the healthy adult, the rate is limited to about 8 g, or 1 UK unit of alcohol per hour in a 70 kg adult, or 120 mg/kg per hour (Fleming, Mihic, & Harris, 2006). The breakdown of alcohol in the liver is largely saturated (i.e., it takes place as quickly as possible) at low BACs. Technically, this is called a *pseudo-zero-order of metabolism*, in which the rate is constant and doesn't vary with alcohol concentrations at the levels generally found during drinking. Breakdown can be faster in the heavier drinker (see later discussion). Alcohol may undergo first-pass metabolism in the stomach, but 90–98 percent of ingested alcohol is metabolized in the liver. The major pathway is oxidation by alcohol dehydrogenase (ADH) to acetaldehyde (Figure 2.2). Acetaldehyde is highly toxic and is usually rapidly oxidized by aldehyde dehydrogenase 2 (ALDH2) to acetate. Acetate is then broken down to water and carbon dioxide.

The enzymes ADH and ALDH are under genetic control. Five classes of ADH have been described, and the class I variety is largely responsible for the first step in alcohol metabolism in the liver (Figure 2.3). Class I consists of enzymes encoded by three different genes that demonstrate up to a 40-fold difference in the maximum speed of the reaction. Complete human genome and expression studies report that there are 19 functional ALDH genes. ALDH2, the isozyme largely responsible for the oxidation of acetaldehyde, exists in two

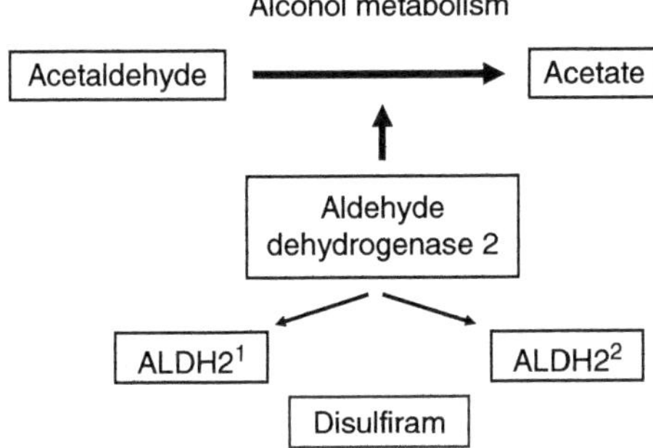

Figure 2.4: Genetic variation in ALDH2. There are two generic variants in ALDH2, one of which is of low activity (ALDH2²). Disulfiram, an aversive drug that is used to aid the maintenance of abstinence, destroys the activity of ALDH2 (effectively blocking the metabolism of alcohol and thereby producing a potentially dangerous reaction).

forms, one of which is virtually inactive (*ALDH2*2* variant). Low-activity ALDH2, which is common in Asian populations, leads to a flushing reaction when alcohol is taken. This reaction is unpleasant and may include nausea, headache, and facial flushing. Individuals with low-activity ALDH2 are less inclined to drink and are thus less vulnerable to developing alcohol problems and dependence (Ball, Pembrey, & Stevens, 2007). Although the toxicity of aldehydes has been long recognized, more recently, there is increasing evidence also linking the low-activity ALDH2 variant with other disorders including stroke, heart failure, and Alzheimer's disease (Chen, Ferreira, Gross, & Mochly-Rosen, 2014). ALDH is also the primary site of action for disulfiram, a drug that acts by suppressing the activity of ALDH2 and is used to help maintain abstinence in alcohol dependence (see Chapter 13). In essence, possessing this low-activity variant is similar to taking disulfiram constantly. The acetate formed from acetaldehyde is released into the circulation and is largely taken up by muscle and heart for oxidation via the tricarboxylic acid cycle (Fleming et al., 2006; see Figure 2.4).

Although ADH is the major pathway for the oxidation of alcohol, it can also be oxidized by two other enzyme systems: the microsomal ethanol-oxidizing system (MEOS) located in the smooth endoplasmic reticulum (SER), and catalase, located in peroxisomes. The contribution of catalase is thought to be minimal. The MEOS is dependent on the cytochrome P450 system, which is located on the SER. It usually plays a small role in the metabolism of alcohol, but this role increases with greater consumption. Chronic alcohol intake enhances MEOS activity by a process of inducing a form of P450 called cytochrome P450 2E1 (CYP2E1). The induction of CYP2E1 leads to an increase in the rate of alcohol metabolism and to an increased tolerance to alcohol and other drugs. Indeed, CYP2E1 may be responsible for up to 10 percent of alcohol metabolism in people with chronic drinking problems.

Extrahepatic alcohol metabolism

It is now accepted that alcohol is subjected to a first-pass metabolism by the ADH isoenzymes, primarily ADH7, in the stomach and that this represents some protection against the systemic effects of alcohol (Birley et al., 2008; Jelski, Chrostek, Szmitkowski, & Laszewicz, 2002).

Acute pharmacological effects

This section describes common acute effects of alcohol ingestion. The chronic effects are described in Chapter 5.

Cardiovascular system

Rarely will acute intoxication have serious consequences for the cardiovascular system. However, an alcohol binge, on top of a history of regular heavy drinking, has been associated with heart arrhythmias, commonly, a supraventricular tachycardia (SVT), and this has been referred to as "holiday heart syndrome." (An SVT is an episode of a fast heartbeat, experienced as palpitations.) Spontaneous recovery typically occurs following abstinence.

Body temperature

Moderate amounts of alcohol can lead to peripheral vasodilatation, which can increase heat loss but is associated with a misleading feeling of warmth. Furthermore, increased sweating can, in turn, lead to heat loss and a fall in body temperature. Large amounts of alcohol can depress the central temperature-regulating mechanism and cause a more pronounced fall in body temperature.

Gastrointestinal tract

Alcohol can stimulate the release of the hormone gastrin, which causes the secretion of gastric acid. Lower alcohol concentration drinks are associated with a greater gastrin release and higher levels of gastric acid. Strong alcoholic drinks, however, cause inflammation of the stomach lining and produce an erosive gastritis.

Kidney

Alcohol produces a diuretic effect independent from the increased flow associated with the ingestion of large volumes of fluid. This diuretic effect is due to the suppression of vasopressin (antidiuretic hormone) release.

Respiration

Moderate amounts of alcohol may either stimulate or depress respiration. Larger amounts (e.g., 400 mg/100 mL or greater) consistently produce depression of respiration.

Central nervous system

The effects of alcohol on the brain are dependent on dose, rate of rise in BAC, and degree of tolerance. Typically, driving skill is affected at 30 mg/100 mL. Ataxia, inattention, and slowed reaction times are evident at levels of about 50 mg/100 mL. Mood and behavioural changes occur at levels of approximately 50–100 mg/100 mL. At levels of 150–300 mg/100 mL, drinkers typically experience loss of self-control, slurred speech, and clumsiness. Individuals unused to heavy drinking are moderately intoxicated at BAC levels of 150–250 mg/100 mL, and obvious intoxication is usually evident at 300 mg/100 mL. At BACs of 300–500 mg/100 mL, individuals are usually severely intoxicated, and stupor and hypothermia may sometimes supervene. Hypoglycemia and seizures are occasionally a feature of BACs in this range. Heavy drinkers become tolerant to the central nervous system effects of alcohol and may on occasion have BAC levels of 500 mg/100 mL without obvious signs of intoxication. However, for nontolerant drinkers, such levels are associated with slowed reflexes and respiration, hypotension, hypothermia, and death.

Understanding how and where alcohol affects brain function is easier when a clinician has some appreciation of the key technologies used in neuroscientific research. We therefore now provide an overview of the different kinds of neuroimaging techniques that have greatly advanced our knowledge about vulnerability to alcohol misuse or development of dependence and the impact of alcohol on the brain and its ability to recover.

Neuroimaging

Broadly speaking, imaging techniques can be broken down into three types: (1) magnetic resonance (MR), (2) radiolabeled tracers and positron emission tomography (PET) or single photon emission computed tomography (SPECT), and (3) measured electrical activity (electroencephalography [EEG], magnetoencephalography [MEG]). All are used clinically (e.g., mapping brain function around a brain tumour) as well as being powerful research tools.

For structural analysis, computed tomography (CT) is no longer used because MR offers greater resolution and the ability to differentiate white matter, grey matter, and cerebrospinal fluid. Recent structural studies suggest that both grey and white matter volumes recover with sustained abstinence (Monnig et al., 2013; Sullivan & Pfefferbaum, 2005). This is consistent with the improvements seen in cognitive functioning. More recently, another MR technique, diffusion tensor imaging (DTI) has been developed to assess white matter integrity by assessing diffusion of water in this tissue. Currently, few studies using DTI have been completed; however, changes consistent with dysregulation in white matter function have been described.

Brain function is commonly measured in terms of blood flow with functional MR imaging (fMRI). fMRI is based on the principle that deoxygenated blood has a different magnetic spin than oxygenated blood, from which blood oxygen level dependent (BOLD) contrast is derived. Therefore, activity in a brain area will alter blood flow, level of oxygenated haemoglobin, and, consequently, BOLD signal. Studies are therefore designed to have a baseline condition followed by a test condition (e.g., presentation of alcohol cues) that is repeated many times over several minutes. Alternatively, the subject may indicate when they are experiencing an "event" (e.g., craving), and the BOLD signal is compared to when they were not. fMRI is commonly used because MR machines are widely available and are a relatively cheap research tool and analytical programmes are available free online. fMRI has good temporal and spatial resolution, and individuals can undergo several scans because it is safe and generally well-tolerated.

PET/SPECT are the most powerful approaches to investigating neuropharmacology in vivo but are in limited use due to their high cost and the requirement of a particular research scanner. Because they require giving a radioactive dose, individuals generally only undergo one or two scans in research studies. Although SPECT is more widely available, PET has higher resolution and therefore is used more commonly for research.

Which neurotransmitter systems can be assessed with PET/SPECT depends on whether there is a tracer available that binds to the target of interest. Tracers are available for dopamine D_2/D_3 receptors and other targets of interest in addiction such as the gamma-aminobutyric acid (GABA)-benzodiazepine receptor, the serotonin transporter, and the mu opiate receptor. For others, such as glutamate N-methyl-D-aspartate (NMDA), tracers are still in development or not widely available. In addition a few tracers are sensitive to neurotransmitters in the brain so that comparing radiotracer binding in two scans provides an index of the change in neurotransmitter levels. For example, one scan acts as a baseline and another may involve either a pharmacological challenge (e.g., amphetamine to increase dopamine) or a behavioural challenge (e.g., cue-induced craving).

Magnetic resonance spectroscopy (MRS) provides biochemical or metabolic information. For example, N-acetyl aspartate (NAA) is reduced in neuronal damage; choline is associated with demyelination; and GABA and glutamate/glutamine alter with metabolism. We know that GABA and glutamate are involved in metabolism and the majority of the MRS signal comes from metabolism rather than neurotransmission.

Last, electrical activity can be measured using EEG or by measuring magnetic fields associated with electrical currents using MEG. MEG is a relatively new technique with high temporal but limited spatial resolution; it can only measure activity in upper layers of the brain.

Sites of action: Brain circuits

We now highlight key findings about brain circuits; more comprehensive reviews of neuroimaging studies in addiction are available elsewhere (Jasinska et al., 2014). Although imaging studies have revealed many similarities between alcohol and other psychoactive substances, differences have also been shown that inform our understanding of substance use disorders. The interaction of neuropharmacology and brain circuitry between nicotine and alcohol is increasingly being studied, whereas the comorbidity of alcohol use disorder and illicit drug use and/or other psychiatric disorders is less frequently investigated.

Brain responses to salient alcohol cues have been widely studied given their importance in alcohol lapse and relapse. Many studies have shown that, compared with neutral cues (such as wildlife videos or household/office objects), salient drug-related cues result in higher levels of brain activity in the mesolimbic system. The mesolimbic system is a dopamine projection from the ventral tegmental area (VTA) in the brainstem to ventral striatum (nucleus accumbens) and orbitofrontal and anterior cingulate cortices within the prefrontal cortex. There have been numerous studies of this pathway in addiction due to its important role in mediating pleasure and the motivation for so-called natural pleasures (food, sex), as well as for many substances of abuse (Figure 2.6). Thus, cue reactivity studies show greater activation in ventral striatum, anterior cingulate, insula, and VTA as well as in the hippocampus and amygdala, which are regions involved in learning and memory (Jasinska et al., 2014; Schacht, Anton, & Myrick, 2013). Such hyperreactivity is consistent with individuals reporting strong responses (such as craving) to salient cues even after years of abstinence.

Other processes of relevance to addiction, such as reward, impulsivity, and decision-making, have been investigated using appropriate psychological tasks during fMRI. For instance, the monetary incentive delay task has been widely used in other conditions to investigate anticipation of a reward. Although blunted responses associated with impulsivity have been reported in alcohol dependence (e.g., Beck et al., 2009), another study failed to replicate this using a different reward task (van Holst et al., 2014). A meta-analysis of imaging studies assessing alcohol-related reward with cue reactivity reported robust activation of a range of brain regions including the ventral striatum and those involved in decision-making, such as the anterior cingulate and ventromedial prefrontal cortex (Schacht et al., 2013). However, there was no difference in activation in these regions between those with alcohol dependence and controls; instead, greater activation was seen in alcohol dependence in areas such as the posterior cingulate. Taking all these studies together, the reward system in alcohol dependence appears dysregulated, and, at the same time, other brain regions outside the ventral striatum are also affected.

Sites of action: Pharmacology

Alcohol is a relatively nonspecific drug that interacts with multiple chemical messengers or neurotransmitter pathways. It does not have an exclusive interaction at one particular brain receptor, as do opioids, nor does it block a reuptake transporter, as does cocaine. Instead, alcohol is thought to bind to a range of regulatory proteins involved in neuronal signalling, such as ion channels or enzymes. The rewarding properties of alcohol are thought to be mediated in part by effects on the dopamine and opioid systems, and alcohol's impact on the GABA and glutamate systems results in many effects such as sedation and respiratory depression as well as tolerance and withdrawal (Lingford-Hughes, Watson, Kalk, & Reid, 2010).

When characterizing neurotransmitter systems and their interaction with alcohol, three stages should be considered: vulnerability or predisposing dysregulation, acute interactions with alcohol, and adaptations that occur with chronic drinking. Such neuroadaptations are likely to contribute to a key feature that Edwards and Gross described as part of the alcohol dependence syndrome: the rapid reinstatement of dependent drinking even after years of abstinence (Edwards & Gross, 1976). Understanding underlying processes such as alcohol-related reward and tolerance/withdrawal informs the development of appropriate strategies from prevention through to treatment of alcohol dependence.

Alcohol and reward

Alcohol and dopamine

As described, the mesolimbic dopamine pathway (VTA → nucleus accumbens) plays a central role in pleasure, motivation, and drug-seeking. In animal models, alcohol has been shown to increase the firing of dopaminergic neurons, which increases dopamine levels in the nucleus accumbens. Firing of the dopaminergic neuron in the VTA is controlled by inhibitory GABA-ergic neurons, which in turn are modulated by a range of inhibitory neurotransmitter receptors such as opioid (mu), nicotinic, and cannabinoid (CB_1) (see Figure 2.5). Thus, alcohol indirectly increases dopamine neuron firing through its effects on these modulators, particularly the GABA and opioid systems. Whereas the dopaminergic mesolimbic pathway has been shown to be involved in motivation, expectation, and drug-seeking for alcohol, nondopaminergic pathways are also involved (Nutt, Lingford-Hughes, Erritzoe, & Stokes, 2015).

There are two families of dopamine receptors, D_1 (D_1 and D_5) and D_2 (D_2, D_3, D_4). Researchers have shown particular interest in the D_2 family as potential therapeutic targets. Neuroimaging studies of the dopaminergic system have been critical in characterizing this system in alcohol use and dependence in humans. In nondependent drinkers, alcohol-induced dopamine release has been observed although not consistently (see Martinez & Narendran, 2010), with one study reporting modulation by mu opiate receptor variants

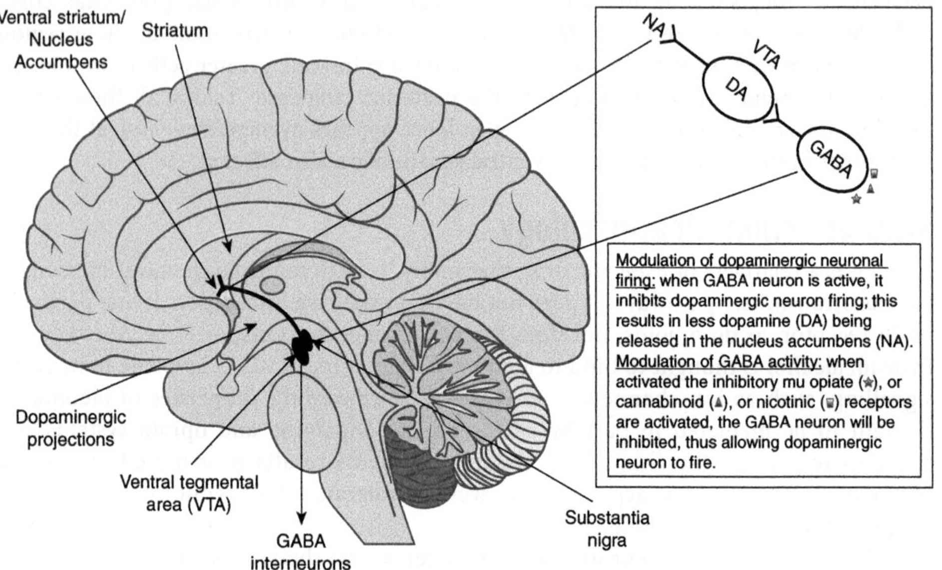

Figure 2.5: Brain reward circuitry relevant to alcohol consumption.

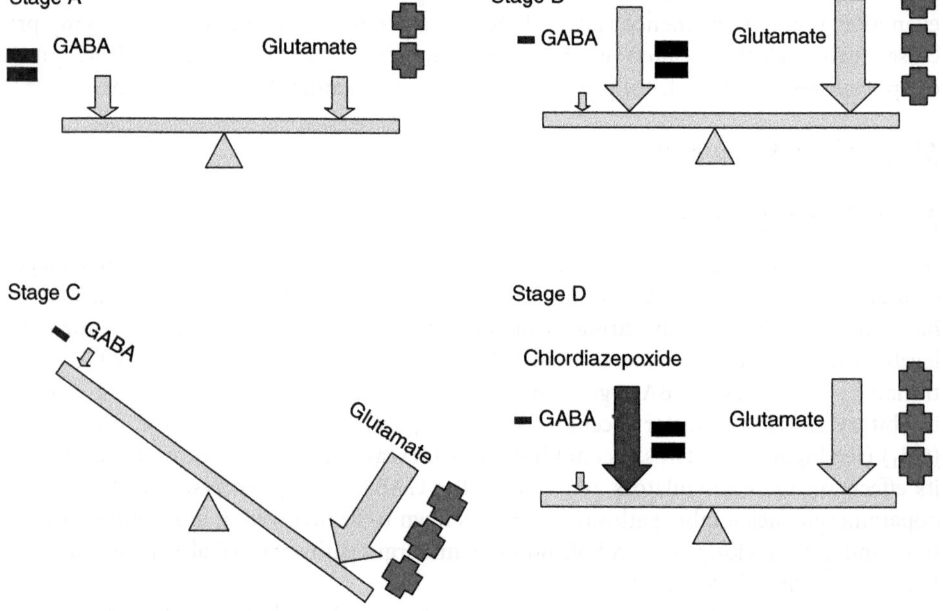

Figure 2.6: Gamma-aminobutyric acid (GABA) and glutamate stages in tolerance and withdrawal. In the brain, there is a balance between the inhibitory GABA systems and the excitatory system (Stage A). Alcohol disrupts that balance, and, with chronic exposure, the brain adjusts and adapts to the presence of alcohol (Stage B). When a physically dependent individual stops drinking or cuts down rapidly, the brain cannot adjust sufficiently quickly, and the individual develops symptoms and signs of physical withdrawal (Stage C). This balance can be restored and the withdrawal symptoms treated using benzodiazepines that are tailed off slowly, thus allowing the brain to re-establish the balance between these two systems (Stage D).

(Ramchandani et al., 2011). In abstinent alcohol dependent individuals, increased dopamine turnover, blunted amphetamine-induced dopamine release, and reduced dopamine D_2/D_3 receptors have been reported in the ventral striatum. These effects appear to persist and are related to craving in some studies. These findings are consistent with dopaminergic hypofunction or "reward deficiency" theories of addiction. However, more recent evidence suggests that the level of dopamine D_3 receptors may be increased in alcohol dependence and that the level of dopamine D_2/D_3 receptors may "normalize" with abstinence (Erritzoe et al., 2014).

Despite the dopaminergic system's key role, medications that modulate it have shown limited clinical effectiveness. For instance, medications that either block dopamine function to reduce pleasure or boost dopamine to address any hypofunction, as well as a partial agonist, have not been found robustly effective (Lingford-Hughes, Welch, Peters, & Nutt, 2012). Disulfiram, although commonly thought of as a liver enzyme blocker, also blocks a similar enzyme in the brain that is involved in dopamine metabolism, dopamine-beta-hydroxylase. Such blockade results in an increase in dopamine as well as a reduction in noradrenaline. It is not clear how much this effect on dopamine and noradrenaline levels contributes to the clinical effectiveness of disulfiram, but a variant of the brain enzyme has been linked with the adverse effects of disulfiram (Mutschler et al., 2012).

Alcohol and opioids

The reinforcing and pleasurable effects of alcohol are mediated, at least in part, by activation of the endogenous opioid system (Figure 2.5). There are three opiate receptor subtypes – mu, kappa, and delta – each of which has an endogenous opioid. beta-endorphins bind to the mu subtype, dynorphins to kappa, and enkephalins to delta. Alcohol increases beta-endorphin release in the VTA, which results in increased dopamine release in the nucleus accumbens by modulating dopaminergic VTA neuronal firing and also through direct stimulation of dopamine cells in the nucleus accumbens (Lingford-Hughes et al., 2010). Whereas the mu receptor is associated with the pleasurable effects of alcohol, the kappa subtype mediates a less pleasant experience (dysphoria) and therefore acts to "counter" mu-related pleasure as alcohol consumption continues to dependent levels. The increased kappa activity is proposed to be maintained during abstinence, with its associated dysphoria increasing the vulnerability to relapse (Butelman, Yuferov, & Kreek, 2012). In addition, the opioid system is involved in impulsivity and in modulating the stress system (hypothalamic-pituitary-adrenal axis) thereby making it a key process to understand in the case of stress-induced alcohol relapse.

PET imaging studies in alcohol dependence have consistently shown that abstinence is associated with higher availability of mu opiate receptors compared with controls; this higher availability appears to persist and is related to craving (Heinz et al., 2005). More inhibitory mu opiate receptors on the inhibitory GABAergic neuron, which modulates dopamine neuron firing, would result in a greater likelihood of dopaminergic activity because the GABAergic neuron would be inhibited (Figure 2.5).

Mu-opioid receptor antagonists such as naloxone and naltrexone block these central effects of beta-endorphins and have been shown to reduce alcohol consumption in animal models and clinical settings (see Chapter 13). Another medication that blocks the mu opioid receptor is nalmefene, but it differs from naltrexone because it behaves like a partial agonist at the kappa receptor, a fact that may be significant in its clinical effectiveness, although, clinically, the two medications have not been directly compared (Walker & Koob, 2008).

Tolerance and withdrawal

Alcohol and GABA

GABA is the main inhibitory neurotransmitter in the brain. There are two receptor systems, $GABA_A$, which is an ion channel (ionotropic), and $GABA_B$, which is linked to G-coupled protein (metabotropic). The $GABA_A$ receptor system is like a ring doughnut that sits in the membrane of the neuron and is composed of five subunits (two alpha, two beta, and one gamma subunit). It has binding sites for several modulators, including barbiturates, benzodiazepines, and neurosteroids (Kumar et al 2009). GABA facilitates the passage of chloride ions through the channel into the cell, making the cell less excitable. Alcohol enhances the coupling between benzodiazepine and GABA thus increasing the GABA-mediated influx of chloride ions and inhibition. $GABA_A$ receptors are named according to their alpha subunit (1–6), which also determines their sensitivity to alcohol (Kumar et al., 2009). The key effects of alcohol on the brain (e.g., reducing anxiety, sedation, memory impairment) are mediated through the $GABA_A$ receptor. These can be linked to specific subtypes, such as $alpha_2$ and $alpha_3$ with anxiety and $alpha_5$ with memory and alcohol liking (Rudolph & Knoflach, 2011).

With continued drinking, changes in the $GABA_A$ receptor result in the reduced sensitivity to alcohol that underpins tolerance (see Figure 2.6). Neuroimaging studies have shown reduced availability of benzodiazepine receptors in abstinent alcoholics, particularly in the frontal lobe (Krystal et al., 2006). Notably, when testing the function of these benzodiazepine receptors, the response to a benzodiazepine challenge was no different between alcohol dependent individuals and controls with regard to increases in beta-EEG, but alcohol dependent individuals were less sensitive to alcohol's sleep-inducing effects (Lingford-Hughes et al., 2005). This reduced sensitivity is consistent with tolerance and also with the common occurrence of sleep problems in alcohol dependence. Understanding more about the roles of these different subtypes is important in characterizing novel targets to treat to reduce the adverse consequences of alcohol.

The $GABA_B$ receptor has received less attention until recently but is now an interesting new target for treatment due to its action of modulating the dopaminergic reward system (Tyacke, Lingford-Hughes, Reed, & Nutt, 2010). We discuss this further in Chapter 13.

Alcohol and glutamate

Glutamate is the main excitatory neurotransmitter system in the brain and, like the GABA system, has both ionotropic and metabotropic receptors. Regarding the effects of alcohol on the brain, the ionotropic NMDA receptor is a key target (Nutt, 1999). Like the $GABA_A$ receptor, the NMDA receptor is like a ring doughnut of subunits sitting in the cell membrane. The NMDA receptor allows calcium ions into the cell, which make the cell more likely to "fire" or be active. A range of compounds including glycine, phencyclidine (PCP), and ketamine bind to and modulate the activity of the NMDA receptor complex. Alcohol acts like a blocker (antagonist) of the NMDA receptor, thus opposing the effects of glutamate (see Figure 2.6). Therefore, alcohol very effectively reduces brain activity by enhancing GABA inhibitory activity and blocking excitatory NMDA glutamate activity. The NMDA receptors adapt to alcohol by increasing the number of receptors to overcome alcohol's blocking actions. Such an increase in NMDA receptors may lead to an excessive influx of calcium, which is damaging to the neuron and is termed *excitotoxic damage.* This mechanism is thought to contribute to alcohol-related neuronal loss (atrophy) and cognitive impairment, including blackouts.

Less is known about the interaction between alcohol and the other two ionotropic receptors, L-alpha-amino-3-hydroxy-5-methyl-isoxazole-4-propionic acid (AMPA) and kainate, although blocking AMPA receptors also reduces alcohol consumption in animal models and therefore is being investigated as a potential treatment target (Holmes, Spanagel, & Krystal, 2013). Regarding the metabotropic receptors, there are several subtypes (mGluR), with mGluR2/3 and mGluR5 linked to alcohol consumption (Holmes et al., 2013).

Glutamate is also critically involved with *synaptic plasticity*, a process whereby particular synapses or connections in the brain are strengthened through repeated use or weakened due to limited use. This process is an important foundation for learning and memory and hence for adapting behaviour to changing environments. Thus, alcohol consumption may interfere with this key process by altering brain connections and strengthening those in circuits activated by alcohol at the cost of "non-alcohol" circuits.

GABA and glutamate in tolerance and withdrawal

As described, both GABA and NDMA glutamate receptor systems adapt with chronic exposure to alcohol (see Figure 2.6). Thus, a compensatory reduction in $GABA_A$ function and an increase in NDMA glutamate function occur to counter the enhancing and blocking effects of alcohol, respectively. These changes underpin tolerance and withdrawal. Many individuals who drink regularly are aware of becoming tolerant to alcohol: alcohol has less of an effect on them (e.g., intoxication or sedation). Although tolerance can occur with nondependent drinking, significant withdrawal symptoms are generally seen when an individual is dependent on alcohol. As alcohol leaves the brain, the reduced GABA and enhanced glutamate activity manifests itself as withdrawal symptoms including tremors, sweats, dry heaves, and, for some, withdrawal seizures and delirium tremens (see Chapter 11).

Medically, these withdrawal symptoms can be prevented or at least significantly reduced by replacing the alcohol with a benzodiazepine, which similarly enhances GABA-induced chloride flux, thereby restoring the balance between these two systems (Figure 2.5). By using a benzodiazepine with a long half-life and/or employing a reducing regime over several days, the brain is allowed the time needed to readjust to the absence of alcohol by restoring the balance between these two opposing systems. Alternatively, reducing glutamate activity with anticonvulsant medication can also treat alcohol withdrawal symptoms (see Chapter 11), reduce brain glutamate levels, and prevent associated toxicity (Hermann et al., 2012; Ward, Lallemand, & de Witte, 2009).

Future directions

Alcohol is a remarkable molecule and a drug whose impact on the brain is not yet fully understood despite humanity's long association with it. Neurobiological and neuropharmacological research has helped to uncover the mechanisms underlying the actions of alcohol, the "appetite" for alcohol, and the biological basis of dependence. This has led to a renewed interest in pharmacotherapies for alcohol dependence, with some promising results. The challenge now is to integrate insights from neuropharmacology, molecular genetics, and clinical science with understanding from other and wider disciplines, particularly psychology. Alcohol consumption is a behaviour with multiple determinants, and the truly crucial questions will, in the long run, yield only to multidisciplinary research. Clinicians should stay abreast of these developments and use emerging scientific knowledge to better detect, assess, and treat drinking problems.

References

Agarwal, D. P., & Goedde, H. W. (1990). *Alcohol metabolism, alcohol intolerance, and alcoholism: Biochemical and pharmacogenetic approaches.* Berlin: Springer.

Ball, D., Pembrey M., & Stevens, D. N. (2007). Genomics. In D. Nutt, T. W. Robbins, G. V. Stimson, M. Ince, & A. Jackson (Eds.), *Drugs and the future* (pp. 89–131). London: Academic Press.

Beck, A., Schlagenhauf, F., Wüstenberg, T., Hein, J., Kienast, T., Kahnt, T., Schmack, K., Hägele, C., Knutson, B., Heinz, A., & Wrase J. (2009). Ventral striatal activation during reward anticipation correlates with impulsivity in alcoholics. *Biological Psychiatry*, **66**(8), 734–742.

Birley, A. J., James, M. R., Dickson, P. A., Montgomery, G. W., Heath, A. C., Whitfield, J. B., & Martin, N. G. (2008). Association of the gastric alcohol dehydrogenase gene ADH7 with variation in alcohol metabolism. *Human Molecular Genetics*, **17**(2), 179–189.

Brick, J. (2004). Characteristics of alcohol: Chemistry, use, and abuse. In J. Brick (Ed.), *Handbook of the medical consequences of alcohol* (pp. 1–6). New York: Haworth.

Butelman, E. R., Yuferov, V., & Kreek, M. J. (2012). κ-Opioid receptor/dynorphin system: Genetic and pharmacotherapeutic implications for addiction. *Trends Neurosciences*, **35**(10), 587–596.

Chen, C. H., Ferreira, J. C., Gross, E. R., & Mochly-Rosen, D. (2014). Targeting aldehyde dehydrogenase 2: New therapeutic opportunities. *Physiological Reviews*, **94**(1), 1–34.

Edwards, G., & Gross, M. M. (1976). Alcohol dependence: Provisional description of a clinical syndrome. *British Medical Journal*, **1**(6017), 1058–1061.

Erritzoe, D., Tziortzi, A., Bargiela, D., Colasanti, A., Searle, G. E., Gunn, R. N., … Lingford-Hughes A. (2014). In vivo imaging of cerebral dopamine D3 receptors in alcoholism. *Neuropsychopharmacology*, **39**(7), 1703–1712.

Fleming, M., Mihic, S. J., & Harris, R. A. (2006). Ethanol. In L. L. Brunton, J. Lazo, & K. L. Parker (Eds.), *Goodman and Gilman's: The pharmacological basis of therapeutics* (11th ed., pp. 591–606). New York: McGraw Hill.

Heinz, A., Reimold, M., Wrase, J., Hermann, D., Croissant, B., Mundle, G., … Mann, K. (2005). Correlation of stable elevations in striatal μ-opioid receptor availability in detoxified alcoholic patients with alcohol craving: A positron emission tomography study using carbon 11-labeled carfentanil. *Archives of General Psychiatry*, **62**(1), 57–64.

Hermann, D., Weber-Fahr, W., Sartorius, A., Hoerst, M., Frischknecht, U., Tunc-Skarka, N., … Sommer, W.H. (2012). Translational magnetic resonance spectroscopy reveals excessive central glutamate levels during alcohol withdrawal in humans and rats. *Biological Psychiatry*, **71**(11), 1015–1021.

Holmes, A., Spanagel, R., & Krystal, J. H. (2013). Glutamatergic targets for new alcohol medications. *Psychopharmacology (Berl)*, **229**(3), 539–554.

Jasinska, A. J., Stein, E. A., Kaiser, J., Naumer, M. J., & Yalachkov, Y. (2014). Factors modulating neural reactivity to drug cues in addiction: A survey of human neuroimaging studies. *Neuroscience & Biobehavioral Reviews*, **38**, 1–16.

Jelski, W., Chrostek, L., Szmitkowski, M., & Laszewicz, W. (2002). Activity of class I, II, III, and IV alcohol dehydrogenase isoenzymes in human gastric mucosa. *Digestive Diseases and Sciences*, **47**(7), 1554–1557.

Krystal, J. H., Staley, J., Mason, G., Petrakis, I. L., Kaufman, J., Harris, R.A., … Lappalainen, J. (2006). Gamma-aminobutyric acid type A receptors and alcoholism: Intoxication, dependence, vulnerability, and treatment. *Archives of General Psychiatry*, **63**(9), 957–968.

Kumar, S., Porcu, P., Werner, D. F., Matthews, D. B., Diaz-Granados, J. L., Helfand, R. S., & Morrow, A. L. (2009). The role of GABA(A) receptors in the acute and chronic effects of ethanol: A decade of progress. *Psychopharmacology (Berl)*, **205**(4), 529–564.

Lingford-Hughes, A., Watson, B., Kalk, N., & Reid, A. (2010). Neuropharmacology of addiction and how it informs treatment. *British Medical Bulletin*, **96**, 93–110.

Lingford-Hughes, A. R., Welch, S., Peters, L., & Nutt, D. J. (2012). BAP updated guidelines: Evidence-based guidelines for the pharmacological management of substance abuse, harmful use, addiction and comorbidity: Recommendations from BAP. *Journal of Psychopharmacology*, **26**(7), 899–952.

Lingford-Hughes, A. R., Wilson, S. J., Cunningham, V. J., Feeney, A., Stevensen, B., Brooks, D. J., & Nutt, D. (2005). GABA-benzodiazepine receptor function in alcohol dependence: A combined 11C-flumazenil PET and pharmacodynamic study. *Psychopharmacology*, **180**, 595–606.

Martinez, D., & Narendran, R. (2010). Imaging neurotransmitter release by drugs of abuse. *Current Topics in Behavioral Neurosciences*, **3**, 219–245.

Mutschler, J., Abbruzzese, E., Witt, S. H., Dirican, G., Nieratschker, V., Frank, J., … Kiefer, F. (2012). Functional polymorphism of the dopamine β-hydroxylase gene is associated with increased risk of disulfiram-induced adverse effects in alcohol-dependent patients. *Journal of Clinical Psychopharmacology*, **32**(4), 578–580.

Monnig, M. A., Tonigan, J. S., Yeo, R. A., Thoma, R. J., & McCrady, B. S. (2013). White matter volume in alcohol use disorders: A meta-analysis. *Addiction Biology*, **18**(3), 581–592.

Nutt, D. (1999). Alcohol and the brain. Pharmacological insights for psychiatrists. *British Journal of Psychiatry*, **175**, 114–119.

Nutt, D., Lingford-Hughes, A., Erritzoe, D., & Stokes, P. R. (2015). The dopamine theory of addiction: 40 years of highs and lows. *Nature Reviews Neuroscience*, **16**, 305–132.

Ramchandani, V. A., Umhau, J., Pavon, F. J., Ruiz-Velasco, V., Margas, W., Sun, H., … Heilig, M. (2011). A genetic determinant of the striatal dopamine response to alcohol in men. *Molecular Psychiatry*, **16**(8):809–817.

Rudolph, U., & Knoflach, F. (2011). Beyond classical benzodiazepines: Novel therapeutic potential of GABAA receptor subtypes. *Nature Reviews Drug Discovery*, **10**(9), 685–697.

Schacht, J. P., Anton, R. F., & Myrick, H. (2013). Functional neuroimaging studies of alcohol cue reactivity: A quantitative meta-analysis and systematic review. *Addiction Biology*, **18**(1), 121–133.

Sullivan, E. V., & Pfefferbaum, A. (2005). Neurocircuitry in alcoholism: A substrate of disruption and repair. *Psychopharmacology*, **180**, 583–594.

Tyacke, R. J., Lingford-Hughes, A., Reed, L. J., & Nutt, D. J. (2010). GABAB receptors in addiction and its treatment. *Advances Pharmacology*, **58**, 373–396.

van Holst, R. J., Clark, L., Veltman, D. J., van den Brink, W., & Goudriaan, A.E. (2014). Enhanced striatal responses during expectancy coding in alcohol dependence. *Drug and Alcohol Dependence*, **142**, 204–208.

Walker, B. M., & Koob, G. F. (2008). Pharmacological evidence for a motivational role of kappa-opioid systems in ethanol dependence. *Neuropsychopharmacology*, **33**(3), 643–652.

Ward, R. J., Lallemand, F., & de Witte, P. (2009). Biochemical and neurotransmitter changes implicated in alcohol-induced brain damage in chronic or "binge drinking" alcohol abuse. *Alcohol and Alcoholism*, **44**(2), 128–135.

Chapter

3

Causes of drinking problems

Why do some people and not others develop drinking problems? Why do some drinking problems dissipate after a brief time, whereas others become entrenched aspects of a person's life? Science points fairly consistently to four broad classes of factors that, on average across people, influence whether a drinking problem emerges and whether it persists (Table 3.1). But because individual lives frequently diverge from average effects, accounting for any individual case of drinking problems will always remain at least partly a matter of speculation not only by the healthcare provider, but by the individual and those around him or her.

Table 3.1 divides the factors that influence drinking problems into three levels, namely the societal, the family/community, and individual. This framework is an oversimplification in a number of respects – most notably because the different factors interact across and within domains – but is useful as an analytic and descriptive convenience.

Availability of the drug

Drinking problems differ in an important respect from many other common health problems in that they can only occur in the presence of a particular environmental feature – namely, alcohol. One can experience chronic back pain, depression, or hypertension anywhere, but one can only have a drinking problem where there is alcohol. And, broadly speaking, the more readily available that alcohol, the more likely drinking problems are to occur, whether one is speaking of a society, a subculture, a community, or an individual.

The most fundamental ways in which societies determine alcohol availability are by laws regulating whether and under what conditions alcohol may be produced, sold, and consumed. Alcohol is de jure or de facto illegal in some regions (e.g., in parts of the Middle East), all of which have an unusually low prevalence of drinking problems. The United States' experience of Prohibition has been represented in many movies and novels as actually having increased problem drinking, and this has become the fashionable view in many circles. However, in fact, the opposite occurred, with alcohol consumption and alcohol-related harm decreasing substantially despite inconsistent enforcement of the law (Hall, 2010). Similarly, the dearth of supply caused by a strike in Finland's nationalized liquor industry led to reduced drinking problems (Mäkelä, 1980).

Societies that allow legal alcohol consumption typically set an age at which individuals are first allowed to purchase alcohol. As this age of purchase rises (e.g., from 18 to 21, as happened in the United States in the 1980s), alcohol consumption and alcohol-related harms decline among young adults.

Table 3.1. Four factors that influence the development of drinking problems

	Level		
Factor	**Societal**	**Community/Family**	**Individual**
Availability of alcohol	Legal status of alcohol	Density of alcohol outlets	Alcohol available at home and at work
	Licensing and sale regulations	Family and social network alcohol availability	Old enough to purchase and drink legally
Economic factors	Influence of drinks industry	Economic shocks	Personal ability to afford alcohol
	Taxation and pricing policy	Class-related drinking patterns	Ability to buy way out of consequences
Values and norms	Cultural drinking patterns	Drinking traditions	Religious beliefs
	Dominant religious traditions	Prominence of youth culture	Beliefs about alcohol
Biological factors	Population risk/protective factors	Parental genes	Individual genes related to alcohol response, anxiety, depression and activity level Neurological vulnerability

Where alcohol is legal, it can be made less available through other policy actions, such as laws restricting sale to particular licensees and times of day. Variations in supply can and do influence demand, just as demand can stimulate greater supply. Policies that expand alcohol availability by reducing restrictions on its supply also tend to increase consumption. Manipulation of policy can therefore have enormous impact on the alcohol consumption of a population. Conversely, failure to utilize such controls can allow alcohol consumption to escalate and related problems to reach epidemic proportions (Alcohol and Public Policy Group, 2010; Anderson & Baumberg, 2006).

At a community level, factors such as the density and distribution of outlets may influence the local incidence of alcohol-related road traffic accidents or violence (Gruenewald & Treno, 2000). Furthermore, particular family and social networks are more or less "wet," with some routinely providing alcohol at social, recreational, and community events and others not doing so.

Individuals also vary in the amount of alcohol available in their daily life context. A well-stocked bar in the home makes heavy drinking easier; living in the country 10 miles from the nearest pub makes it harder. Certain occupations also offer unusually high access to alcohol, including working in a restaurant, bar, or in the drinks industry itself.

Economic factors

In trying to explain why societies increase alcohol availability, it is informative to ask *who benefits*? Almost invariably, the answer is producers and sellers of alcoholic beverages.

The presence of a drinks industry, which can mass produce alcohol and then aggressively market and sell it, causes a wide-scale increase in alcohol consumption and drinking problems. A number of undeveloped societies that had only locally made, low-strength, hard-to-create alcoholic beverages (e.g., the Haya Indians who, through an elaborate process, made low-strength banana wine for ceremonial events [Carlson, 2006]), have seen a sharp rise in drinking problems with the arrival of stronger, attractively packaged, more easily acquired commercial alcoholic beverages such as the industry can provide.

The distribution of alcohol consumption is typically skewed in a population. For example, in the United States, the top 10 percent of drinkers account for the majority of national alcohol consumption (Cook, 2007). Alcohol producers and sellers are thus economically dependent on the existence of a large pool of problem drinkers: without those individuals who consume the equivalent of two or more bottles of wine a day, they would lose the bulk of their revenue. As a result of this economic reality, the industry tends to oppose any measure that would reduce the size of this heavy drinking group.

From the same observation flows the recognition that increases in the effective price of alcohol are potent drivers of reduced alcohol problems because of their concentrated influence on the heaviest drinkers. For example, a 10 cent per unit tax might cost a typical drinkers a few dollars a year, but cost heavy drinkers $500 a year or more, thus providing a powerful incentive to reduce consumption.

Taxes are not the only effective way to use price to reduce problem drinking. Canadian provinces have adopted a minimum unit pricing policy that prevents the sale of the high-strength, low-cost beverages favoured by heavy consumers who contribute disproportionately to alcohol-related harm. Remarkably, from 2002 to 2009, a mere 10 percent increase in the average minimum price of alcoholic beverages predicted a 32 percent decrease in fully alcohol-attributed mortality (Zhao, Stockwell et al., 2013).

The United Kingdom has been considering minimum unit pricing, but the effort has thus far been successfully stopped by the drinks industry and its political allies in England and Wales. Scotland, in contrast, passed such a policy and was immediately sued in International Court by the Scotch Whisky Association and other wine and spirits producers, who claimed that minimum unit pricing violates European laws governing trade. The European Court of Justice produced a murky ruling in 2015 that left ambiguous whether Scotland can go forward with its policy, which would significantly reduce alcohol-related crime, hospital admissions, morbidity, and mortality.

Economic factors also shape drinking because different forms of alcohol are linked in the public mind (often through advertising) with different economic classes. A well-off person may therefore drink wine rather than beer, not out of genuine liking but based on a sense that wine is what well-off people drink. These class distinctions are often socially reinforced: the factory worker who goes to the pub with his friends after work and orders a glass of sherry may endure substantial derision.

Economic upheaval in a community can also stimulate problem drinking. Multiple studies have shown that economic shocks (e.g., the closing of a factory and associated mass redundancy in the community) tend to be followed by increases in family problems, psychiatric care-seeking, and disorder, all of which seem likely to have reciprocally positive relationships with problem drinking (Kiernan, Toro, Rappaport, Seidman, 1989). At an individual level, some would argue that the stress of being unable to pay bills and otherwise make ends meet drives people to drink; others would disagree and assert instead that, far from being victims of circumstance, problem drinkers bring such financial woes upon themselves. As usual, data have cast doubt on such one-sided explanations. Longitudinal research shows that although problem drinking does indeed generate economic strains for drinkers and their families, these strains in turn lead to a subsequent worsening of the drinking problem (Humphreys, Moos, & Finney, 1996).

In the wake of the popular book *The Spirit Level*, the idea that economic inequality caused drinking problems (indeed, virtually all human problems) enjoyed a lengthy European vogue. The evidence, however, is unkind to this proposition: indices of a society's level of problem drinking either show no relationship or a positive relationship to economic inequality (Cameron, 2013).

Personal finances may shape the nature of drinking problems. Drink-driving arrests and boating accidents are more common among those who can afford such modes of transportation. Money may, to some extent, also allow a person to buy his or her way out of some drinking problems, at least in the short term; for example, by hiring a skilled barrister to have charges reduced or dismissed after an alcohol-involved mishap.

Values and norms

Across countries with similar legal regimes, the prevalence and amount of drinking varies substantially. Because drinking is often a social activity, and drinkers tend to make judgments about how much drinking is normal based on social comparisons, cultural norms of higher prevalence (i.e., few abstainers) and heavier volume drinking tend to reproduce themselves. This in turn leads to more drinking problems (Alcohol and Public Policy Group, 2010).

The quantity of alcohol consumed is not the only characteristic of drinking that affects the occurrence of drinking problems. Norms regarding patterns of alcohol consumption are also important. For example, different drinking problems are likely to arise in the woman who drinks four glasses of wine every day, as compared with the woman who drinks three bottles of wine in two days but who then drinks nothing for two or three weeks. Whereas the former is at greater risk of damage to the liver, brain, and other organs, the latter is at greater risk of marital disharmony and other social problems.

Cultural norms can influence the pattern of drinking just as much as the amount. In France, habitual consumption of wine with meals is associated with a relatively high but constant per capita consumption that predisposes toward chronic medical complications such as cirrhosis and certain cancers. In urban centres in the United Kingdom and North America, particularly among working-class men, alcohol is more likely to be consumed away from the home and often in relatively large quantities at a sitting. This pattern of drinking to intoxication is often accompanied by adverse consequences such as marital disharmony, accidents, interpersonal violence, and myocardial infarctions.

Both health professionals and the drinks industry attempt to influence alcohol consumption norms. Both have engaged in educational approaches, such as programmes informing young people of the risks of heavy alcohol consumption. In general, such programmes have a minimal impact, particularly in comparison to commercial marketing initiatives that portray drinking as glamorous, fun, and sexy. As a result, the drinks industry tends to endorse educational programmes, whereas health professionals are more keen on restricting pro-alcohol marketing, which seems more likely to reduce alcohol consumption (Alcohol and Public Policy Group, 2010).

Cultural norms may also influence the ways in which people behave when intoxicated. Drunken behaviour is shaped not only by the biological effects of alcohol as a drug, but also by social and cultural expectations as to how people will behave whilst intoxicated (MacAndrew & Edgerton, 1970). This may influence, for example, the likelihood of drunken antisocial behaviour.

One important element of culture is religious practice. Virtually all of the factors described thus far had some bearing on this (e.g., the Protestant religious groups who supported U.S. Prohibition, the Islamic prohibition on alcohol affecting anti-alcohol values in the Middle East). People with alcohol problems are far less likely to engage in religious practices than are the general population. In contrast, being raised in any mainstream religion is a potent protective factor against a young person developing an alcohol problem (Humphreys & Gifford, 2006).

Cultural norms around drinking often vary by gender, with drinking and heavy drinking much more tolerated in males than females in most of the world. However, along with many others changes in women's social and economic status in Western countries has come changes in drinking norms. This has included a substantial increase in heavy drinking by women in developed nations and, with it, an increase in alcohol-related consequences for health and well-being. In light of the fact that the same amount of ethanol may affect women more profoundly than men, the old rule that any alcohol treatment programme will have a patient population that is two-thirds to three-quarters male may well be overturned.

Values and norms also are potent forces on drinking problems at the community level. For example, some neighbourhoods (usually but not always due to the presence of universities) are part of a youth culture in which drinking, dating, mating, and dancing are prevalent and intertwined. Communities also have drinking traditions, such as one can find on Newcastle's Quayside or in the Irish ethnic bars of Boston's Southie district, or, at the other extreme, the largely dry counties of parts of the U.S. Deep South.

Families, too, have their drinking traditions, which children observe and from which they learn. In some families, drinking heavily is a matter of pride and identity (e.g., "He could hold his drink like a real McAllister!"). Children raised by parents who personally provide them alcohol are particularly likely to engage in heavy drinking in their adolescence (Aiken et al., in press).

At an individual level, personal religious beliefs and values, as well as specific beliefs about alcohol, also may affect an individual's likelihood of developing drinking problems. In general, these effects are intuitive (i.e., more religious beliefs and more anti-alcohol beliefs lessen drinking problems). But, for a small portion of people, these same beliefs may make drinking more exotic and hence an appealing forbidden fruit.

Biological factors

Biological factors that influence risk comprise two broad areas. The first is genetic/epigenetic and the second is neurological vulnerabilities of either nongenetic or unknown origins (some of which may someday be revealed as genetic/epigenetic). We discuss each factor in turn in this section.

Genetics

Many years of research into the genetics of alcohol use disorders identified no single causal "gene." Rather, risk for disorder involves many possible genetic variants and their interactions with each other and the environment (Ducci & Goldman, 2008; NIAAA, 2013). For instance, genetic variation may contribute to differences in alcohol metabolism, reward/intoxication sensitivity, and withdrawal seizure potential as well as to the likelihood of developing dependence.

We now briefly describe which genes are involved in alcohol dependence and the various approaches used to study them. More comprehensive reviews are available (e.g., Hirschorn & Daly, 2005; NIAAA, 2013).

A gene is made of *alleles*, of which there can be different types or *polymorphisms*, thus resulting in heterogeneity. Common research approaches include *genomics*, which aims to identify genetic polymorphisms, and *proteomics*, which examines changes in function of the protein for which a gene codes (e.g., an enzyme or receptor). Much of recent research developments occurred due to technological advances and associated reduction in costs, as well as greater sample sizes and improved characterization of populations. As with neuroimaging, the aim of genetic studies is to improve understanding of the underlying neurobiology of alcohol use, misuse, and dependence as well as to identify novel targets for prevention and treatment.

Alcohol dependence, like many other disorders, tends to run in families. Studies have examined those families with monozygotic or dizygotic twins where at least one is affected by alcohol dependence. If the risk for alcohol dependence is associated with genetic factors, then monozygotic twins with identical genomes would have higher concordance than would dizygotic twins, who share only 50 percent of their genomes. Such an approach has indeed shown higher concordance in monozygotic twins, thus supporting a genetic influence to alcohol dependence. Through such twin studies and those involving adoption, the genetic component of the variance or heritability of alcohol dependence is estimated at around 50 percent (Enoch, 2013; Rietschel & Treutlein, 2013). Therefore, the interaction with environmental risk factors is equally as important.

To investigate which specific genes or areas of genome may underlie alcohol dependence, genetic markers have been compared in affected and nonaffected family members. In these family-based linkage studies, either a few markers or a genome-wide set of up to a few thousand markers are characterized or genotyped. The markers must segregate with the gene for the disorder. This approach has the advantage of being an unbiased, comprehensive search across the genome for markers. However, it depends on the size and number of families (generally needing hundreds) and the quality of the characterization of the individuals (phenotyping), as well as on the frequency and penetrance of the allele and links with markers. And findings may not generalize to other families or populations. Such an approach was undertaken in the Collaborative Study on the Genetics of Alcoholism.

An alternative research approach involves association studies in which genetic markers for a disease (e.g., alcohol dependence) or individual trait (e.g., impulsivity) are characterized across a population rather than within a family. Such a case-control approach involves comparing common allelic variants in cases (e.g., alcohol dependence) and controls and requires prior knowledge of the gene or area of genome of interest. This candidate gene approach is therefore simpler in design and cheaper to undertake, thus making it widely used. It has more power to detect the impact of a common genetic variant than do linkage studies.

Rather than a candidate gene approach, technological advances mean that the entire genome can now be interrogated using *genome-wide association studies* (GWAS) to identify genes or at least areas of the genome associated with disorders or traits (Hirschhorn & Daly, 2005; Rietschel & Treutlein, 2013). A variation may involve only a single DNA building block (i.e., nucleotide), and these variations are therefore known as *single-nucleotide polymorphisms* (SNPs). GWAS do not require an *a priori* hypothesis or knowledge about a particular gene or gene region, and they have been widely applied to understand the genetic contributions to many common complex disorders and behaviours. Several thousand individual subjects are required since most genetic variants have a modest effect on disease or contribution to a trait. In addition, given the large number of variants in the genome (up to 1 million), large samples are required for statistically appropriate analysis and interpretation. GWAS has led to a number of inconsistent findings and false positives, and thus any reported findings should be viewed with a healthy degree of scepticism until robustly replicated.

An alternative to identifying a single variant or gene is to study how genes work together in a network and/or interact with the environment. Such analysis will be necessary to characterize how individual genes and networks contribute to a complex disorder such as alcohol dependence. Due to the multiple comparisons involved, large datasets are required, with collaboration between centers or the use of publicly held databases (e.g., a connectome). One such approach, *convergent functional genomics*, integrates human and animal data to prioritize candidate genes to increase the ability to distinguish signal from noise even with limited size cohorts and datasets. In alcohol dependence, 10 genes were identified including for neurotransmitter receptors DRD2 and GABRA2 as well as SNCA, a presynaptic chaperone implicated in brain plasticity and neurogenesis, and GFAP, an astrocyte intermediate filament-type protein involved in neuron–astrocyte interactions, cell adhesion, and cell–cell communication (Levey et al., 2014).

Alcohol metabolism

The influence of genetic heritability on alcohol metabolism is well known, with variants of the alcohol dehydrogenase (ADH) and aldehyde dehydrogenase (ALDH) genes associated with alcohol dependence and alcohol-related traits. For instance, one variant, ALDH2, is responsible for a "flushing syndrome" in East Asian populations, which is manifested by an unpleasant physiological response to the ingestion of alcohol. Carriers of the mutant gene tend to drink little or no alcohol because they feel unwell when they do so. The gene therefore dramatically reduces the incidence of heavy drinking and alcohol-related problems in the populations that carry it. Similar but subtler effects in the way that the body "handles" alcohol may influence the amount that Caucasian individuals drink.

Genes encoding neurotransmitter pathways and treatment response

As described, variations in the gamma-aminobutyric-A ($GABA_A$) receptor confer sensitivity to alcohol, and therefore, not surprisingly, several associations with genes encoding for subunits of this receptor and alcohol dependence. Candidate gene approaches have often, although not consistently, implicated alleles of the *GABRA2* gene, which encodes the $alpha_2$ subunit of the $GABA_A$ receptor, in risk of alcohol dependence (Edenberg & Foroud, 2013).

Less consistent or robust links with genes for other $GABA_A$ receptor subunit have also been found such as *GABRG1, GABRA1, GABRG3, GABRR1, GABRR2*, and *GABRB3.*

Other genetic variations in neurotransmitter pathways have been reported in alcohol dependence. These include the mu and kappa opioid receptors, the neuropeptide Y receptor, the muscarinic M_2 receptor, and corticotrophin-releasing hormone (CRHR1) (Enoch, 2013; Edenberg & Foroud, 2013).

In other areas of medicine, genetic information is used to "personalize" treatment, particularly in the presence of a potentially adverse side-effect profile. A similar approach therefore might be helpful to guide choice of treatment in alcohol dependence despite the lack of evidence from other approaches for "treatment matching." The strongest candidate is a polymorphism of the *ORPM1* gene that encodes the mu opioid receptor, which has been shown to be associated with response to naltrexone treatment in different cohorts (e.g., Anton et al., 2008). However, in a prospective study, this polymorphism did not modulate response to naltrexone (Oslin et al., 2015). Another study investigated a number of genes encoding a range of neurotransmitter systems with response to acamprosate and naltrexone (Ooteman et al., 2009). Associations were found between *DRD2, GABRA6, and GABRB2* genes and treatment response, but limited differences were found between the two medications. The genotype of the serotonin transporter and the $5HT_3$ receptor have also been shown to influence treatment outcome with ondansetron, a $5HT_3$ antagonist (Johnson et al., 2014). More recently, a polymorphism of the *GRIK1* gene that codes the $GluK_1$ subunit of kainate glutamate receptors has been found to modulate response to topiramate in heavy drinkers (Kranzler et al., 2014).

Epigenetics

Epigenetics is a more recent development and refers to changes in gene expression due to modifications of the genome that modulate transcription and/or translation without affecting the underlying DNA sequence. It is an important mechanism through which function adapts to environmental impacts, and it involves processes such as DNA methylation and histone modification. For instance, alcohol exposure can induce changes to synaptic plasticity-associated gene expression and result in the enrichment of immature synapses, aberrant synaptic plasticity, and dysfunctional dendritic spine formation (Kyzar & Pandey, 2015).

Neurobiological vulnerabilities

Neuroimaging techniques (see Chapter 2) are increasingly applied alongside epidemiological approaches to characterize what kind of brain responses may be linked to risk of substance misuse. Such characterization could help resolve a common dilemma for findings of imaging studies in humans: determining whether any pattern seen is a cause or a consequence of substance use. A few cohort studies being conducted around the world should be informative, including IMAGEN (http://www.imagen-europe.com/en/imagen-europe.php?hs=id3&display=none), which has assessed and is following 2,000 adolescents with regard to their mental health and risk-taking behaviour, including substance use. One surprising finding has already emerged: a family history of alcohol dependence is not associated with altered reward anticipation in teenagers aged 13–15, whereas dysregulation is generally seen in older individuals. This suggests that family history does not affect the developing reward system until later in life (Müller et al., 2015). It may be that young people who drink excessively are at risk of functional and structural brain damage that has enduring consequences for the brain reward system later in life (Hermens et al., 2013.

In addition, having a family history of alcohol dependence is associated with differences in the brain that suggest delayed maturation. Neural circuitry, including the frontal cortex, is less developed in adolescents with a family history of alcohol dependence compared with those without such a family history (Spadoni, Simmons, Yang, & Tapert, 2013). Another study reported a smaller amygdala in those at high risk of alcohol dependence (Hill et al., 2001). Such reports are important to consider when interpreting imaging studies in alcohol dependent individuals since such a family history is commonly present. How, then, can the evidence supporting the importance of both genetic and environmental causes for heavy drinking and drinking problems be brought together? The truth is, of course, that a behaviour such as alcohol consumption cannot be totally understood either on the basis of genes or environment alone, but only as a product of the interaction between a variety of genetic and environmental influences (Ducci & Goldman, 2008).

Thus, one might see an individual as being more or less disposed to heavy drinking, to particular alcohol-related problems, or to dependence on alcohol. This level of predisposition determines the risk, or probability, of being a heavy drinker or of suffering from a particular drink-related problem. If a combination of environmental and genetic risk factors exceeds a certain hypothetical threshold, then that individual will drink heavily or suffer a particular problem associated with his or her drinking.

We now understand more about the individual who drinks heavily and escapes harm or of the person who drinks moderately and suffers various complications. In the former case, the individual may be predisposed to heavy drinking by a combination of hereditary and environmental factors. However, at the same time, they may have a (genetic) constitutional resilience that protects them from liver damage, and they may learn (from their environment) social controls and patterns of behaviour that avoid public drunkenness, drink-driving, or other alcohol-related problems. In the latter case, the reverse may be true. Thus, an individual may drink moderately as a result of minimal genetic and environmental predisposition toward heavy drinking and yet be subject to, say, liver disease owing to a genetic susceptibility of the liver to damage by alcohol.

Does "self-medication" cause drinking problems?

Table 3.1 might be argued to have a sizable lacuna: where is psychological suffering among the causes of drinking problems? After all, we commonly speak of people "drinking to relieve stress" and people with depression, schizophrenia, and other psychological challenges are often said to be "self-medicating" their affliction. Can we not therefore assert, as classic psychoanalytic theory has it, that drinking problems are symptoms of underlying psychological suffering that is being self-medicated with alcohol?

Unquestionably, drinking problems are prevalent among individuals who have other mental health problems and among individuals who are experiencing substantial stress (e.g., job loss, divorce). However, it has to be said that drinking problems cause all these same problems, and although the drinker may frame his or her life narrative in an exculpatory way, what "drove the person to drink" very often came about because of drinking rather than the other way round (Lembke, 2012).

It should be remembered as well that if alcohol were truly a self-medication for disorders like depression and social anxiety disorder, it would have a salubrious impact. Yet depressed and anxious individuals who drink heavily have a worse prognosis than those who do not (Lembke, 2012).

Finally, if drinking problems were merely symptoms of underlying psychological disorders, they would deliquesce when the mental health problem was adequately treated. But Nunes and Levin's (2004) meta-analysis showed that of patients with comorbid depression and substance use disorder who were treated with antidepressant medications, few achieved sustained remission of the substance use problem even in the subset of studies where the impact of the medication on depression was large. This suggests that drinking problems have an independent existence in people with comorbid psychiatric problems, rather than being a side effect of symptom self-medication.

References

Aiken, A., Wadolowski, M., Bruno, R., Najman, J., Kypri, K., Slade, T., … Mattick, R. P. (in press). Cohort profile: The Australian Parental Supply of Alcohol Longitudinal Study (APSALS). *International Journal of Epidemiology*.

Alcohol and Public Policy Group. (2010). Alcohol: No ordinary commodity – a summary of the second edition. *Addiction*, **105**, 769–779.

Anderson, P., & Baumberg, B. (2006). *Alcohol in Europe*. London: Institute of Alcohol Studies.

Anton, R. F., Oroszi, G., O'Malley, S., Couper, D., Swift, R., Pettinati, H., & Goldman, D. (2008). An evaluation of mu-opioid receptor (OPRM1) as a predictor of naltrexone response in the treatment of alcohol dependence: Results from the Combined Pharmacotherapies and Behavioral Interventions for Alcohol Dependence (COMBINE) study. *Archives of General Psychiatry*, **65**(2), 135–144.

Cameron, D. (2013). Thoughts (and some data) on *The Spirit Level. New Directions in the Study of Alcohol*, **35**, 21–24.

Carlson, R. G. (2006). Ethnography and applied substance misuse research: Anthropological and cross-cultural factors. In W. R. Miller & K. Carroll (Eds.), *Rethinking substance abuse: What the science shows and what we should do about it* (pp. 97–114). New York: Guilford.

Cook, P. J. (2007). *Paying the tab: The costs and benefits of alcohol control*. Princeton, NJ: Princeton University Press.

Ducci, F., & Goldman, D. (2008). Genetic approaches to addiction: Genes and alcohol. *Addiction* **103**, 1414–1428.

Edenberg, H. J., & Foroud, T. (2013). Genetics and alcoholism. *Nature Reviews Gastroenterology and Hepatology*, **10**(8), 487–494.

Enoch, M. A. (2013). Genetic influences of the development of alcoholism. *Current Psychiatry Reports*, **11**, 412.

Gruenewald, P. J., & Treno, A. J. (2000). Local and global alcohol supply: Economic and geographic models of community systems. The supply side initiative: International collaboration to study the alcohol supply. *Addiction*, **95**(Suppl 4), 537–549.

Hall, W. (2010). What are the policy lessons of National Alcohol Prohibition in the United States, 1920–1933? *Addiction*, **105**, 1164–1173.

Hermens, D. F., Lagopoulos, J., Tobias-Webb, J., De Regt, T., Dore, G., Juckes, L., …. Hickie, I. B. (2013). Pathways to alcohol-induced brain impairment in young people: A review. *Cortex*, **49**, 3–17.

Hill, S. Y., De Bellis, M. D., Keshavan, M. S., Lowers, L., Shen, S., Hall, J., & Pitts, T. (2001). Right amygdala volume in adolescent and young adult offspring from families at high risk for developing alcoholism. *Biological Psychiatry*, **49**(11), 894–905.

Hirschhorn, J. N., & Daly, M. J. (2005). Genome-wide association studies for common diseases and complex traits. *Nature Review: Genetics*, **6**, 95–108.

Humphreys, K., & Gifford, E. (2006). Religion, spirituality and the troublesome use of substances. In W. R. Miller & K. Carroll (Eds.), *Rethinking substance abuse: What the science shows and what we should do about it* (pp. 257–274). New York: Guilford.

Humphreys, K., Moos, R. H., & Finney, J. W. (1996). Life domains, Alcoholics Anonymous, and role incumbency in the 3-year course of problem drinking. *Journal of Nervous and Mental Disease*, **184**, 475–481.

Johnson, B. A., Seneviratne, C., Wang, X. Q., Ait-Daoud, N., & Li, M.D (2014). Determination of genotype combinations that can predict the outcome of the treatment of alcohol dependence using the 5-HT3 antagonist ondansetron. *American Journal of Psychiatry*, **170**(9), 1020–1031.

Kiernan, M., Toro, P. A., Rappaport, J., & Seidman, E. (1989). Economic predictors of mental health services utilization: A time-series analysis. *American Journal of Community Psychology* **17**, 801–820.

Kranzler, H. R., Covault, J., Feinn, R., Armeli, S., Tennen, H., Arias, A. J., ... Kampman, KM. (2014). Topiramate treatment for heavy drinkers: Moderation by a GRIK1 polymorphism. *American Journal of Psychiatry*, **171**(4), 445–452.

Kyzar, E. J., & Pandey, S. C. (2015). Molecular mechanisms of synaptic remodeling in alcoholism. *Neuroscience letters*, **601**, 11–19.

Lembke, A. (2012). Time to abandon the self-medication hypothesis in patients with psychiatric disorders. *American Journal of Drug and Alcohol Abuse*, **38**, 524–529.

Levey, D. F., Le-Niculescu, H., Frank, J., Ayalew, M., Jain, N., Kirlin, B., ... Niculescu, A. B. (2014). Genetic risk prediction and neurobiological understanding of alcoholism. *Translational Psychiatry*, **20**, e391.

MacAndrew, C., & Edgerton, R. B. (1970). *Drunken comportment*. London: Nelson.

Mäkelä, K. (1980). Differential effects of restricting the supply of alcohol: Studies of a strike in Finnish liquor stores. *Journal of Drug Issues*, **10**, 131–144.

Müller, K. U., Gan, G., Banaschewski, T., Barker, G. J., Bokde, A. L., Büchel, C., ... IMAGEN Consortium. (2015). No differences in ventral striatum responsivity between adolescents with a positive family history of alcoholism and controls. *Addiction Biology*, **20**, 534–545.

NIAAA. (2013). Update on the genetics of alcoholism. *Alcohol Research: Current Reviews*, **34**(3), 261–380.

Nunes, E. V., & Levin, F. R. (2004). Treatment of depression in patients with alcohol or other drug dependence: A meta-analysis. *JAMA*, **291**, 1887–1896.

Ooteman, W., Naassila, M., Koeter, M. W., Verheul, R., Schippers, G.M., Houchi, H., ... van den Brink, W. (2009). Predicting the effect of naltrexone and acamprosate in alcohol-dependent patients using genetic indicators. *Addiction Biology*, **14**(3), 328–337.

Oslin, D. W., Leong, S. H., Lynch, K. G., Berrettini, W., O'Brien, C. P., Gordon, A. J., & Rukstalis, M. (2015). Naltrexone vs placebo for the treatment of alcohol dependence: A randomized clinical trial. *JAMA Psychiatry*, **72**, 430–437.

Rietschel, M., & Treutlein, J. (2013). The genetics of alcohol dependence. *Annals of the New York Academy of Sciences*, **1282**(1), 39–70.

Spadoni, A. D., Simmons, A. N., Yang, T. T., & Tapert, S. F. (2013). Family history of alcohol use disorders and neuromaturation: A functional connectivity study with adolescents. *American Journal of Drug and Alcohol Abuse*, **39**(6), 356–364.

Zhao, J., Stockwell, T., Martin, G., Macdonald, S., Vallance, K., Treno, A., ... Buxton, J. (2013). The relationship between minimum alcohol prices, outlet densities and alcohol-attributable deaths in British Colombia. *Addiction*, **108**, 1059–1069.

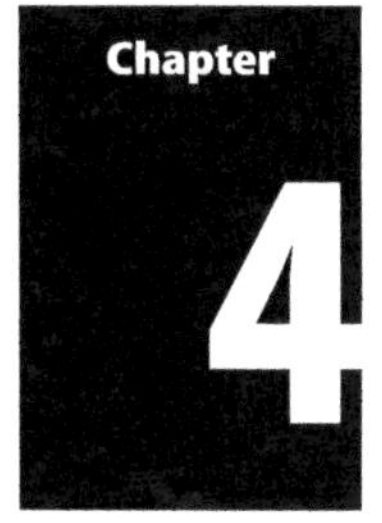

Social complications of drinking problems

When problem drinkers are standing before them, clinicians can directly observe the problems that these patients might "carry with them": neurological impairment, medical complications, psychopathology, and illegal drug dependence. These are all serious disorders worthy of clinical attention and are accordingly addressed in other chapters of this book. But this chapter is about what cannot typically be directly observed in the consulting room: the web of family interactions, social networks, and institutional responses that problem drinkers encounter in their daily lives. This surround can have a profound influence on the course of treatment and on the drinker's life course as well. A drink-driving (drunk-driving) arrest can shock one patient into productive action but send another into drunken despair. A network of drinking mates can undermine treatment, whereas a supportive but firm family can be a major aid to therapeutic progress. And a single alcohol-fuelled act of violence can have life-long consequences, both for the perpetrator and the victim.

Before proceeding to specific social contexts in which drinking problems reverberate, we consider four important conceptual issues. Each shapes our understanding of how drinking problems unfold and therefore has implications for clinical intervention.

Pinpointing the "complications" of drinking problems in individual lives is rarely simple

Chapter 3 discussed the causes of drinking problems, which logically must precede them in time. This chapter addresses the complications, which logically must follow drinking problems in time. Yet the discerning reader will note that some problems (e.g., marital conflict, difficult economic circumstances) are mentioned under both headings. Likewise, in the treatment of individual patients, clearly distinguishing putative causes from consequences can be quite challenging.

Marilyn is a 28-year-old estate agent who has been married to a carpenter for 3 years. The couple planned a traditional family arrangement in which Marilyn would keep her job only until she became a mother and then focus entirely on rearing children. After 2 years of marriage, the relationship began to sour when the couple discovered that Marilyn was infertile. Marilyn reacted to this news by feeling like "a failure as a woman" and suspected that her husband secretly held the same view. Until this point in her life, Marilyn had rarely consumed alcohol for fear that she would end up like her bullying, frequently drunk parents. Nonetheless, Marilyn began to drink regularly when she was alone, despairing: "What difference does it make?" She describes her husband as having steadily withdrawn attention and affection. During this period, her drinking increased, as did her depression and loneliness. She began missing appointments with clients and eventually lost her job. She is now typically severely intoxicated by 3 p.m. and has headaches and vomiting most mornings. Her sexual relationship with her husband has all but ceased in the past year, starting when he called her "repulsive" after finding her extremely intoxicated and naked on the bedroom floor. She has lately had the persistent anxiety that he is having an extramarital affair, and she states that alcohol is the only thing that stops this fear from racing through her mind.

One could argue that the lesson of this sad situation is that Marilyn's drinking problems created complications for her marriage and her emotional well-being. Yet one could also hypothesize that it was actually health problems and personal tragedy – infertility in someone who desperately wanted a child – that caused Marilyn's problem drinking. Alternatively, perhaps Marilyn's depression and anxiety accelerated the course of her incipient drinking problem, which otherwise would have been transient. Or perhaps Marilyn acquired a genetic liability from her alcoholic parents and that is the true cause of her current misery. One could even argue that this married couple's perceptions of a woman's proper role (i.e., that her worth is tied ultimately to being a mother) is causing drinking problems, marital unhappiness, and depression. Even from this short case description, a number of other conjectures on the causes versus the complications of Marilyn's drinking could be made, much as one could stand in a river and speculate endlessly about which particular rivulet, eddy, rock, and overturned tree stump is truly defining the water's course.

The question of whether causes and complications can be clearly made out in a complex life seems less academic when one recognizes how commonly patients want to know the answer to the "big questions"; for example, "Did something make me drink?" "Is this suffering my fault?" "What else will change if I get my drinking under control?" For the clinician to say "there is no way to know for sure if all of your problems would have befallen you even if you had never had a drink" is philosophically correct, but clinically inept because it potentially destroys the patient's incentive to change. At the other extreme, for the clinician to hang every bad event in the patient's life on problem drinking could induce crushing guilt, inappropriate self-blame, and false hope that life will be a bed of roses as soon as the cork is in the bottle.

Clinicians needn't pretend to have perfect understanding of what caused what in an individual's past nor shield the patient from the fundamental uncertainties that are part and parcel of human existence. In general, focusing on what can be changed – the future – is more likely to motivate behaviour change than is trying to assign responsibility for the past. Speaking probabilistically to patients is often the best course (i.e., "Neither of us can know for sure if your marriage became unhappy because you started drinking heavily or the reverse, but I hope we can agree that it's more likely to get better in the future if you get your drinking under control"). As authors, we adopt precisely the same probabilistic stance in this book. We highlight problems that we consider social "complications" because scientific evidence shows that they are prevalent in the drinking population and that they are usually made worse by drinking. These two facts make them worthy of the clinician's attention. Yet in using the term "complication," we unhesitatingly acknowledge that, in any individual life, the complication may actually have been a cause of problem drinking or, for that matter, both a complication and a cause.

One person's curse is another person's blessing

Inexperienced clinicians sometimes assume that problem drinkers invariably define an adverse consequence of drinking as would those around them. A patient losing a job from problem drinking may distress the clinician, as well as the patient's partner and children, but the patient may enjoy the newfound free time and lack of responsibility. Another spouse, to the clinician's surprise, may be perfectly satisfied that her otherwise demanding and tiresome husband slowly passes out from heavy drinking each evening, granting her peace, quiet, and the run of the house. For these reasons, the experienced clinician will always assess the drinking surround neutrally, rather than subtly cuing the patient as to which drinking-related consequences should be considered problematic. After all, therapeutic leverage often comes more from what the drinker considers the complications of drinking than from what others view as its downsides.

The social contexts of problem drinking are to some extent selected and to some extent select

Problem drinkers do not choose the liver with which they were born, nor can their liver seek greener pastures when heavy alcohol consumption imposes added strain. In contrast, problem drinkers can often choose the social environments in which they will and will not participate. In like fashion, the people who compose the drinker's social environment can chose whether or not they wish to associate with the drinker. For example, one of the interesting observations of social epidemiology is that people who drink heavily tend to have social networks in which heavy drinking is common. This comes about in part through selection by the drinker (e.g., choosing to hang around in pubs or to drink at hours of the day that most people consider "too early for a drink"). It also comes about through the choices made by other people; for example, the light-drinking relatives who slowly reduce contact so as to avoid exposure to a couple's drunken rows. This phenomenon helps explain why many heavy drinkers do not see themselves as above average in their alcohol consumption: they drink about as much as those around them.

Clinicians are therefore well-advised to conduct a "higher level" review of social complications beyond that needed for medical or psychiatric consequences. Specifically, one must consider not only the consequences of problem drinking in the drinker's social environment, but also how drinking got that person into that specific environment in the first place. This awareness can help patients see new possibilities in life that are not apparent because they have drifted into their current range of social environments in order to support their drinking. For example, a problem drinker may be pleased to hear that, rather than worry about how to get along with a demeaning boss and cope more effectively with menial pay as a warehouse worker (a job chosen because it allows drinking), bringing drinking under control may open better job opportunities in which such concerns are irrelevant. The same principle often applies in romantic relationships (e.g., rather than attempt to divine which of the habitués at a dive bar might be asked out on a date, a problem drinker can start seeking dates in locations not centred on heavy drinking).

In addition, this "higher level review" can guard against any tendency in the clinician to regard the patient as a passive victim of social environments, which is a "story" that some patients like to tell and may even believe themselves. For example, the man who says he drinks heavily because he has no wife or friends, or because his children never visit, isn't acknowledging that his drinking may be causing others to drop him from their social networks in the first place.

A person's resources moderate the strength of the link between drinking problems and social complications

Consider two women with identical drinking problems. Each drives her car home from a late-night party while intoxicated and encounters a roadside sobriety checkpoint. The police officers' breathalyzer test indicates that each woman's blood alcohol level is just barely over the legal limit. In theory, the fates of these two women – their "complications of drinking" – should also be identical, but, in practice, they may not be. If one of the women is a well-known author and the other is a short-order cook, or if one drives a Mercedes and the other a shambling jalopy, or if one is toothsome and charming and the other rudely stamped and verbally clumsy, the policeman may use his discretion differently. In the case of the more successful, wealthier, or more appealing woman, a warning may suffice in his mind, "Just this once," but for the less successful, poorer, less-appealing woman no such mercy may be forthcoming.

Some people, whether through social standing, money, guile, good looks, charm, or connections are unusually good at evading what would otherwise be the consequences of their drinking problems. The high-profile parade of spectacular drinking disasters among rich and famous people is often attributed to the media's obsession with celebrity. But an alternative explanation is equally plausible: because such people are often insulated from the more minor complications of their drinking when their problem is less severe, they (ironically enough) may be more likely to progress to the point at which they experience a complication that no amount of influence, money, or fame can make disappear.

Clinicians, like anyone else, can have their judgement affected by a patient's affluence, wit, and the like and must guard against the tendency to buy into the patient's narrative that drinking cannot really be that serious because consequences have been largely eluded thus far. At the other end of the continuum, the therapeutic relationship can suffer if a clinician ignores the fact that social complications can come down unusually harshly on certain individuals (e.g., the higher odds that a patient from a racial minority group will be pulled over in "random" traffic stops by police).

We now turn to domains in which social complications of drinking are commonly experienced: family, work/education, crime, and financial stability/housing.

Family complications of problem drinking

Drinking problems can reverberate throughout a person's social network, including to friends and to distant in-laws who may be in contact only a few times a year. But in almost all cases, the most profoundly affected people are the drinker's partner and children, upon whom we focus here.

The partner

A "partner" could be the problem drinker's legally recognized spouse (of a different or the same sex) or a significant nonmarital romantic relationship. Because clinical writings in prior eras often took as read that "partners" were female and problem drinkers male, we emphasize here that we use "partner" to refer to men as well as women, consistent with the rise of heavy drinking among women in recent decades (Grucza, Bucholz, Rice, & Bierut, 2008).

A history from the partner as an individual

Some clinicians take a history from the partner solely to obtain independent information on the problem drinker. This approach ignores an important reality: partners of problem drinkers are people in their own right. When this is not recognized in the assessment process, weeks can go by before it is suddenly realized that treatment is proceeding on the basis of much being known about the patient while the partner remains a cipher, and their interaction is hence inexplicable. Treatment of the patient is handicapped, and the fact that the partner may also need help is overlooked.

Interviewing a person about their personal life when they have come to the clinic in support of someone else can feel overly forward to clinicians, a traducing of reasonable social constraints. For their part, partners may sometimes feel defensive about any clinical enquiries and raise an objection (e.g., "I'm not the one with the problem!"). Clinicians must persist gently but firmly through their own hesitations and any partner resistance for the mutual benefit of the patient and partner. How to take an initial history from the partner in respectful, comfortable terms is fully discussed in Chapter 10.

How drinking problems affect the partner and the relationship

As mentioned, social networks to some extent select their members. In the case of couples in which one member has a drinking problem, this can result in social isolation as outsiders withdraw out of embarrassment, discomfort, or fear. The nondrinking partner may encourage this isolation, either out of shame or from a desire to protect the drinking partner from criticism.

A frequent additional stressor is the unpredictability of the drinker's behaviour. A wife may not know whether, when her husband gets back from the pub, he will be docile and drowsy or in a raging temper. A man readying himself for an evening on the town might worry that this will be one of the occasions when his partner gets drunk and humiliates them both in a social situation by being loud, crude, or sexually inappropriate. The exhaustion that can be engendered by the experience of dealing with continuing distress and peaks of crisis over a period of years may be the partner's dominant complaint.

Historically, clinical writings with a sexist cast attributed much of the behaviour of wives of problem drinking husbands to psychopathology (e.g., a secret joy or sense of superiority that their husband was alcohol dependent). Yet a more direct explanation of the behaviour of many wives – and husbands as well – is that they continue to love the problem drinker despite it all. Cross-culturally, the allowing of second and third chances, the tolerance of abuse and disappointment, and the efforts to control drinking are very commonly motivated by the fact that the partner worries about, cares for, and wishes to help the problem drinker (Orford et al., 2005). In this stressful situation, the partner suffers from having to watch a loved one harm him- or herself and agonizes over where love ends and damaging overindulgence begins.

In addition to emotional strain, partners of problem drinkers often face concrete realities that can be tangibly threatening; there is the risk of eviction if the rent is not paid, or violence may result in serious physical injury. Divorce, which often has significant adverse economic and psychological effects, can also result from problem drinking. More commonly, problem drinking creates a host of minor tangible problems that have to be coped with: electricity shut off for a day until the bill is belatedly paid, the neighbours complaining about doors being slammed when the drinker got home last night, frequently rowing, the smell of vomit in the toilet, or the drinker being unkempt or wetting the bed.

It would, however, be a mistake always to picture such relationships only in extreme terms. Intense suffering certainly occurs with sad frequency, but infinite gradations exist. Sometimes the problem drinker's deportment when inebriated causes little distress. Perhaps the drinker becomes a bit silly and argumentative or simply nods off and is difficult to drag up to bed.

On a more positive note, partners can benefit substantially from the problem drinker's successful treatment. Spouses of remitted alcohol dependent patients score similarly or somewhat better on mental health measures as do controls and substantially better than spouses of actively drinking alcoholics (Moos, Finney, & Cronkite, 1990). Much of what is sometimes put down to enduring psychopathology in partners of problem drinkers is therefore actually a reaction to a difficult situation that dissipates when the drinking problem is resolved.

The types of hardship that the partner may encounter are discussed in more detail in relation to taking the "independent history" from the partner (see Chapter 10).

Relationships in which both partners have a drinking problem

This extraordinarily difficult situation is encountered more often than might be guessed from the prevalence rate of drinking problems. Heavy drinkers are unusually likely to initiate romantic relationships with other heavy drinkers, and drinking together can be a central activity in such relationships.

The story is usually that of a person with a drinking problem marrying someone else with an established and evident drinking problem. For one or both partners, it may be a second marriage. They met perhaps in a bar or even in a hospital ward and formed a marriage of convenience between drinkers. They have no knowledge of each other's sober beings and are, sadly, likely to drag each other down further. Alcohol-related problems do sometimes develop in both partners in an already established marriage. Quite often, the development is not simultaneous, with one partner following in the other's footsteps, perhaps justifying his or her own drinking as a reaction to understandable stress. Both partners may tell themselves that if they have a drinking problem, at least it's less severe than that of their partner. A markedly different type of relationship involves former drinkers who have met at Alcoholics Anonymous or in treatment and are both committed to "recovery" and able to give each other much support.

In general, when both partners have a serious problem, it can be difficult to reach them with effective help. If they met in a pub and each purposefully attached to a problem-drinking partner, the clinician may encounter a baffling pack of pathological motivations. In such instances, all that may be possible is to make the offer of help, try to maintain some sort of monitoring contact, and wait for the occurrence that can provide the therapeutic opening; for example, one partner going into hospital with a physical illness. Where the heavy drinking has developed during the relationship, rather than being its foundation, the prospects for treatment are usually more hopeful. Both partners may simultaneously be able to seek help, or it may be necessary to start with the partner who is more motivated, or with any children who could benefit from the support of a treatment professional. If treatment can capture the potential for mutual understanding, which can exist between partners who have shared the same problem, an initially difficult situation can be turned to special advantage.

Experiences to which children are exposed

The experiences of the child of a problem-drinking parent are varied depending on the degree of emotional support provided by either parent, the variety of other social and emotional supports that may be available, the age of the child when the parent developed the drinking problem, and the child's level of ability to understand the problem drinker's behaviour and moods (Steinglass, Bennett, Wolin, & Reiss, 1987). Of great importance is the actual behaviour of the parent when intoxicated; continued rowdiness, arguments, or violence have far more adverse impact than do instances when drunkenness is not associated with verbal, physical, or sexual aggression.

Families with drinking problems are often places of which the social worker will report that "you know there is something wrong as soon as you walk in the door." A drinking problem, of whatever degree or nature, that as its end-result produces what can be summarized as a bad home atmosphere is attacking the centre of what family life should be able to give to a child. Whether children are more damaged when the problem drinker is of their same sex and therefore a likely role model is uncertain, but, in any event, the impact of problem-drinking parents can differ between boys and girls in the same family. If a parent when drunk continuously picks on a particular child, scolding them, finding fault, demeaning or hitting them, then that child is immensely at risk. Likewise, if an intoxicated parent is flirtatious or seductive with a child, the long-term effect on the child's psychological development can be severe even if these abusive behaviours never progress to physical contact.

In some families, a parent's drinking behaviour results in the parent's permanent removal from the home through separation, divorce, or even premature death. Temporary absences are also common, for example due to drinking benders, hospitalizations, or incarcerations. Children may have to suffer criticism of their parents from family, neighbours, or friends, and the behaviour of their parents may lead to embarrassment or shame. The drinking parent may be unreliable regarding familial responsibilities, and the behaviour of the sober parent may also be adversely affected – even to the point where the child views this parent less favourably than the problem drinker (Velleman & Orford, 1999).

Although the risks of parental drinking problems just described are significant, not all families end up in such evil case. Some problem drinkers are able to continue parenting fairly effectively, or at least to refrain from grossly destructive behaviour (Reich, Earls, & Powell, 1988). Furthermore, even given some poor parental behaviour, within the same family, one child may be adversely affected but another may be unperturbed. The clinical challenge is to be open to these possibilities while at the same time not being fobbed off by a "happy family" cover story that has been adopted in what in fact is a deeply distressing situation.

Problems that children may develop

Children of parents who have drinking problems are at risk for a range of adverse effects (Table 4.1). These effects may be alcohol-specific: for example, a child following the parent's model of heavy drinking (Jacob & Johnson, 1997). They can also be non–alcohol related: for example, a lack of consistent limit-setting by the parent enabling defiant behaviour in the child (Jacob & Johnson, 1997).

Table 4.1. Problems frequently experienced by children of problem drinkers

- Anxiety
- Depression
- Low self-esteem
- Relationship difficulties
- Poor school performance
- Antisocial behaviour
- Physical and sexual abuse
- Accidental injury
- Risk of alcohol-related problems in later life

The psychological damages and the social disabilities that can result will interact. In the school setting, anxiety may lead to social disability, poor academic performance, and other problems. Antisocial behaviour in school can lead to expulsion, thus setting the stage for poor unemployment prospects, criminal behaviour, and run-ins with the police.

The absence of emotional regard within the home can mean that an adolescent will develop particularly rejecting attitudes toward the parents. The fortunate adolescent will find other positive individuals with whom to identify, perhaps a teacher, grandparent, or member of the clergy. However, more commonly, the adolescent enters precipitously into identification with an adolescent peer group. Such an extreme version of a normal process is not necessarily harmful, but the children from this disturbed home can be vulnerable to involvement with groups that are themselves disturbed and engaging in unhealthy and antisocial behaviour, including binge-drinking or other drug-taking. These deviant peer attachments may in part represent a revenge on the parents or substitute comfort or excitement to replace the good inner feelings that are so lacking.

There can, however, be no fixed predictions as to how a child from a drinking home will meet adolescence. Rather than becoming highly peer-oriented, some adolescents become desperately clingy and anxiously involved in the home, tied to protecting the nondrinking parent and unable to make any identification with other young people. Still another outcome is the adolescent who heroically and at significant emotional cost takes up abandoned parental responsibilities (e.g., quasi-parenting the younger children, balancing the checkbook and buying the groceries, taking a job to make ends meet) and attempts to "redeem the family's name" by working assiduously to excel outside the home (e.g., academically or at sports).

At any stage of childhood, the possibility of actual physical damage must be considered. There is an association between drinking problems and nonaccidental injury, and, in childhood and adolescence, the risk of physical assault may continue; the damage is often no more than bruising, but the risk of more serious injury is not to be discounted. Sexual abuse of children is substantially more likely (Velleman & Orford, 1999). Accidental injury may occur due to inadequate supervision.

Although the idea that "adult children of alcoholics" suffer from a unique syndrome is popular in some clinical circles, no psychiatric problems are unique to this population (Griffin et al., 2005). Recent, painstaking work suggests that, with the possible exception of an increased risk of drinking problems, the damaging effects of parental alcoholism on adults are mediated through stressors also found in other disturbed, nonalcoholic home environments: sexual abuse, physical violence, parental psychopathology, and a conflictual family environment characterized by low cohesion, organization, and expressiveness (Griffin et al., 2005). It also bears mentioning that many adult children of alcoholics are well-adjusted and even find ways to use their painful experiences to their advantage.

Holiday celebrations were frequently spoiled during Kate's childhood, as a result of her father's invariable drunkenness. Even the normal routine of daily life had accommodated his unpredictable behaviour after "a drink with colleagues" on the way home from work. When Kate married and started a family of her own, she and her husband therefore determined that they would never let drinking spoil their home life. They translated this into agreed family expectations on what would constitute acceptable drinking and the occasions when drinking might be done.

Work and education

I wrote 30 job applications to various firms and told them I had been treated for a drink problem, was now sober, and wanted to find my way back with everything in the open. I didn't get a single interview. So the next time I kept quiet about my drinking, spun a yarn about that year off work, handed in two out-of-date references, lied on the medical form, and got the job. And then? They checked things out. I was fired on Friday, and yes, it's stupid, but I've been drinking. Just what they expected.

The difficulty that a person with a drinking problem may encounter when seeking employment has just been instanced, and the example shows how stigmatization may compound the objective difficulties. The varieties of adverse influence that excessive drinking may have on work performance are many and costly (Babor et al., 2010; Jones, Casswell, & Zhang, 1995). The impact is not limited to any one level of seniority in the employment hierarchy. Drinking problems are as likely to do damage in the boardroom as on the shop floor.

Drinking can be particularly destructive in work settings and professions in which the lives and well-being of others are in the problem drinker's hands. For the bus or train driver, the airplane pilot, or the naval ship commander, the effects of intoxication or hangover carry enormous dangers for the public. In senior positions in industry or the armed services, in the diplomatic service, or in the legal profession (Goodliffe, 1994), drunken indiscretion, irascibility, or bad judgment at a crucial moment can have far-ranging repercussions. Legal authorities recognize the tremendous damage alcohol dependent physicians can do, which is why extensive disciplinary and monitoring procedures are quite rightly called into action if a doctor's drinking comes to official attention (DuPont et al., 2009). For teachers and clergy, the hint of scandal may be especially damaging, although it is surprising how tolerant or blind-eyed those in the individual's environment often appear to be. These more dramatic examples may not be relevant to many cases, yet they serve to underscore that, whoever the individual the clinician is trying to assess and help, the analysis of their alcohol-related social complications requires a job-specific enquiry.

A social complication of drinking that deserves greater note is the long-term handicap that results when an educational or training opportunity is partly wasted or totally lost. Being dismissed from a university, failing to complete a postgraduate degree, the abandonment of an apprenticeship because of a drinking problem, may all have serious long-term consequences. The consequences may include not only objective career damage, but enduring feelings of self-blame and regret that dog the individual even if the drinking problem has long since been resolved.

Crime

Crime and drinking problems often co-occur, but the association is not unidirectional, nor need it in all cases be causal (Graham & West, 2001). For example, growing up in a violent neighbourhood filled with taverns and off-licenses could increase an individual's risk of engaging in crime and becoming a problem drinker without these two behaviours being causally related to each other.

At the same time, alcohol consumption can clearly contribute directly to crime. Experimental research in humans and animals indicates that alcohol consumption can disinhibit aggressiveness (Heinz et al., 2011). This effect is not limited to the laboratory: quasi-experimental studies of labour strikes that disrupted national alcohol production show that population rates of violent and nonviolent crime drop when the alcohol supply is restricted (Mäkelä, Rossow, & Tryggvesson, 2002).

The variations on the alcohol–crime connection are legion, and, over time, clinicians will encounter all of them because pressure from the legal system is a common motivator for problem drinkers to seek treatment. There is no type of offence that will not sometimes be related to drinking and many types of offence that will often be so related. The problems load at the low-severity end of the spectrum: petty theft, minor assault, traveling on public transport without a ticket, failing to pay for the meal in the cheap café, urinating in the subway, panhandling aggressively. The person with a drinking problem may know that when they are drunk (and only when they are drunk), they are apt to engage in their own particular offence; for example, taking cars for joy rides, "going burgling" in a clumsy sort of fashion, or passing dud cheques.

By definition, problem drinking is a risk factor for drink-driving offences (Hingson & Winter, 2003). Individuals with alcohol problems should be reminded about their responsibility to inform the regulatory authorities as appropriate (e.g., Driving and Vehicle Licensing Authority in the UK) about this health issue; although this can be tricky to raise in a therapeutic setting, it is nonetheless the clinician's responsibility to inform the patient. Estimates for the proportion of subjects among drink-driving offenders variously defined as "alcoholics" or "problem drinkers" range from 4 to 87 percent across samples and jurisdictions, with prevalence rates influenced by operational definition. Repeat offenders are particularly likely to have serious alcohol problems (Miller & Fillmore, 2014), as are individuals with unusually high blood alcohol content at the time of arrest.

From the clinical angle, the conclusion must be that enquiry into driving behaviour and drink-driving offences should be an integral part of any assessment. Not everyone who has been convicted of driving while intoxicated will have an otherwise manifest drinking problem (Miller & Fillmore, 2014), but among clinical populations there will be a significant proportion of individuals whose driving poses a threat to themselves and other people, a fact that puts distinct responsibility on the clinician.

Although heavy drinking in no way excuses physical aggression morally, it can be a contributing cause of it because normally inhibited impulses are set free: a skid row drinker hits a fellow member of a bottle-gang on the head with an iron bar, a drunken man follows a woman out of a pub and gropes her in the car park, two intoxicated yobs begin an argument that ends in a brutal assault.

Finally, although most people are aware that drinking problems can lead to crime perpetuation, few consider that drinking problems are also associated with being a *victim* of crime, including violent assault by a partner (Devries et al., 2013). A grossly intoxicated person will easily fall prey to having their pockets turned out, or be unable to outrun a mugger. Sociopathic criminals may target visibly drunken individuals as easy marks or even ply an individual with drinks for the purposes of robbing or sexually assaulting him or her later. A partner may exploit an opportunity to take long-sought revenge against a currently intoxicated and helpless partner who has abused them in the past.

Financial and housing stability

An awareness of the possible financial complications of drinking problems and of the family's financial position is necessary for any complete case assessment. To maintain a major drinking habit is expensive, and large additional sums are often spent without the drinker knowing where the money has gone – drinks grandly offered to strangers, banknotes stuffed into a stripper's garter, meals out and taxis home, coins and bills that fall unnoticed as keys are fumbled for, massive cigarette consumption, gambling, and so on. As with housing problems and many other social complications, the well-moneyed will be better protected for a longer time.

The financial balance is determined not only by the cost of the drinking and associated spending, but also by whether drinking affects the inflow of cash. Demotion, sickness, and unemployment add to the stringencies. Complicated and devious stratagems may be engaged in to maintain income. "Moonlighting" or the second job is common (perhaps in a bar to further aid drinking), loans are negotiated on preposterous terms, possessions are pawned, houses remortgaged. The employee "works a bit of a racket," and a load of bricks disappear from the builder's yard. It becomes vital to evade income tax and to defraud Social Security. The rent is not paid, and credit card payments fall behind.

The family may have reached the stage where financial chaos has become the central and pressing pain. From the social work angle, sorting out that chaos may be the necessary first aid, but it will convey no lasting benefit if the drinking problem is not radically met.

When financial complications are extreme, they may result in a substandard housing situation or, indeed, no housing at all. Cases are frequently encountered where drinking is leading directly to a housing problem. In this latter type of instance, the patient's claim that they are "drinking because of their unsatisfactory surroundings" has a hollow ring – theirs is the only house in the street that is shabby and unpainted and with an old sofa lying in the front garden. Housing problems of this kind will be more acute the more marginal the family's income. Bad relationships with neighbours, gross evidence of poor house maintenance, failure to meet the rent, services cut off, eviction, the sojourn in "temporary accommodation," and multiple changes of address are familiar elements in the housing history as the drinking problem becomes more extreme.

Literal homelessness due to problem drinking tends to result from a combination of financial distress as well as exhaustion of family and social supports (i.e., the drinker is kicked out of the house and has become so intolerable that no one else will take him in). Heavy drinking is a lifestyle among a subgroup of homeless people, and entry into this social environment may reinforce continued heavy consumption, particularly of the binge variety. On the other hand, those homeless problem drinkers who can be helped into "sober housing," meaning a setting in which continued housing is contingent on abstinence and alcohol is not available, can evince remarkable turnarounds in their life situations.

References

Babor, T., Caetano, R., Casswell, S., Edwards, G., Giesbrecht, N., Graham, K., ... Room, R. (2010). *Alcohol: No ordinary commodity: Research and public policy* (2nd edition). Oxford: Oxford University Press.

Devries, K. M., Child, J. C., Bacchus, L. J., Mak, J., Falder, G. Graham, K., ... Heise, L. (2013). Intimate partner violence victimization and alcohol consumption in women: A systematic review and meta-analysis. *Addiction*, **109**, 379–391.

DuPont, R. L., McLellan, A. T., White, W. L., Merlo, L. J., & Gold, M. S. (2009). Setting the standard for recovery: Physicians health programs. *Journal of Substance Abuse Treatment*, **36**, 159–171.

Goodliffe, J. (1994). Alcohol and depression in England and American lawyer disciplinary proceedings. *Addiction*, **89**, 1237–1244.

Graham, P., & West, P. (2001). Alcohol and crime: Examining the link. In N. Heather, T. J. Peters, & T. Stockwell (Eds.), *International handbook of alcohol dependence and problems* (pp. 439–470). Chester, UK: John Wiley & Sons.

Griffin, M. L., Amodeo, M., Fassler, I., Ellis, M. A., & Clay, C. (2005). Mediating factors for the long-term effects of parental alcoholism in women: The contribution of other childhood stresses and resources. *American Journal on Addictions*, **14**, 18–34.

Grucza, R. A., Bucholz, K. K., Rice, J. P., & Bierut, L. J. (2008). Secular trends in the lifetime prevalence of alcohol dependence in the United States: A re-evaluation. *Alcoholism: Clinical and Experimental Research*, **32**(5), 763–770.

Heinz, A. J., Beck, A., Meyed-Lindenberg, A., Sterzer, P., & Heinz, A. (2011). Cognitive and neurobiological mechanisms of alcohol-related aggression. *Nature Reviews Neuroscience*, **12**, 400–413.

Hingson, R., & Winter, M. (2003). *Epidemiology and consequences of drinking and driving.* Bethesda, MD: National Institute on Alcohol Abuse and Alcoholism. http://pubs.niaaa.nih.gov/publications/arh27-1/63-78.htm

Jacob, T., & Johnson, S. (1997). Parenting influences on the development of alcohol abuse and dependence. *Alcohol Health and Research World*, **21**, 204–209.

Jones, S., Casswell, S., & Zhang, J. F. (1995). The economic costs of alcohol-related absenteeism and reduced productivity among the working population of New Zealand. *Addiction*, **90**(11), 1455–1461.

Mäkelä, P., Rossow, I., & Tryggvesson, K. (2002). Who drinks more and less when policies change? The evidence from 50 years of Nordic studies. In R. Room (Ed.), *The effects of Nordic alcohol policies*. Helsinki: Nordic Council for Alcohol and Drug Research.

Miller, M. A., & Fillmore, M. T. (2014). Cognitive and behavioral preoccupation with alcohol in recidivist DUI offenders. *Journal of Studies on Alcohol*, **75**, 1018–1022.

Moos, R. H., Finney, J. W., & Cronkite, R. C. (1990). *Alcoholism treatment: Context, process and outcome*. New York: Oxford University Press.

Orford, J., Natera, G., Mora, J., et al. (2005). *Coping with alcohol and drug problems: The experiences of family members in three contrasting cultures*. Hove, UK: Routledge.

Reich, W., Earls, F., & Powell, J. (1988). A comparison of the home and social environments of children of alcoholic and non-alcoholic parents. *British Journal of Addiction*, **83**, 831–839.

Steinglass, P., Bennett, L. A., Wolin, S. J., & Reiss, D. (1987). *The alcoholic family*. London: Hutchinson.

Velleman, R., & Orford, R. (1999). *Risk and resilience: Adults who were the children of problem drinkers*. Amsterdam: Harwood.

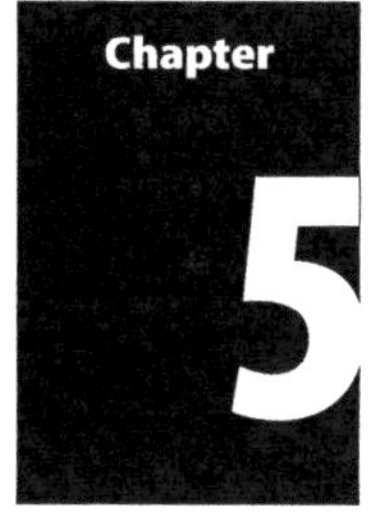

Physical complications of excessive drinking

The physical element is an important part of a comprehensive approach to drinking problems. Helping services should be organized to cope effectively with diagnosis and treatment in the physical domain and, whatever the particular professional affiliation of the clinician who is working with the problem drinker, there is need for an alertness toward possible physical pathologies. Social workers in a counseling service are, of course, practising their own special types of skill, and no one would suggest that they should also cultivate highly specialized knowledge of liver pathology. It is, however, a reasonable expectation that they should know enough about the liver to understand the significance to their client of a diagnosis of cirrhosis, rather than their being mystified by this term and consequently deflecting that client from talking about something of vital importance. A polite conspiracy can be set up in which both parties pretend that the body does not exist.

Why physical complications matter

Excessive alcohol consumption is a major contributor to mortality and ill health, and "it is a causal factor in more than 60 major types of diseases and injuries and results in approximately 2.5 million deaths each year" (World Health Organization, 2011, p. 20) (Table 5.1). This translates into 4 percent of all deaths worldwide and to approximately 4.5 percent of the global burden of disease and injury attributable to alcohol.

Burden of disease is quantified in terms of disability adjusted life years (DALYs), a summary measure that combines years of life lost to premature death with years of life lost due to disability. Males have a higher alcohol-related disease burden than do females. Alcohol is the world's leading risk factor for deaths in males aged 15–59, and the deaths of young people in particular contribute to loss of many years of life (Whiteford et al., 2013).

There are large variations in the alcohol-attributable disease burden in different regions of the world, with injuries accounting for a higher proportion of the burden in lower income countries and cancers accounting for a higher proportion in higher income countries. For any given level of pattern of drinking, the harm is greater in poorer societies than in more affluent ones. In addition, homemade alcoholic beverages in some parts of the world may be contaminated with methanol or lead that also adversely affect health (World Health Organization, 2011).

Alcohol is the third largest risk factor for mortality in developed countries after tobacco and hypertension, and it accounts for 9.2 percent of DALYs lost. This compares with figures of 12.2 percent and 10.9 percent for tobacco and hypertension, respectively (Rehm et al., 2004; World Health Organization, 2007). The burden from liver cancer has increased between 1990 and 2010 by more than 45 percent, in part due to alcohol; cirrhosis accounted

Table 5.1. Major disease and injury conditions related to alcohol and proportions attributable to alcohol worldwide (%)

	Men	Women	Both
Malignant neoplasms			
Mouth and oropharynx cancers	22	9	19
Oesophageal cancer	37	15	29
Liver cancer	30	13	25
Breast cancer	N/A	7	7
Neuropsychiatric disorders			
Unipolar depressive disorders	3	1	2
Epilepsy	23	12	18
Alcohol use disorders	100	100	100
Diabetes mellitus	−1	−1	−1
Cardiovascular diseases			
Ischaemic heart disease	4	−1	2
Haemorrhagic stroke	18	1	10
Ischaemic stroke	3	−6	−1
Gastrointestinal diseases			
Cirrhosis of the liver	39	18	32
Unintentional injury			
Motor vehicle accidents	25	8	20
Drownings	12	6	10
Falls	9	3	7
Poisonings	23	9	18
Intentional injury			
Self-inflicted injuries	15	5	11
Homicide	26	16	24

Source: Room, Babor, & Rehm (2005).

for 1.2 percent of global DALYs, with a nearly equal share related to hepatitis B, hepatitis C, and alcohol (Murray et al., 2012). Within mental and behavioural disorders that accounted for 7.4 percent of DALYs, alcohol use (0.7 percent) was in the top five after depressive disorder (2.5 percent), anxiety disorders (1.1 percent), and drug use disorders (0.8 percent). Notably, though, whereas the prevalence of alcohol, opioid, and cocaine dependence increased between 1990 and 2010, prevalence of other mental disorders did not (Whiteford et al., 2013).

Although physical complications are common in any population of heavy drinkers, early detection and cessation of drinking can lead to recovery from the medical comorbidity. Continued drinking, on the other hand, is likely to exacerbate the alcohol-related problem and may seriously threaten life. Physical complications impinge on all aspects of the problem drinker's life, and it is unrealistic to compartmentalize psychological, social, and physical disability. Therefore, any assessment, even if done by someone without medical training, should include questions about physical health. If there are any concerns or queries, these should be referred to an appropriate individual or service.

Often, physical complications are the main reason for seeking help. If information about the physical symptoms is imparted clearly, so that the patient can understand their significance, this information can be used to consider the patient's position. Thus, an understanding of the physical symptoms may have the potential to influence drinking behaviour. As ever, the clinician is the informant, the person who brings up the issue, and who shares and reflects the patient's feelings and concerns, rather than the disembodied pronouncer of facts. The way in which information on physical problems is presented to the patient can be part of treatment. Here are two dialogues that illustrate different ways in which the patient's concern over his physical health can be met at interview. First, and very briefly, a dialogue that is not to be dismissed as caricature:

PATIENT: What does the doctor mean when he said my liver had been hit by the drinking?

COUNSELLOR: You will have to ask the doctor to explain.

PATIENT: But he never explains anything.

COUNSELLOR: Well, he's the person to ask.

Second, and more constructively:

PATIENT: What did the doctor mean when he said my liver had been hit by the drinking?

COUNSELLOR: That's something pretty important to talk about. What did you think he meant?

PATIENT: I suppose I was very scared. Not sure I believe him, though. He may just be trying to frighten me. But if what he's really saying is that I'm going to die of cirrhosis? I'll go out on the crest of the all-time greatest booze-up.

COUNSELLOR: I don't think anyone wants to scare you in a horror-story sort of way, but it's your own liver and you have a right to know about it.

PATIENT: So what's the score?

COUNSELLOR: I spoke to your doctor on the phone. You have undoubtedly done your liver some harm, and if you go on drinking you would be risking cirrhosis, and that's a miserable way to die. If you stop drinking, your liver disease will not progress and may improve. Even cutting back significantly on your drinking would likely benefit you. You've a right to know all the facts. It's reasonable to be anxious, but at least there are positive steps you can take toward repairing the damage.

PATIENT: When I was getting that pain, I guessed it must be my liver, but I suppose I have been shutting my eyes, doing the "it can't happen to me" trick.

The vital question is what any information on physical consequences means to the patient. Patients and their families are concerned about their physical health and deserve to be given the facts. Explaining and talking through this information is an opportunity for the therapist to facilitate behavioural change in the patient.

Some patients stop drinking abruptly or greatly reduce their consumption when persuaded that alcohol is posing a tangible threat to their physical health. Even if the news of physical damage constitutes the turning point, in reality, this is only the final event to tip a decision when the moment for change has been set up by many previous occurrences. That said, using the results of the physical examination or the laboratory tests for crude scare tactics is likely to be counter productive. Patients may dismiss what they are being told simply because the information is too frightening to accept, or they may decide that all is lost and that they may as well drink themselves to death.

Physical complications

The medical conditions associated with alcohol consumption can be broken down into those directly due to alcohol and those due to acute and chronic conditions to which alcohol is a contributory factor (World Health Organization, 2011). Physical conditions directly attributable to alcohol include alcoholic polyneuropathy, alcoholic gastritis, alcoholic liver disease, and ethanol toxicity. Acute conditions to which alcohol is a contributory cause include road injuries (drivers and pedestrians), injuries from falls, fires, drownings, occupational injuries, other accidents, suicide, and assault. Whilst amount consumed is linked to ill-health, heavy drinking events are particularly linked with injuries, intentional and unintentional. Chronic alcohol-attributable conditions include various cancers, liver cirrhosis, acute and chronic pancreatitis, spontaneous abortion, and psoriasis (World Health Organization, 2011).

Heavy drinking in pregnancy can lead to foetal alcohol spectrum disorders. Heavy drinking in adolescents and young people is likely to affect brain development (see Chapter 2). In some conditions, both the toxic element and disturbance of nutritional status may be implicated as causes of damage. Less is known about the risks associated with different beverage types, although it has been suggested that the risk of developing certain physical disorders is higher for drinkers of spirits (Chou, Grant, & Dawson, 1998).

What level of alcohol intake constitutes a threshold for physical dangers? The answer must vary according to the particular condition, but, in general, the evidence points to a dose–response relationship, with higher consumption being associated with a higher risk of disease. Even individuals who drink "socially" but above the daily guidelines are at risk.

Binge drinking puts individuals at higher risk of developing alcohol dependence syndrome, injuries, and brain trauma. There is considerable individual variation in the effects of alcohol consumption: not every chronic heavy drinker develops liver cirrhosis.

However, whatever the risks at the relatively lower ranges of intake, by the time someone is drinking in the fashion characteristic of the dependence syndrome, the question of whether their level of intake carries dangers hardly needs to be asked. The answer is resoundingly "yes" for nearly every tissue of the body. And, quite apart from any specific tissue damage discussed in this chapter, it should be remembered that, as a consequence of heavy drinking and dietary neglect, almost every aspect of the body's chemistry may in some circumstances be put out of balance; even such seemingly obscure aspects as serum zinc or magnesium levels may be disturbed.

Table 5.2. Major alcohol-related disorders and harms to health

- **Acute intoxication**
- **Cancers:** head and neck cancers, cancers of the gastrointestinal tract, liver cancer, and female breast cancer
- **Cardiovascular disorders:** arrhythmias, ischaemic heart disease, cardiomyopathy, cerebrovascular disease
- **Gastrointestinal disorders:** alcoholic liver disease, acute and chronic pancreatitis, gastritis and peptic ulceration, Mallory–Weiss syndrome
- **Endocrine and metabolic disease:** type II diabetes, alcohol-induced pseudo-Cushing's syndrome, male hypogonadism, hypoglycaemia, alcoholic ketoacidosis, gout, hyperlipidaemia
- **Immune system disorders**
- **Alcoholic muscle, bone, and skin disease**
- **Respiratory disease:** respiratory tract infection; acute respiratory distress syndrome (ARDS)
- **Haematological effects:** anaemia, macrocytosis, iron deficiency, neutropaenia, thrombocytopaenia
- **Accidents**
- **Surgical complications**
- **Neurological disorders:** alcohol withdrawal seizures, peripheral neuropathy, alcoholic cerebellar degeneration, Wernicke–Korsakoff syndrome, alcoholic pellagra encephalopathy, alcohol-related brain damage, central pontine myelinolysis, Marchiafava–Bignami disease, alcohol amblyopia, hepatic encephalopathy
- **Foetal alcohol spectrum disorders (FASD)**

The physical complications that can result from excessive drinking will now be described. As far as possible, technical language is explained, but, as noted in the Introduction, this is a chapter where the nonmedical reader will have to show some forbearance. However as stated before, at the very least, initial and continuing assessments should include questions about physical health, and, if there are any concerns or queries, these should be referred to an appropriate individual or service. Table 5.2 lists the major alcohol-related health conditions contributing to morbidity and mortality. The presence of these conditions should alert the clinician to the possibility of an underlying drinking problem. In any case, basic inquiry into the patient's drinking history should be absolutely routine in medical practice.

Acute alcohol intoxication and coma

The effects of intoxication vary according to a number of factors including the amount of alcohol consumed, how rapidly it has been consumed, and whether the drinker has a degree of tolerance to alcohol or rarely drinks. A life-threatening overdose with alcohol is unlikely to occur in the alcohol dependent person, both because of their experience in handling their drinking and their raised tolerance. That is not to deny the possibility of such a patient at times getting very drunk or drinking to unconsciousness. Drinking to the point of collapse and "passing out" is more likely to be the result of a casual drinking binge or a Saturday night celebration, and it is this type of patient who is the familiar late-night visitor to the Emergency Room. Drug overdoses are often taken in the context of intoxication, intentionally or otherwise. Occasionally, a child will overdose accidentally with alcohol: this is discussed in relation to hypoglycaemia (see the section on Hypoglycaemia).

Intoxication can usually be dealt with on a sensibly conservative basis and patients left to sleep off their binge, with due care taken to ensure that they do not inhale their vomit: examination must of course also ensure that there is no other cause for unconsciousness. A stomach wash-out may sometimes be indicated. With higher levels of intoxication, there is a risk of respiratory depression and death. The blood alcohol concentration (BAC) likely to be associated with such a tragedy will vary with the individual, but a BAC of 400 mg/100 mL is usually quoted as the threshold for very serious danger. Because of the occasional risk of death from respiratory paralysis, the more common danger from inhaled vomit, and the many possibilities of being unwarily overwhelmed by some underlying or complicating condition (head injury, hypoglycaemia, ketoacidosis, systemic infection, overdose of other licit or illicit drugs, for example), the problem set by alcoholic overdose and by the often rather unwelcome visitor to the Emergency Room should not be too casually dismissed as "routine." When coma is thought to be due to alcohol, it is important that a high alcohol concentration is shown by measurements of breath or blood alcohol. Skull radiography, neuroimaging, and urine toxicology are other fundamental investigations. Alcoholic coma has a mortality rate of approximately 5 percent.

Acute poisoning with methyl alcohol (methanol) is a rarer and a much more threatening condition than intoxication with ordinary beverage alcohol. There are substantial risks of blindness or death, and intensive emergency medical care will be required, possibly with dialysis.

Cancers

Evidence has mounted over recent years that the more alcohol an individual drinks over time, particularly regularly, increases the risk of developing a number of cancers (Bofetta & Hashibe, 2006; Department of Health, 2016; International Agency for Research on Cancer, 1998; World Cancer Research Fund/American Institute for Cancer Research, 2007). Greater alcohol consumption increases the risk of cancers of the mouth, pharynx, larynx, and oesophagus (gullet); liver cancer (either directly or indirectly via chronic infection with hepatitis B or C); and colo-rectal (men) and breast (women) cancers.

There appears to be "no safe threshold below which no effect on any cancer risk is observed" which influenced the recent changes to advice in the UK to drink no more than 14 units per week (Department of Health, 2016, p. 7). (British Medical Association Board of Science, 2008, p. 29). In addition, because many who drink alcohol excessively also smoke tobacco, this is an added risk, particularly for head and neck cancers. Genes involved in metabolizing (breaking down) alcohol likely moderate cancer risk. For instance, some forms of aldehyde dehydrogenase 2 (ALDH2) (see Chapter 2), which metabolizes toxic acetaldehyde to nontoxic substances, are associated with increased risk of head and neck cancers (Druesne-Pecollo et al., 2009).

Cardiovascular disease

The hypothesized protective or beneficial effects to the heart of one to two drinks per day have been the subject of much interest and debate about what contributes to this so-called J-shaped curve (Department of Health, 2016; O'Keefe et al., 2014; Thompson, 2013). Claims regarding this J-shaped relationship have often been oversimplified and oversold, as we explore in the next section. In any event, it should be remembered that because noncardiovascular adverse outcomes rise linearly with increased drinking, there is no case for nondrinkers to begin drinking in order to lower their overall risk of disease (Department of Health, 2016).

Alcohol-related arrhythmias

Arrhythmias, or disturbances of the normal heart rhythm, can occur as a result of episodic heavy drinking and heavy consistent alcohol use; these arrhythmias are often called "holiday heart" because of their association with binge drinking on weekends and holidays. The mildest presentation is that of palpitations caused by a few extra and irregular beats (extrasystoles). Palpitations can also be caused by an alcohol-induced tachycardia (fast heart rate): either atrial fibrillation or atrial flutter or a supraventricular tachycardia. Atrial fibrillation is the most common arrhythmia associated with alcohol use. These arrhythmias typically resolve with abstinence, but some individuals will require antiarrhythmic medication. Ventricular arrhythmias have also been reported.

Several studies have now documented an association between alcohol use and sudden coronary death in both heavy drinkers and occasional drinkers, even in people without any evidence of preexisting heart disease (Mukamal et al., 2005*a*).

Hypertension

Alcohol raises blood pressure and increases the risk of hypertension in a dose-dependent manner in both men and women, independent of age, body weight, and cigarette smoking (Corrao, Bagnardi, Zambon, & Arico, 1999). Consumption exceeding 30 g/d is associated with higher blood pressure, and binge drinking may be particularly implicated (Beilin & Puddey, 2006). A meta-analysis of 15 randomized controlled trials showed that reducing alcohol consumption was associated with reduced systolic and diastolic pressures (Xin et al., 2001). In addition, trials in alcohol dependent patients show that blood pressures are lower in those who cut down or abstain (Stewart et al., 2008). Individuals presenting with hypertension to a general practitioner or physician should always have an alcohol history taken, together with appropriate laboratory investigations, and should be advised to reduce their alcohol consumption.

In the absence of the possibility of conducting a randomized trial to understand the impact of alcohol consumption on cardiovascular health, an alternative approach, Mendelian randomization, has been used. This takes a large epidemiological population to compare those with and without a variant of an ALDH enzyme that is associated with alcohol-related flushing and lower levels of alcohol consumption (see Chapter 2). A meta-analysis of studies found that those individuals with the variant of *ALDH2* associated with lower alcohol consumption also had lower blood pressure (Chen et al., 2008).

Stroke

There are two broad categories of stroke. These are *haemorrhagic stroke*, due to ruptured blood vessels on the surface of the brain (subarachnoid haemorrhage) and in the substance of the brain (intracranial haemorrhage), and *ischaemic stroke*, due to blockage of brain blood vessels by clot formation or emboli to the brain from the heart or elsewhere, or blockage of blood vessels outside the brain (mainly the carotid arteries). Alcohol increases the risk of haemorrhagic stroke in a dose-dependent fashion (Corrao et al., 1999). Episodic heavy drinking is a risk factor for both haemorrhagic and ischaemic stroke, particularly in adolescents and people under the age of 40 years. The risk of heavy drinking leading to ischaemic stroke is moderated by a gene that influences high density lipoprotein (HDL) cholesterol, one of the mediators of the cardioprotective effect. In the absence of this gene effect, there is no statistical relationship between alcohol consumption and risk of ischaemic stroke. When the gene is present, alcohol consumption increases the risk of ischaemic stroke

(Mukamal et al., 2005*b*). Moderate drinking has been shown to have some beneficial effect in reducing the risk of ischaemic stroke; however, the effect is small and present only at lower levels compared with coronary heart disease (Klatsky, Armstrong, Friedman, & Sidney, 2001; O'Keefe et al., 2014)

Coronary heart disease

Observational data suggest that light to moderate alcohol consumption is associated with significant decreases in cardiovascular-related death, with maximum protection derived from ½ to 1 drink per day for women and 1–2 drinks for men (O'Keefe et al., 2014). Drinking more than 2½ drinks per day for women and 3 drinks for men is associated with higher death rates in a dose-dependent manner. However, the greatest benefits appear in middle-aged (>50 years) and older individuals (Hvidtfeldt et al., 2010). In addition, light to moderate alcohol consumption has been shown to improve outcomes in those with established coronary heart disease (Constanzo Di Castelnuovo, Donati, Iacoviello, & de Gaetano, 2010).

The "cardioprotective effect" has been proposed to derive from alcohol itself and frequency of drinking rather than from any specific beverage type. Alcohol may have a partial inhibitory effect on atherosclerosis by increasing levels of HDLs, which carry cholesterol to different parts of the body. This is because HDLs are associated with a reduced risk of coronary heart disease and are thought to protect the arteries from a build-up of cholesterol. However, the effect of alcohol on HDL appears small. Alcohol also reduces platelet stickiness and aggregation, lowers plasma fibrinogen, and increases fibrinolysis.

However, associations identified in observational research may not be causal. The Mendelian randomization approach (explained earlier) has also been used to explore the relationship between alcohol consumption and coronary heart disease. Those with a variant of the ALDH 1B gene (*ALDH1B)* associated with alcohol-related flushing and lower levels of alcohol consumption (see Chapter 2) had a lower risk of coronary heart disease and a more favourable cardiovascular profile (Holmes et al., 2014).

Therefore, the latest evidence suggests that alcohol consumption increases coronary heart disease among all drinkers, including those who drink "moderately." It is therefore no longer appropriate to advise drinking alcohol to improve cardiovascular health, particularly because heavy drinking episodes are associated with increased rates of heart attacks. The number of years of life lost attributable to drinking outweighs the years saved attributable to protective factors.

Cardiomyopathy

Chronic excessive alcohol consumption (more than 90 g/d for 5 years or more) can lead to cardiomyopathy and heart failure (Rubin & Urbano-Marquez, 1994). In the United States, alcohol accounts for about a third of nonischaemic dilated cardiomyopathy. In addition to the direct toxic action of alcohol on heart muscle, other consequences of heavy alcohol consumption such as hypertension, altered metabolism, and increased acetaldehyde also contribute to damage of the heart muscle (Walker et al., 2013), although a genetic predisposition may also be an important factor. Alcoholic cardiomyopathy was formerly attributed to thiamine deficiency, but this is probably not the case because it occurs in heavy drinkers who are well nourished. The disorder usually manifests itself between the ages of 30 and 60 years. Although more common in men because of their heavier consumption, women seem to be particularly vulnerable (Urbano-Marquez et al., 1995). Whilst complete abstinence improves outcomes, cardiomyopathy and heart failure are a common cause of death in heavy drinkers (O'Keefe et al., 2014).

Alcoholic cardiomyopathy is characterized by an enlarged, hypertrophied heart. The left ventricle is dilated, and there is dysfunction in cardiac contractility, leading to a depressed output (ejection fraction). In the early stages of hypertrophy and dilatation, there may be few symptoms. However, as the disorder progresses, patients develop arrhythmias, including atrial and ventricular tachyarrhythmias and atrioventricular conduction defects. Congestive cardiac failure (heart failure) is another typical form of presentation (breathlessness on exertion, breathlessness at night, and peripheral edema).

Subclinical forms of alcoholic cardiomyopathy can be identified in problem drinkers using noninvasive procedures such as echocardiography. Early detection and abstinence may halt or reverse the progress of this disorder.

Gastroenterological disorders

Alcoholic liver disease

Alcohol misuse is the commonest cause of liver damage in the United Kingdom, Europe, the United States, and Australia. Rates of liver disease vary enormously from country to country but appear to be highest where alcohol consumption is highest. Many studies suggest that women are at greater risk than men for a given level of alcohol consumption. In the UK, attention has recently been drawn to the fact that the improvements in other chronic disorders such as stroke, heart disease, and many cancers have not been seen in liver disease (Williams et al., 2014). Liver disease has become the third most common cause of premature death in the UK, and mortality rates have increased by 400 percent since 1970. The UK situation is worse than in other western European countries, where reductions in alcohol-related liver disease are evident. Chronic liver disease can be a silent killer (i.e., the individual is unaware of any difficulties until liver impairment is significant from hepatitis or cirrhosis and he or she presents with jaundice, gastric bleeding, or encephalopathy [confusion]).

The liver is vulnerable to alcohol-related injury because it is the primary site of alcohol metabolism. Three types of alcoholic liver disease have been described: fatty liver, alcoholic hepatitis, and alcoholic cirrhosis (see Table 5.3). All three may coexist. Fatty liver is present in up to 90 percent of persistent heavy drinkers at some time. Alcoholic hepatitis is seen in approximately 40 percent of individuals with a history of persistent heavy drinking. About a third of patients with alcohol-related liver disease are alcohol dependent, and about a third of lifelong heavy drinkers will develop cirrhosis (Williams et al., 2014). Important contributing factors to greater severity of liver disease with excess alcohol consumption include genetic and environmental factors such as obesity and viral hepatitis (e.g., hepatitis B and C). Genetic factors that increase the oxidation of alcohol to acetaldehyde or reduce the

Table 5.3. Alcohol and the liver

- Fatty liver rarely causes illness and is reversible with abstinence.
- Alcoholic hepatitis may be fatal but can be reversible with abstinence.
- Alcoholic cirrhosis is often progressive and fatal but can stabilize with abstinence.
- Abstinence is the single most important component of treatment for alcoholic liver disease.

rate of acetaldehyde clearance will increase acetaldehyde levels in the liver and cause greater injury. Women develop cirrhosis at lower levels of alcohol consumption than men. In women, a reduced "first pass" metabolism of alcohol in the stomach by gastric alcohol dehydrogenase (ADH) leads to increased blood alcohol levels. The ratio of water to fat is lower in women than in men. Alcohol is distributed in water, so, for a given body weight, the concentration of ethanol in water and thus in the bloodstream tends to be higher in women than in men. Alcohol dependent individuals with hepatitis C infection develop liver injury at a younger age and at a lower cumulative dose of alcohol than do those without hepatitis C. Continuing heavy alcohol consumption is associated with accelerated progression of liver disease associated with cirrhosis and a higher risk of hepatocellular carcinoma in patients with hepatitis B and C. Cigarette smoking and coffee consumption also appear to increase the risk of developing cirrhosis in alcohol dependent individuals, although the reasons for this are not known. Smoking more than 20 cigarettes per day and drinking four or more cups of coffee per day is associated with a greater risk.

Fatty liver

The first histological change seen in persistent heavy drinkers is deposition of fat in the liver. Although this is usually asymptomatic, patients may present with nonspecific symptoms such as malaise, tiredness, nausea, an enlarged and tender liver, or abnormal liver function tests. Occasionally, very severe fatty liver can lead to jaundice (obstructive jaundice), liver failure, or death due to a fatty embolism (globules of fat getting into the circulation and obstructing arteries to the brain). Fatty liver is reversible with abstinence.

Alcoholic hepatitis

Minor degrees of alcoholic hepatitis may be asymptomatic and clinically indistinguishable from fatty liver. More severe episodes reflect inflammation and destruction of liver tissue. Inflammation underpins alcoholic liver disease either from the direct impact of alcohol and withdrawal, as well as from indirect responses to gut microflora (bacteria). Scar tissue may begin to replace liver tissue. This process is called *fibrosis*. Symptoms of alcoholic hepatitis include loss of appetite, abdominal pain, nausea, weight loss, jaundice, and fever. Severe alcoholic hepatitis has a mortality rate of around 30–40 percent after 28 days (Hazeldine & Sheron, 2014). Corticosteroids, which suppress the inflammation process, may improve survival rate in the early stages, but abstinence is the best treatment and is essential for long-term survival. Abstinence leads to reversal of the histological changes, but alcoholic hepatitis almost always progresses to cirrhosis in women, even following abstinence.

Alcoholic cirrhosis

Cirrhosis may arise de novo in some cases, without passing through the intermediate state of hepatitis. Here, liver tissue becomes scarred by the development of fibrous septa that link the hepatic veins to portal tracts. This scarring, together with the regeneration of liver tissue, disturbs the normal liver architecture, and the consequences are twofold. First, the actual loss of functioning liver tissue causes a range of metabolic disturbances, and, ultimately, liver failure may occur. Second, and very importantly, the scarring and disorganization lead to the squeezing and blocking off of blood vessels. This physical damming causes a build-up of pressure in the portal venous system (the veins that carry blood from the gastrointestinal tract to the liver), a condition called *portal hypertension*. This can, in turn, cause bleeding from veins at the lower end of the oesophagus (oesophageal varices), and this bleeding can be severe and fatal.

Cirrhosis can exist in degrees. If the condition is not too advanced, abstinence may lead to stabilization and enhance life expectancy. From the patient's point of view, they may know nothing of this insidious condition until they suddenly become jaundiced, find their abdomen swelling up with fluid (ascites), or have a massive bleed. More often, the diagnosis is picked up at an earlier stage on clinical examination and liver toxicity tests, with confirmation coming from various special investigations. Ultrasound scanning is a relatively easy and noninvasive investigation.

Treatment for cirrhosis is largely directed at relieving symptoms and complications. Liver transplantation can be used as a treatment for end-stage alcoholic cirrhosis. Outcomes are as good as for other liver disease and superior to those with hepatitis C, although worse survival is seen with combined hepatitis C and alcohol-related liver disease (Lucey, 2014). Psychiatric and specialist alcohol assessment has become an important element of the screening process in many transplant centres, because of the risks of anxiety, depression, and relapse to drinking in the postoperative period. If individuals do drink alcohol, the majority (~80 percent) only consume small amounts. If the individual relapses (as opposed to lapses), survival is reduced with progressive episodes of hepatitis.

Acute pancreatitis

Alcohol misuse and biliary disease are the two main causative factors in acute pancreatitis. As with the liver, more recently, a contribution from an inflammatory response to gut bacteria has been recognized. Individuals with acute alcoholic pancreatitis are likely to be young men drinking in excess of 80 g of alcohol per day. About 5–15 percent of alcoholics will ever experience pancreatitis. The most common form of presentation is a sudden onset of severe upper abdominal pain, typically penetrating through to the back and associated with vomiting. The pain lessens in severity over the first 72 hours. Patients with severe acute pancreatitis may be feverish, hypotensive, have rapid breathing, and suffer with acute ascites, pleural effusions, and paralytic ileus (paralysis of the intestines). The diagnosis is usually made from the clinical presentation and confirmed by gross elevations of amylase and lipase in the blood. The mortality rate is between 10 and 40 percent.

> A businessman, aged 52, had a long history of alcohol dependence. On occasion, he would stop drinking for a few months, but he was never willing to consider long-term abstinence as the goal. One weekend, he relapsed once more into drinking with a very heavy binge. On Sunday night, he was admitted as an emergency to his local hospital with appalling abdominal pain radiating through to the back. A raised serum amylase confirmed the diagnosis of acute pancreatitis. Despite the hospital's best efforts, he died in shock 36 hours later. Postmortem examination showed extensive necrosis of the pancreas and some old scarring. There was also evidence of early liver cirrhosis.

Chronic pancreatitis

Heavy drinking is the most frequent contributor to chronic pancreatitis in adults in the Western world, particularly the calcifying form. However, it is now thought that alcohol alone is not a sufficient cause, but rather sensitizes the pancreas to other insults. Smoking is an independent risk factor for chronic pancreatitis, and genetic (e.g., variants of enzymes) and environmental factors also modify the disease (Brock, Nielsen, Lelic, & Drewes, 2013).

It mainly affects men who have been drinking heavily. Although the quantity and duration of alcohol consumption are related to the development of this condition, it rarely occurs alongside cirrhosis. The main presenting symptom is severe dull epigastric (abdominal) pain radiating to the back, which may be partly relieved by leaning forward. The pain is often associated with nausea and vomiting. Steatorrhoea (fat in the faeces making them pale, loose and difficult to flush away), diarrhoea, and weight loss also occur. These symptoms occur when more than 90 percent of the functioning exocrine tissue (the tissue that secretes digestive enzymes) is destroyed. Damage to the Islets of Langerhans, with consequent failure of insulin secretion and diabetes mellitus, occurs more slowly. Treatment is focused on the management of acute attacks of pain and other complications, such as diabetes mellitus and fat malabsorption. Abstinence from alcohol is the mainstay of treatment and is essential if attacks of pain are to be stopped. Managing chronic severe and intractable pain may be challenging and involve long-term opiate use, which carries its own risks.

Gastritis, peptic ulceration, and intestinal symptoms

Alcohol alters the tone of the sphincter between the oesophagus (gullet) and stomach, stimulates gastric juice secretion, and increases mucosal permeability. This combination leads to increased risk of oesophageal reflux (i.e., acidic stomach contents in the oesophagus that is experienced as heartburn or indigestion). It can also cause acute erosive ulcers in the stomach and duodenum (first part of small bowel). Studies of the interaction between alcohol consumption and *Helicobacter pylori*, another cause of gastritis, have shown that heavy consumption may sustain infection but moderate consumption (e.g., <75 g/week) may be protective (Franke, Teyssen, & Singer, 2005).

Patients presenting to alcohol services commonly suffer from intestinal symptoms, such as diarrhoea and malabsorption. The general malnutrition and weight loss seen in these patients are usually due to dietary neglect. Alcohol dependent individuals are therefore at risk of vitamin deficiencies (especially of folic acid, B_1/thiamine, and B_{12}). Deficiencies of minerals and trace elements (zinc, selenium) are also possible, again as a result of malabsorption and malnutrition.

Mallory-Weiss syndrome

This syndrome is associated with heavy alcohol consumption and alcohol dependence, and it occurs as a result of acute intense vomiting that leads to a build-up of pressure within the oesophagus. This, in turn, causes a longitudinal tear in the mucosa at the gastro-oesophageal junction, with consequent vomiting of blood.

Endocrine and metabolic disorders

Alcohol is a source of calories, each gram being equivalent to 7.1 kcal (Lieber, 1988). Why, then, are alcohol dependent individuals not all overweight? It would appear that, in alcohol dependence, this excess energy is largely used by the induced microsomal ethanol-oxidizing system (MEOS). Alcohol dependent people also tend to neglect their diet, so the two factors taken together mean that the excess energy does not translate into weight gain.

Type II diabetes

Alcohol consumption is associated with type II diabetes in a U-shaped fashion, with 24 g/d in women or 22 g/d in men providing the most "protection" (Baliunas et al., 2009). This is probably due to the fact that alcohol increases insulin sensitivity in low doses. However, consumption of more than 50 g/d in women and 60 g/d in men is harmful. Individuals with diabetes are recommended to drink moderately.

Alcohol-induced pseudo-Cushing's syndrome

Alcohol-induced pseudo-Cushing's syndrome is a term used to describe heavy drinkers who present with a clinical picture similar to that seen in Cushing's syndrome: truncal obesity with thin extremities, ruddy appearance, "moon-face," bruising, striae (stretch marks), muscle wasting, and hypertension. Biochemical abnormalities include elevated urinary and plasma cortisol levels (the latter failing to suppress with dexamethasone), reduced circadian rhythm of plasma cortisol, and normal or suppressed adrenocorticotropic hormone (ACTH). The biochemical abnormalities rapidly revert to normal with abstinence from alcohol. The mechanism underlying this disorder is poorly understood.

Fertility

Although alcohol alters the level of oestrogen and progesterone, it is not clear if or at what level alcohol consumption has an adverse impact on fertility in women. Nevertheless, women trying to conceive are advised not to drink alcohol, although this is more related to the adverse effects of alcohol on the foetus (foetal alcohol syndrome). Alcohol causes a lowering of plasma testosterone concentrations through a direct toxic effect on the Leydig cells in the testis where testosterone is synthesized. This effect occurs independently of liver disease and may be related to the total lifetime dose of alcohol consumed. Alcohol also is toxic to sperm.

Hypoglycaemia

Alcohol-induced hypoglycaemia (lowering of the blood sugar) can occur as a result of alcohol intoxication or after a modest intake of alcohol in individuals who are malnourished or fasting. Clinically, the patient may present as flushed and sweaty with a rapid pulse and the appearance of being drunk and uncoordinated. An alternative presentation is in coma and hypothermic, without obvious features of hypoglycaemia. Children and adolescents are particularly susceptible to alcohol-induced hypoglycaemia, and the condition is much more dangerous for them than for adults (Lamminpaa, 1995).

Alcoholic ketoacidosis

This is a rare condition, one that usually arises when an episode of heavy drinking has been followed by vomiting or cessation of eating. Patients can present in a drowsy and collapsed state, with a blood alcohol level of zero. Metabolic acidosis is a more typical presentation: this responds to rehydration and glucose. A metabolic alkalosis may also be evident if there has been vomiting.

Gout

Gout is a metabolic disorder characterized by episodic painful swelling of peripheral joints, especially the fingers and toes. Individuals with gout have high levels of uric acid, which is deposited in the joints and causes inflammation and swelling. Most gout occurs in middle-aged men who often have a family history of the disorder and drink heavily (Choi et al., 2004). Beer is particularly liable to produce hyperuricacidaemia because of its high purine content. Other conditions predisposing to gout include obesity, hyperlipidaemia, and hypertension, all of which are independently associated with heavy drinking. Heavy drinking can bring out a latent tendency toward gout or aggravate established gout.

Hyperlipidaemia

Heavy drinking is associated with a rise in circulatory blood fats (serum triglycerides). This will only be picked up by laboratory tests but probably carries implications for enhanced risk of arteriosclerosis.

Immune system disorders

It has been known for many years that chronic excessive alcohol use is associated with suppression of the immune system, leading to high rates of infectious disease in this group (Estruch, 2001). Autoimmunity is also triggered by heavy alcohol consumption, contributing to organ damage such as alcoholic liver disease and skin disorders.

Heavy drinkers are at particular risk of respiratory infections, including pneumonia (Cook, 1998). They are also vulnerable to septicaemia secondary to pneumonia, urinary tract infections, bacterial peritonitis, and biliary infections. There is a strong association between alcohol consumption, HIV infection and other sexually transmitted diseases (Baliunas, Rehm, Irving, & Shuper, 2010). The combination of alcohol dependence and HIV/AIDS puts individuals at particular risk for tuberculosis, including drug-resistant strains. In addition, alcohol abuse may interfere with antiretroviral medication effectiveness as well as medication compliance (Hendershot, Stoner, Pantalone, & Simoni, 2009).

There is some evidence that alcohol dependence predisposes individuals in some way to develop hepatitis C infection, the increased incidence being on the order of 10 percent. This might reflect an increased susceptibility to hepatitis C in this group, increased risk behaviours, or both.

Although alcohol dependent individuals have increased serum immunoglobulins, this does not reflect a strong immune system. Rather, the increase is due to an abnormal regulation of the synthesis of antibodies (Estruch, 2001). Alcohol dependent individuals have reduced cell-mediated immunity. Lymphocyte (white cell) numbers are reduced in those with liver disease; although numbers are normal in those without liver disease, alterations in the percentage of various types are seen. B cells are normal or slightly reduced, and natural killer cells show reduced functional activity.

More recently, however, the underlying mechanisms involving effects on adaptive and innate immunity, increased circulating immunoglobins, alterations in cytokine expression, and impaired phagocytic functions are receiving increasing attention. These processes provide more targets for treatment. Neuropsychiatric disorders such as "sickness behaviour" or symptoms commonly seen in depression (loss of appetite, sleep disturbance, etc.) and dementia are also likely to have a neuroinflammatory component (consider, for example, the impact of flu on mood and cognition).

Alcoholic muscle, skin, and bone disease

Effects of alcohol on skeletal muscle

Acute myopathy produced by alcohol poisoning is a condition occurring in less than 5 percent of alcohol misusers. It is characterized by severe pain, tenderness, swelling, and weakness of the skeletal muscles. In its severe form, acute rhabdomyolysis is associated with myoglobinuria, renal damage, and hyperkalaemia (raised potassium levels). Alcohol consumption reduces the normal metabolic responses of skeletal muscle to the action of insulin by causing acute insulin resistance.

Chronic alcoholic myopathy occurs in up to 60 percent of individuals with long-standing alcohol problems and is easily overlooked or misattributed to poor nutrition. As is the case with alcoholic liver disease and brain damage, women are more susceptible than men. Individuals typically present with proximal muscle weakness, pain and abnormal gait, and show evidence of atrophy and loss of muscle fibre in the shoulder and pelvic girdle region. Histology reveals a reduction in the diameters of white (fast-twitch) fibres. The weakness and atrophy tend to improve with abstinence or a substantial reduction in consumption.

Here is a case abstract that illustrates a fairly typical picture:

> A 45-year-old storekeeper who was severely alcohol dependent complained that he had developed "terrible rheumatics." There was severe pain and some tenderness and swelling of both upper arms, and he could no longer lift his stock down from the shelves. It took about 2 months for him to make a reasonable recovery.

Effects of alcohol on skin

Heavy drinkers and individuals misusing alcohol are prone to a variety of skin disorders including psoriasis, discoid eczema, and superficial cutaneous fungal infections, such as tinea pedis and pityriasis versicolor. Rosacea and acne may be exacerbated by alcohol.

Psoriasis is an alcohol-related skin condition that deserves special note. The daily alcohol consumption of men with psoriasis is higher than in men with other skin diseases, and heavy drinking appears to be related to the severity of the disease. In heavy drinkers, psoriasis mainly affects the palms of the hands and the soles of the feet. Alcohol-induced psoriasis responds poorly to treatment unless the patient stops drinking.

Effects of alcohol on bone

Heavy drinkers have increased rates of osteoporosis (reduction in the amount of bone per unit volume without a change in its composition) and osteopenia and an increased frequency of fractures and avascular necrosis. The association between alcohol consumption and osteoporosis is dose-dependent and independent of nutritional status (Preedy, Mantle, & Peters, 2001). The association between alcohol consumption and decreased bone mass may be weaker in women than in men.

The reduced bone density in individuals with alcohol dependence is thought to arise as a result of impaired bone formation (reduced osteoblastic function) and increased bone resorption (increased numbers of osteoclasts). These effects of alcohol on bone metabolism appear to be reversible with abstinence. Heavy drinkers are therefore at risk of fractures even after minimal trauma. Symptoms of back pain indicative of osteoporosis and possible vertebral collapse should not be overlooked. Postmenopausal women may be particularly susceptible to the effects of alcohol on bone.

Respiratory disease

Respiratory tract infection

As mentioned, heavy alcohol consumption is associated with defects in the body's immune responses. Clinically, this is reflected in an excess of lower respiratory tract infections with

Streptococcus pneumoniae, *Mycobacterium tuberculosis*, and *Klebsiella pneumoniae*. Self-neglect and an associated way of life, particularly in skid row drinkers, are also important factors predisposing to infections. Because heavy drinkers may both vomit and become stuporose, they are prone to inhale material into their lungs and hence develop lung abscesses or bronchiectasis (dilation and infection of the smaller bronchi).

Many problem drinkers also smoke heavily. A carcinoma of the lung is not, therefore, an uncommon coincidental finding, sometimes confusing the diagnostic picture: what is thought to be an alcoholic dementia turns out, for instance, to be a secondary cancer of the brain, or a severe alcoholic peripheral neuropathy turns out to be a cancer-related (carcinomatous) neuropathy. The simple message is that if a problem drinker presents for an assessment and has not had a recent chest X-ray, such an examination should be arranged.

Adult respiratory distress syndrome

Adult respiratory distress syndrome (ARDS) is a severe form of lung injury that results from blood infections, trauma, pneumonia, and blood transfusions. Alcohol predisposes the lung to the inflammatory stresses of infection and trauma.

Haematological effects

Problem drinking gives rise to anaemia, macrocytosis, simple iron deficiency, neutropaenia and thrombocytopaenia.

Anaemia

Anaemia is common in problem drinkers and can be caused by a variety of factors including malnutrition, chronic blood loss, liver disease, malabsorption, chronic infections, and the direct toxic effect of alcohol on the bone marrow.

Macrocytosis

Macrocytosis (enlarged red blood cells) is also common in problem drinkers, and an unexplained macrocytosis should always alert clinicians to the possibility of an alcohol problem. If nutrition is adequate, it is probably caused by the direct toxic action of alcohol on the bone marrow. Folate deficiency in malnourished problem drinkers can give rise to a megaloblastic anaemia. However, alcohol may interfere directly with folate metabolism.

Iron deficiency

Iron deficiency among heavy drinkers will probably reflect a poor diet or chronic blood loss due to gastritis or bleeding varices. It may be associated with folate deficiency.

Neutropaenia and thrombocytopaenia

Heavy drinking may cause a neutropaenia (lowering of white cells), either by a toxic effect on the bone marrow or as a result of folate deficiency, and thereby render patients susceptible to infections. Alcohol may also interfere with neutrophil function. Thrombocytopaenia (decrease in platelets) is frequent in heavy drinkers and can account for a susceptibility to bruising. The platelet count usually returns to normal with abstinence.

Accidents/trauma

Alcohol is an underlying and frequently overlooked risk factor for accidents in the general population, not just in individuals with alcohol problems or alcohol dependence. Ingestion of alcohol causes diminished coordination and balance; slower reaction times; and impaired attention, perception, and judgment, all of which increase the risk of accidental injury. Road traffic accidents in which alcohol is implicated are more serious than accidents in which it is not, and the risk of being involved in an accident rises as a function of the increased BAC. Alcohol-related accidents in particular contribute to high mortality rates in young men. Approximately one-third of pedestrians killed in road traffic accidents by day have measurable BACs. Although the literature on alcohol-related accidents has historically been focused largely on road traffic accidents and drink-driving (drunk-driving), accidents in the home, workplace, and civil aviation, and also leisure accidents such as drowning, now receive more prominence. Positive blood alcohol levels have been obtained in 40 percent of fatal industrial accidents and 35 percent of nonfatal work-related accidents. The consumption of more than 60 g of alcohol within a 6-hour period is associated with a significant risk of injury. Alcohol consumption may put women at particular risk for injury because of the greater physiological impact of a given dose of alcohol (McLeod, Stockwell, Stevens, & Phillips, 1999).

Studies from various countries suggest that drinking is involved in 26–54 percent of home and leisure injuries (Babor et al., 2010). It is particularly associated with violent family incidents and is implicated in child abuse.

Surgical complications

Heavy drinking is associated with an increased risk of postoperative complications. This risk is evident in consumption levels of about five drinks (≥60 g) per day (Tønnesen, 1999). Complications include prolonged hospital stay, the need for further surgery, infections, cardiopulmonary insufficiency, and bleeding. A Danish study has shown that a period of preoperative abstinence lasting for 1 month (treatment with disulfiram 800 mg twice weekly) reduced postoperative complications in heavy drinkers with colorectal disease (Tønnesen et al., 1999).

It is worth entering a brief general reminder as to the potential importance of the patient's heavy drinking to the work of the anaesthetist both operatively and postoperatively. Emergency surgery may in particular run into difficulties if intoxication is overlooked and recovery is complicated by a seizure or by other unexpected withdrawal symptoms. Tolerance to alcohol may result in cross-tolerance to certain anaesthetics, notably thiopentone.

Neurological disorders

Alcohol withdrawal seizures

Alcohol withdrawal seizures occur in about 2–5 percent of alcohol dependent individuals and are responsible for one-third of seizure-related admissions (Bråthen et al., 2005). The seizures occur approximately 7–48 hours after cessation of drinking; are generalized, tonic-clonic (*grand mal*); and are thus associated with a loss of consciousness followed by convulsive movements in all four limbs. During a particular withdrawal episode, the patient may have only one seizure, but more commonly there will be three or four seizures over a couple of days. Very rarely, status epilepticus will supervene. This is a continuous run of seizures, one merging into another, which is associated with risk to life. Alcohol withdrawal seizures have sometimes been termed "rum fits," but they are not associated with any one type of beverage.

Predisposing factors to alcohol withdrawal seizures include hypokalaemia, hypomagnesaemia, a previous history of withdrawal seizures, and concurrent epilepsy. An electroencephalogram (EEG) is generally unhelpful, but a brain scan will help to rule out intracranial lesions since these may also be associated with a seizure occurring "out of the blue."

Alcohol dependent individuals who have experienced seizures due to alcohol withdrawal may be more prone to developing further seizures in future withdrawal episodes. A seizure also may precede delirium tremens (see Chapter 11). Therefore, an in-patient setting may be preferable for any proposed subsequent planned detoxification for this group (see Chapter 11 for management). Patients at risk of alcohol withdrawal seizures should be advised not to stop drinking suddenly, but to continue at the same level of consumption until they are in a medical care setting. If they refuse to seek care but wish to detoxify on their own, this should be an extremely slow reduction of consumption. Tragedies have sometimes occurred when a severely dependent patient has stopped drinking on their own initiative and sustained a withdrawal seizure. This can be hazardous in any case, but particularly so in certain situations (e.g., when driving a vehicle).

Seizures of other origin

A number of other possible reasons for seizures in patients with drinking problems must be borne in mind, as well as the fact that seizures may be entirely coincidental. Heavy drinking may, for example, lower the threshold in a person with an underlying epileptic tendency of any origin. A patient with epilepsy who is being treated with anticonvulsants may simply forget to take his or her tablets when he or she goes on a drinking binge. Heavy drinking can also lead, as a result of liver enzyme induction, to increased metabolic clearance of anticonvulsant medication.

Heavy drinkers are often heavy cigarette smokers, and a seizure may on occasion be the first and tragic signal of the secondary spread to the brain (metastases) from a carcinoma of the lung. Problem drinkers are prone to accidents, and a seizure may be symptomatic of an old or more recent head injury. Heavy drinkers may also be on antidepressants, many of which cause seizures in overdose. Alcoholic "dementia" may sometimes be accompanied by seizures. Other causes of seizures are coincidental withdrawal of sedative or hypnotic drugs, particularly benzodiazepines, alcohol-related hypoglycaemia (lowered blood sugar; see the earlier section on Hypoglycaemia), and fatty emboli lodging in the brain.

Peripheral neuropathy

Alcoholic peripheral neuropathy is a sensorimotor neuropathy detectable to some degree in approximately 10 percent of chronic heavy drinkers. The main causal factors are thought to be vitamin B deficiency and the toxic effect of alcohol. The lower limbs are more frequently affected than the upper limbs, and the typical presentation is with an insidious onset of weakness, pain, parasthesia, and numbness in the feet, which progresses proximally and symmetrically in a "glove-and-stocking" distribution. Bilateral foot drop and weakness of the small hand muscles and finger extensors may occur. Distal reflexes are usually absent. Treatment includes B-group vitamins and abstinence. Recovery is usually slow and incomplete, with some residual sensory loss, and, in some, continued analgesia is required.

Alcoholic cerebellar degeneration

The cerebellum plays a key role in balance and motor integration, and its role in cognitive processing (e.g., problem-solving, working memory) is increasingly recognized. It is sometimes the focus for alcohol-related brain damage. Alcoholic cerebellar degeneration usually develops insidiously and is characterized by ataxia of gait (unsteadiness) and incoordination of the legs. It is thought to be due to thiamine deficiency, but alcohol neurotoxicity may also be an important factor. Abstinence and treatment with thiamine (vitamin B_1) may halt the progress of the disorder, but the patient may still be left with a disabling condition.

Wernicke–Korsakoff syndrome

Although Wernicke's encephalopathy and Korsakoff's syndrome were originally described as different entities (in 1881 and 1887, respectively), both are caused by thiamine (vitamin B_1) deficiency. Thiamine is a critical co-factor for brain metabolism; its deficiency results in Wernicke's encephalopathy, which is the acute or subacute manifestation of the syndrome, and in Korsakoff 's syndrome, the chronic form. They show the same underlying pathological lesions in deep midline and midbrain regions (i.e., the diencephalon) involving periventricular and periaqueductal grey matter, walls of the third and fourth ventricles, and cerebellum involving rupture and abnormal changes in the lining of blood vessels and loss of neurons and white matter (Victor, Adams, & Collins, 1971). Cortical abnormalities have also been reported in a proportion of cases. Prevalence rates of the Wernicke–Korsakoff syndrome vary, with autopsy studies reporting rates of about 1.5 percent (Cook, Hallwood, & Thomson, 1998). The condition is more common in autopsy studies of alcoholics. Incidence rates are reported to have increased in Scotland over recent years (Ramayya & Jauhar, 1997). Both Wernicke's and Korsakoff's are essentially clinical diagnoses based on good examination in the absence of tests or pathognomic features on neuroimaging.

Wernicke's encephalopathy

Wernicke's encephalopathy occurs in individuals with alcohol misuse and dependence and in a variety of other disorders associated with a poor intake or absorption of thiamine. These other disorders include gastric carcinoma, other malignancy, hyperemesis in pregnancy, anorexia nervosa, and haemodialysis, as well as post-bariatric surgery. In alcohol dependent individuals, Wernicke's encephalopathy is often precipitated by alcohol withdrawal or the stress of an intercurrent illness that results in an increased metabolic load to the brain. Some individuals may have a particular susceptibility to developing the condition.

The encephalopathy usually has an abrupt onset, although it may take a few days for the full picture to develop (Lishman, 1998; Thomson et al., 2008). Mental confusion or unsteady gait (ataxia) are often the first features to be seen. Patients may be aware of ocular abnormalities – they complain of wavering vision or double vision on looking to the side. The classic triad of confusion, ataxia, and ocular abnormalities (nystagmus, an oscillatory movement of the eyeballs, and ophthalmoplegia, a paralysis of the eye muscles that might cause a squint) is diagnostic, but is only present in 10 percent of patients. Therefore, because many heavy drinkers present with confusion and ataxia, and the symptoms and signs may only be present in part or not at all, the diagnosis is often missed. There must always, therefore, be a high index of suspicion, particularly in cases of unexplained confusion. Other common features include anorexia, nausea, and vomiting (Thomson et al., 2008). There is usually a degree of memory disorder. Lethargy and hypotension have also been described.

Rarely, the disorder presents with hypothermia, stupor, or coma. About 17–20 percent of sufferers die in the acute stage (Cook et al., 1998).

Given the difficulties in making a definitive diagnosis, there should be a low threshold for making a presumptive diagnosis and initiating treatment.

Wernicke's encephalopathy is a medical emergency. Treatment with high-dose parenteral thiamine should be given promptly to offset the risk of death or irreversible brain damage. Parenteral thiamine is itself associated with a very small risk of an anaphylactic reaction and should only be given when appropriate anaphylaxis treatment (e.g., as for Hep B vaccination) is available; it can be given safely in the community. Up to 1 g of thiamine may be needed initially to achieve a clinical response. Thereafter, 500 mg of thiamine should be given once or twice daily for 3–5 days (Thomson & Marshall, 2006; see Chapter 11).

Hypomagnesaemia may impair the clinical response to treatment, and it is therefore worth checking serum magnesium levels. Electrolyte imbalance and dehydration must be avoided, and any intercurrent infection treated.

Ocular abnormalities usually recover quite quickly (days to weeks), and the ataxia usually responds within the first week but takes about 1–2 months to resolve (Lishman, 1998). Some patients are left with a residual nystagmus and ataxia. Improvements in acute confusion or delirium usually occur within 1–2 days. Global confusion begins to improve after 2–3 weeks but may take 1–2 months to clear. As it improves, so the amnesic (memory) defects become more obvious.

A milder, subclinical form of Wernicke's encephalopathy exists in which patients do not manifest the clinical signs and symptoms just outlined. Undiagnosed and untreated episodes are experienced, resulting in chronic pathological changes at autopsy. The existence of subclinical Wernicke's encephalopathy has important implications for the prophylactic use of high-dose parenteral vitamin B therapy in alcohol dependent patients, as well as in those who are thought to be at risk of thiamine deficiency (see Chapter 11).

Korsakoff's syndrome

Korsakoff's syndrome often emerges as a chronic disorder following an episode of Wernicke's encephalopathy. It can, however, develop insidiously, with no clear prior history of a Wernicke episode. The main defect in Korsakoff's syndrome is in recent memory (Kopelman, Thomson, Guerrini, & Marshall, 2009; Lishman, 1998). New learning is impaired. In some instances, there is no new learning and an anterograde amnesia is evident (this is an inability to lay down new memories). However, the immediate memory span is unimpaired, so performance on a test of digit span (ability to repeat a list of numbers) is usually normal. Some retrograde amnesia (loss of memory for events occurring before the onset of the syndrome) is usually evident, and this may be of long duration. Individuals with Korsakoff's syndrome also manifest a disturbance in time sense; for instance, some recent memory is allocated to the past, or a past event is brought up as a recent happening. Remote memory for matters beyond the retrograde gap is better preserved but may also be impaired. Confabulation (the fabrication of ready answers and fluent descriptions of fictitious experiences compensating for gaps in memory) has been described. However, confabulation is not pathognomic, and it may come and go and seems to be commoner in the early stages (i.e., during the Wernicke phase; Lishman, 1998).

Other cognitive functions may appear to be superficially intact but are often found to be impaired when examined carefully. These individuals therefore find it difficult to sustain mental activity, have an inflexible mindset, and have a reduced capacity to shift attention from one task to another. Their thinking is often stereotyped, perseverative, and facile (Lishman, 1998). There are marked disturbances in personality, with a degree of apathy and self-neglect. Some patients are chatty, but the content of the conversation is superficial and repetitive. They often lack interest in their surroundings and may show little interest in alcohol. They show a remarkable lack of insight, with few realizing that they have memory deficits. It is likely that Korsakoff's syndrome is misdiagnosed in clinical practice and that there is some overlap between it and "alcoholic dementia."

In Korsakoff's syndrome, the pathology at the base of the brain is usually associated with cortical thinning, atrophy, and dilatation of the cerebral ventricles (Zahr, Kaufman, & Harper, 2011). Neuroimaging studies report a range of subcortical lesions in mammillary bodies, thalamus, pons, and hippocampus, as well as in the cerebellum. Dysfunction in the mammillo-thalamic tract is linked with memory impairment; however, recent evidence show that mammillary body atrophy is not pathognomic for Korsakoff's syndrome. Functional imaging studies with positron emission tomography (PET) and functional magnetic resonance imaging (fMRI) also report reduced function in the mammillo-thalamic tract and hippocampal connections, as well as in frontal cortex and cerebellum. Neuropsychological studies also reveal frontal lobe deficits, which could explain certain aspects of the syndrome, such as lack of insight and apathy.

The amnesia of Korsakoff's syndrome does not generally respond to treatment with thiamine. This raises the question that thiamine deficiency may not be the sole factor contributing to the development of the disorder. Alcohol neurotoxicity must also be considered, either alone or in association with thiamine deficiency.

These rather strange-sounding eponyms should not deflect the nonspecialist from trying to understand what is being talked about, and the following case abstract illustrates both how the acute element can present very suddenly and the type of chronic disorder that may occur when the Wernicke–Korsakoff syndrome supervenes.

> A woman, aged 48, who had been drinking a bottle of whisky each day for 10 or more years, was admitted to a psychiatric hospital for detoxification. It was noted that she was suffering from severe peripheral neuropathy (weakness, tingling, and pain in the legs). On the evening of admission, she was found to be rather confused, to be complaining of double vision, and to be staggering. By the next evening, she was stuporose, and her eye movements were uncoordinated (external ocular palsies). At this stage, and much too late, she was started on massive doses of thiamine – the classical picture of confusion, staggering gait, and ocular palsies should have alerted the staff to the dangerous onset of Wernicke's encephalopathy. After 5 days of the acute illness, the confusion cleared and the patient was then found to have a grossly impaired memory for recent events, a tendency to make things up to fill her gaps in memory (confabulation), and very little ability to remember new information, as witnessed by her difficulty in finding her way around the ward. This amnesic syndrome (Korsakoff's syndrome) showed little recovery over the ensuing months, and arrangements had to be made for the patient's transfer to long-term residential care.

This is a story of a tragedy that might have been averted, and there is a good argument for giving thiamine prophylactically to any patient who is in danger of this sort of complication.

Alcoholic pellagra encephalopathy

This is caused by a deficiency of the B vitamin, nicotinic acid, and its precursor tryptophan in association with chronic alcohol misuse. It is rarely reported in the British and American literature, perhaps because of the routine use of parenteral multivitamin therapy (Lishman, 1981). However, this also may be due to underdiagnosis because it is still evident in other countries, such as Japan. Clinical features include a fluctuating confusional state with global memory loss, visual hallucinations, restlessness alternating with apathy, and other neurological signs including myoclonic jerks and hyperreflexia. Differential diagnosis can be difficult, and it can be misdiagnosed as delirium tremens. Treatment with thiamine and pyridoxine can aggravate the condition. The condition responds to treatment with nicotinic acid.

Alcohol-related brain damage

The mechanisms underlying alcohol-related brain damage are complex (Zahr et al., 2011). Poor nutrition and diminished vitamin reserves predispose to thiamine and nicotinic acid depletion. Alcohol is neurotoxic, and acetaldehyde, its main metabolite, may have a similar action; thus, liver impairment also contributes to brain damage. Neuroadaptations with reduced GABAergic inhibition and increased glutamatergic excitation result in less neuroplasticity. Metabolic factors resulting from acute and chronic intoxication and withdrawal, such as hypoxia, electrolyte imbalance, and hypoglycaemia, are also important, as are alcohol withdrawal seizures, hepatic encephalopathy, subarachnoid haemorrhage, haemorrhagic stroke, and head injury. Their impact may depend on the brain's state of development: young people who drink excessively are at risk of functional and structural brain damage that may have long-lasting adverse consequences (Hermens et al., 2013).

Many individuals with a history of chronic alcohol misuse have mild to moderate impairment in short- and long-term memory, learning, visuospatial organization, visuoperceptual abstraction, maintenance of cognitive set, and impulse control. Performance on neuropsychological testing improves with abstinence, but some impairment may still be evident even 5 years later. Neuropathological studies have shown that, in comparison with controls, brain weight is significantly reduced in heavy drinkers at autopsy, with selective neuronal loss. With the advent of computed tomography (CT) scanning, cortical shrinkage (particularly in the frontal area) and ventricular enlargement were confirmed in about two-thirds of alcoholics compared with age-matched controls (Lishman, 1998).

Neuroimaging studies with MRI have shown reduced volume in cortical regions, particularly in the frontal lobe in uncomplicated alcoholism (Sullivan & Pfefferbaum, 2005; Zahr et al., 2011). Studies have highlighted damage in the hippocampus (a key area in learning and memory) that appeared related to a history of seizures, with the impact of alcohol increasing with age. Crucially, however, longitudinal studies have shown that abstinence is associated with increased volume in grey and white matter, as well as with improved activity and connectivity between brain regions. This is consistent with improvements seen in cognitive performance.

Cognitive deficits likely represent one possible factor contributing to poor treatment outcome. Therapeutic programmes may be too complex for these individuals to grasp. Clinicians should therefore be familiar with the risk factors and early signs of cognitive impairment in their patients. Simple objective feedback about neuropsychological test results and neuroimaging of the brain may help to motivate the patient to abstinence. Patients with moderate to severe brain damage who appear cognitively intact may not be able to understand the principles of motivational interviewing or cognitive behavioural therapy (see Chapter 13). Their initial needs are more basic and likely to include good nutrition, treatment with parenteral and oral thiamine, and residential placement in a supervised setting. The repetitive structure and routine of Alcoholics Anonymous (AA) is well-suited to those with mild to moderate brain damage. AA, of course, also has within it much complexity, but the cognitively handicapped patient will perhaps be able to focus on the simpler aspects of the AA programme.

Central pontine myelinolysis

This is a rare disorder of cerebral white matter in the brainstem, one that is usually seen in alcohol dependent individuals but that can also occur in malignancy, nonalcoholic liver disease, chronic renal disease, rapid correction of hyponatraemia, hypokalaemia and other debilitating diseases. Clinical features include a pseudobulbar palsy and spastic or flaccid quadriplegia that evolves over a few days or weeks, often resulting in coma or death. Lesions are often picked up on MRI scans. Postmortem examination reveals demyelination of the pons.

Marchiafava–Bignami disease

This rare disorder of the corpus callosum and adjacent white matter is not confined to problem drinkers. A nutritional deficiency or a contaminant of alcohol have been postulated as causes. Presentation can either be acute with agitation, apathy, hallucinations, epilepsy, and coma, or insidious, with dementia, spasticity, dysarthria, and inability to walk. Lesions can be visualized on brains scans, but the diagnosis is usually made only at postmortem. Treatment with thiamine has been shown to improve outcome.

Alcohol amblyopia

This uncommon condition presents as a gradual bilateral blurring of vision in association with alcohol misuse. It can be accompanied by difficulty in distinguishing red from green. Most patients are also smokers. Testing reveals a central blind spot (scotoma), with the peripheral field of vision intact. The most likely cause is a deficiency of both thiamine and vitamin B_{12}. It responds to treatment with thiamine and B-complex vitamins. The same picture sometimes occurs as "tobacco amblyopia."

Hepatic encephalopathy

In heavy drinkers with alcoholic liver disease, the predominant clinical picture can be that of hepatic encephalopathy. This is a chronic organic reaction with psychiatric and neurological abnormalities that come and go and are extremely variable. The typical features include impaired consciousness (ranging from hypersomnia to coma), delirium, impaired recent memory, mood swings, a flapping tremor, muscular incoordination, foetor hepaticus (a characteristic smell on the breath), upgoing plantar responses, and hypo- or hyperactive reflexes (Krige & Beckingham, 2001). Liver function tests are usually abnormal, and an EEG shows a picture that can be extremely helpful in diagnosis (initial slowing of the alpha rhythm, followed by appearance of 5–7 per second theta waves, and later theta activity replacing alpha activity). Hepatic encephalopathy is a sign of deteriorating liver function. It can be precipitated by alcohol withdrawal and benzodiazepine use.

Foetal alcohol spectrum disorders

That the mother's drinking could cause damage to the unborn baby was widely believed in the nineteenth century, but was later to be forgotten or dismissed as temperance scare mongering. It is only over the past four decades or so that firm evidence has accumulated for the reality of the danger, and, even so, there are questions remaining as to the level of maternal drinking that carries risk. There is currently no reliable evidence on the incidence of foetal alcohol spectrum disorders (FASD) in the UK because in England and Scotland data are only collected on foetal alcohol syndrome (FAS), not the full spectrum of disorders (British Medical Association Board of Science, 2007). Records from hospital admissions found 128 cases in 2002/03 in England, with little increase over the next 5 years (unlike the rise seen in other alcohol-related disorders).

In the United States, the incidence estimates for FAS range from 0.5 to 2.0 per 1,000 live births (Abel & Sokol, 1991; British Medical Association Board of Science, 2007). Rates of FASD vary with ethnicity and socioeconomic and medical status, as well as because of stigma, thus resulting in underreporting and underdiagnosis. Nutrition, licit and illicit drug use, and smoking all contribute to variability in studies. Some populations are more likely to have children affected by these disorders, particularly indigenous populations in Australia, the United States, and Canada. A systematic review reported that mothers of FASD children tended to be older and have low educational levels, family members with alcohol abuse, and other children with FASD. They usually received little prenatal care and drank before and during pregnancy, with frequent episodes of binge drinking (Esper & Furtado, 2014).

Diagnostic criteria for FAS are well-established. The fully developed picture includes (1) prenatal and postnatal growth retardation, (2) craniofacial abnormalities of the face and head (a small head, shortened eyelids, underdeveloped upper lip, and flattened wide nose), and (3) central nervous system dysfunction. Associated abnormalities include limb deformities and congenital heart disease. As they mature, these children remain small for their age and often have significant cognitive impairment. Cognitive deficits, together with concentration, attention, and behavioural problems, may handicap education or employment.

The clinical features of partial foetal alcohol syndrome (PFAS), alcohol-related birth defects (ARBD), and alcohol-related neurodevelopmental disorders (ARND) are less well-defined (British Medical Association Board of Science, 2007). Children with PFAS usually have minor facial anomalies, intellectual deficits, hyperactivity with attention deficit, impulsivity, short attention span, and developmental delay. Children with ARND typically have prominent neurocognitive deficits but do not have facial anomalies or growth problems. Children with ARBD are characterized by behavioural problems or structural abnormalities; these children have no facial anomalies (British Medical Association Board of Science, 2007).

Evidence from animal studies indicates that the critical periods of exposure occur during the first and third trimesters in humans. The very early stages of embryogenesis are critical periods for damage to the developing brain and development of craniofacial anomalies. Prenatal alcohol exposure during the third trimester is associated with damage to the cerebellum, hippocampus, and prefrontal cortex (British Medical Association Board of Science, 2007).

The crucial public health question relates to what is meant by "heavy drinking" in this context. It is not known what levels of prenatal alcohol exposure produce what intensity of developmental problems. However, there is no doubt that a woman who is drinking at a level that implies her having developed alcohol dependence is at risk of damaging her baby. Women who drink heavily during pregnancy also have increased rates of complications of pregnancy and delivery, and of spontaneous abortion, preterm delivery, and stillbirth.

For any alcohol treatment service, the practical message must be that a woman of child-bearing age who has a serious drinking problem requires very special counseling and should be discouraged from having a baby until her drinking has been dealt with successfully. One has to think not only of the potential damage to an unborn child, but also of the lifetime emotional effects on the parents.

What is the safe upper limit of drinking for a pregnant woman or a woman intending to have a child? Although there is no robust evidence that a small amount of alcohol consumption is associated with harm to the fetus or mother, neither is there sufficient evidence to determine the threshold for harm. As for other adverse outcomes of alcohol consumption, it may depend on the measures being used, such as neuropsychological or cardiac functioning or birthweight. The British Medical Association report recommends that pregnant women or women considering pregnancy should abstain absolutely from alcohol (British Medical Association Board of Science, 2007). The National Institute for Health and Clinical Excellence (NICE) advises that women should abstain from alcohol completely during the first 3 months of pregnancy due to the risk of miscarriage and, for the rest of the pregnancy, drink only 1–2 units once or twice a week (National Institute for Health and Clinical Excellence, 2008). Binge drinking should be avoided completely. Women trying to conceive are advised to limit their alcohol consumption to no more than 1–2 standard drinks once or twice per week. It might be sensible for them to consider abstinence. The latest advice from both the UK Chief Medical Officer and the US Surgeon General is that pregnant women should abstain from alcohol.

The need for two kinds of alertness

This chapter started with the plea that everyone working with problem drinkers should be more aware of the physical element within the assessment and treatment plan. It should similarly be pleaded that everyone who works in the medical field be vigilant to the possibility of an undeclared drinking problem underlying any one of a host of clinical presentations.

Medical problems sometimes emerge during abstinence, and the clinician should be alert to this reality. When patients finally stop drinking, they often become aware of lingering injuries, pains, tiredness, and a host of other problems. What they perceive as depression may, in fact, be hypothyroidism. The wise clinician will keep a watchful eye on the newly abstinent patient and will not attribute every symptom and sign to alcohol.

References

Abel, E. L., & Sokol, R. J. (1991). A revised conservative estimate of the incidence of FAS and its economic impact. *Alcoholism: Clinical and Experimental Research*, **15**, 514–524.

Babor, T., Caetano, R., Casswell, S., Edwards, G., Giesbrecht, N., Graham, K., … Room, R. (2010). *Alcohol: No ordinary commodity* (2nd ed.). Oxford: Oxford University Press.

Baliunas, D., Rehm, J., Irving, H., & Shuper, P. (2010). Alcohol consumption and risk of incident human immunodeficiency virus infection: A meta-analysis. *International Journal of Public Health*, **55**, 159–166.

Baliunas, D. O., Taylor, B. J., Irving, H., Roerecke, M., Patra, J., Mohapatra, S., & Rehm, J. (2009). Alcohol as a risk factor for type 2 diabetes. *Diabetes Care*, **32**, 2123–2132.

Beilin, L. J., & Puddey, I. B. (2006). Alcohol and hypertension: An update. *Hypertension*, **47**, 1035–1038.

Bofetta, P., & Hashibe, M. (2006). Alcohol and cancer. *Lancet Oncology*, 7, 149–156.

Bråthen, G., Ben-Menachem, E., Brodtkorb, E., Galvin, R., Garcia-Monco, J. C., Halasz, P., ... EFNS Task Force on Diagnosis and Treatment of Alcohol-Related Seizures. (2005). EFNS guideline on the diagnosis and management of alcohol-related seizures: Report of an EFNS task force. *European Journal of Neurology*, **12**, 575–581.

British Medical Association Board of Science. (2007). *Fetal alcohol spectrum disorders – A guide for healthcare professionals*. London: British Medical Association.

British Medical Association Board of Science. (2008). *Alcohol misuse: Tackling the UK epidemic*. London: British Medical Association.

Brock, C., Nielsen, L. M., Lelic, D., & Drewes, A. M. (2013). Pathophysiology of chronic pancreatitis. *World Journal of Gastroenterology*, **19**(42), 7231.

Chen, L., Davey Smith, G., Harbord, R. M., & Lewis, S. J. (2008). Alcohol intake and blood pressure: A systematic review implementing a Mendelian randomization approach. *PLoS Medicine*, **5**(3), e52.

Choi, H. K., Atkinson, K., Karlson, E. W., Willett, W., & Curhan, G. (2004). Alcohol intake and risk of incident gout in men: A prospective study. *Lancet*, **363**, 1277–1281.

Chou, S. P., Grant, B. F., & Dawson, D. A. (1998). Alcoholic beverage preference and risks of alcohol-related medical consequences: A preliminary report from the National Longitudinal Alcohol Epidemiologic Study. *Alcohol: Clinical and Experimental Research*, **22**, 1450–1455.

Cook, C. C., Hallwood, P. M., & Thomson, A. D. (1998). B vitamin deficiency and neuropsychiatric syndromes in alcohol misuse. *Alcohol and Alcoholism*, **33**(4), 317–336.

Cook, R. T. (1998). Alcohol abuse, alcoholism, and damage to the immune system – a review. *Alcoholism: Clinical and Experimental Research*, **22**, 1927–1942.

Corrao, G., Bagnardi, V., Zambon, A., & Arico, S. (1999). Exploring the dose-responsive relationship between alcohol consumption and the risk of several alcohol-related conditions – a meta analysis. *Addiction*, **94**, 1551–1573.

Costanzo, S., Di Castelnuovo, A., Donati, M. B., Iacoviello, L., & de Gaetano, G. (2010). Alcohol consumption and mortality in patients with cardiovascular disease: A meta-analysis. *Journal of the American College of Cardiology*, **55**(13), 1339–1347.

Druesne-Pecollo, N., Tehard, B., Mallet, Y., Gerber, M., Norat, T., Hercberg, S., & Latino-Martel, P. (2009). Alcohol and genetic polymorphisms: Effect on risk of alcohol-related cancer. *Lancet Oncology*, **10**(2), 173–180.

Esper, L. H., & Furtado, E. F. (2014). Identifying maternal risk factors associated with fetal alcohol spectrum disorders: A systematic review. *European Child & Adolescent Psychiatry*, **23**(10), 877–889.

Estruch, R. (2001). Nutrition and infectious disease. In N. Heather, T. J. Peters, & T. Stockwell (Eds.), *International handbook of alcohol problems and dependence* (pp. 185–204). Chichester, UK: John Wiley & Sons.

Franke, A., Teyssen, S., & Singer, M. V. (2005). Alcohol-related diseases of the esophagus and stomach. *Digestive Diseases*, **23**(3–4), 204–213.

Hazeldine, S., & Sheron, N. (2014). Current treatment options for alcohol-related liver disease. *Current Opinion in Gastroenterology*, **30**(3), 238–244.

Hendershot, C. S., Stoner, S. A., Pantalone, D. W., & Simoni, J. M. (2009). Alcohol use and antiretroviral adherence: Review and meta-analysis. *Journal of Acquired Immune Deficiency Syndrome*, **52**, 180–202.

Hermens, D. F., Lagopoulos, J., Tobias-Webb, J., De Regt, T., Dore, G., Juckes, L., ... Hickie, I. B. (2013). Pathways to alcohol-induced brain impairment in young people: A review. *Cortex*, **49**(1), 3–17.

Holmes, M. V., Dale, C. E., Zuccolo, L., Silverwood, R. J., Guo, Y., Ye, Z., ... InterAct Consortium. (2014). Association between alcohol and cardiovascular disease: Mendelian randomisation analysis based on individual participant data. *British Medical Journal*, **349**, g4164.

Hvidtfeldt, U. A., Tolstrup, J. S., Jakobsen, M. U., Heitmann, B. L., Grønbaek, M., O'Reilly, E., … Ascherio, A. (2010). Alcohol intake and risk of coronary heart disease in younger, middle-aged, and older adults. *Circulation*, **121**(14), 1589–1597.

International Agency for Research on Cancer. (1998). *Alcohol drinking*, IARC Monographs on the Evaluation of Carcinogenic Risks to Humans (vol. 44). Lyon, France: International Agency for Research on Cancer.

Klatsky, A. L., Armstrong, M. A., Friedman, G. D., & Sidney, S. (2001). Alcohol drinking and risk of hospitalization for ischemic stroke. *American Journal of Cardiology*, **88**(6), 703–706.

Kopelman, M. D., Thomson, A. D., Guerrini, I., & Marshall, E. J. (2009). The Korsakoff syndrome: Clinical aspects, psychology and treatment. *Alcohol and Alcoholism*, **44**(2), 148–154.

Krige, J. E. J., & Beckingham, I. J. (2001). ABC of diseases of liver, pancreas, and biliary system: Portal hypertension – 2. Ascites, encephalopathy, and other conditions. *British Medical Journal*, **322**(7283), 416.

Lamminpaa, A. (1995). Alcohol intoxication in childhood and adolescence. *Alcohol and Alcoholism*, **30**, 5–12.

Lieber, C. S. (1988). The influence of alcohol on nutritional status. *Nutrition Review*, **46**, 241–254.

Lishman, W. A. (1981). Cerebral disorders in alcoholism. *Brain*, **104**, 1–20.

Lishman, W. A. (1998). *Organic psychiatry: The psychological consequences of cerebral disorder*, 3rd ed. Oxford: Blackwell Scientific Publications.

Lucey, M. R. (2014). Liver transplantation for alcoholic liver disease. *Nature Reviews Gastroenterology & Hepatology*, **11**(5), 300–307.

McLeod, R., Stockwell, T., Stevens, M., & Phillips, M. (1999). The relationship between alcohol consumption patterns and injury. *Addiction*, **94**, 1719–1734.

Mukamal, K. J., Chung, H., Jenny, N. S., Kuller, L. H., Longstreth, W. T., Mittleman, M. A., … Siscovick, D. S. (2005b). Alcohol use and risk of ischaemic stroke among older adults: The cardiovascular health study. *Stroke*, **36**, 1830–1834.

Mukamal, K. J., Tolstrup, J. S., Friberg, J., Jensen, G., & Grønbaek, M. (2005a). Alcohol consumption and risk of atrial fibrillation in men and women: The Copenhagen City Heart Study. *Circulation*, **112**, 1736–1742.

Murray, C. J. L, Vos, T., Lozano, R., Naghavi, M., Flaxman, A. D., Michaud, C., … Memish, Z. A. (2012). Disability-adjusted life years (DALYs) for 291 diseases and injuries in 21 regions, 1990–2010: A systematic analysis for the Global Burden of Disease Study 2010. *Lancet*, **380**(9859), 2197–2223.

National Institute for Health and Clinical Excellence. (2008). National Collaborating Centre for Women's and Children's Health. *Antenatal care: Routine care for the healthy pregnant woman*, 2nd ed. London: RCOG Press.

O'Keefe, J. H., Bhatti, S. K., Bajwa, A., DiNicolantonio, & Lavie, C. J. (2014, March). Alcohol and cardiovascular health: The dose makes the poison … or the remedy. *Mayo Clinic Proceedings*, **89**(3), 382–393.

Preedy, V. R., Mantle, D., & Peters, T. J. (2001). Alcoholic muscle, skin and bone disease. In N. Heather, T. J. Peters, & T. Stockwell (Eds.), *International handbook of alcohol problems and dependence* (pp. 169–184). Chichester, UK: John Wiley & Sons.

Ramayya, A., & Jauhar, P. (1997). Increasing incidence of Korsakoff's psychosis in the east end of Glasgow. *Alcohol and Alcoholism*, **32**, 281–285.

Rehm, J., Room, R., Monteiro, M., Gmel, G., Graham, K., Rehn, N., … Jernigan, D. (2004). Alcohol use. In M. Ezzati, A. D. Lopez, A. Rodgers, & C. J. L. Murray (Eds.), *Comparative quantification of health risks: Global and regional burden of disease due to selected major risk factors* (vol. **1**., pp. 959–1109). Geneva: World Health Organization

Room, R., Babor, T., & Rehm, J. (2005). Alcohol and public health. *Lancet*, **65**, 519–530.

Rubin, E., & Urbano-Marquez, A. (1994). Alcoholic cardiomyopathy. *Alcoholism: Clinical and Experimental Research*, **18**, 111–114.

Stewart, S., Latham, P. K., Miller, P. M., Randall, P., & Anton, R. E. (2008). Blood pressure reduction during treatment for alcohol dependence: Results from the Combining Medications and Behavioural Interventions for Alcoholism (COMBINE) study. *Addiction*, **103**, 1622–1628.

Sullivan, E. V., & Pfefferbaum, A. (2005). Neurocircuitry in alcoholism: A substrate of disruption and repair. *Psychopharmacology*, **180**(4), 583–594.

Thomson, A. D., Cook, C. C. H., Guerrini, I., Sheedy, D., Harper, C., & Marshall, E. J. (2008). Wernicke's encephalopathy: "Plus ca change, plus c'est la meme chose." *Alcohol and Alcoholism*, **43**, 180–186.

Thomson, A. D., & Marshall, E. J. (2006). The natural history of Wernicke's encephalopathy and Korsakoff 's psychosis. *Alcohol and Alcoholism*, **41**, 151–158.

Thompson, P. L. (2013). J-curve revisited: Cardiovascular benefits of moderate alcohol use cannot be dismissed. *Medical Journal of Australia*, **198**(8), 419–422.

Tønnesen, H. (1999). The alcohol patient and surgery. *Alcohol and Alcoholism*, **34**, 148–152.

Tønnesen, H., Rosenberg, J., Nielsen, H. J., Rasmussen, V., Hauge, C., Pedersen, I. K., & Kehlet, H. (1999). Effect of preoperative abstinence on poor postoperative outcome in alcohol misusers: Randomised controlled trial. *British Medical Journal*, **318**, 1311–1316.

Urbano-Marquez, A., Estruch, R., Fernandez-Sola, J., Nicolas, J. M., Pare, J. C., & Rubin, E. (1995). The greater risk of alcoholic cardiomyopathy and myopathy in women compared with men. *Journal of the American Medical Association*, **274**, 149–154.

Victor, M., Adams, R. D., & Collins, G. H. (1971). *The Wernicke-Korsakoff syndrome*. Philadelphia, PA: F. A. Davis.

Walker, R. K., Cousins, V. M., Umoh, N. A., Jeffress, M. A., Taghipour, D., Al-Rubaiee, M., & Haddad, G. E. (2013). The good, the bad, and the ugly with alcohol use and abuse on the heart. *Alcoholism: Clinical and Experimental Research*, **37**(8), 1253–1260.

Whiteford, H. A., Degenhardt, L., Rehm, J., Baxter, A. J., Ferrari, A. J., Erskine, H. E., ... Vos, T. (2013). Global burden of disease attributable to mental and substance use disorders: Findings from the Global Burden of Disease Study 2010. *Lancet*, **382**(9904), 1575–1586.

Williams, R., Aspinall, R., Bellis, M., Camps-Walsh, G., Cramp, M., Dhawan, A., ... Smith, T. (2014). Addressing liver disease in the UK: A blueprint for attaining excellence in health care and reducing premature mortality from lifestyle issues of excess consumption of alcohol, obesity, and viral hepatitis. *Lancet*, **384**, 1953–1997.

World Cancer Research Fund/American Institute for Cancer Research. (2007). *Food, nutrition, physical activity, and the prevention of cancer: A global perspective*. Washington DC: American Institute for Cancer Research.

World Health Organization. (2007). *WHO Expert Committee on Problems Related to Alcohol Consumption. Second Report*. WHO Technical Report Series 944. Geneva: World Health Organization.

World Health Organization. (2011). *Global status report on alcohol and health*. Geneva, Switzerland: World Health Organization.

Xin, X., He, J., Frontini, M. G., Motsamai, O.I., & Whelton, P.K. (2001). Effects of alcohol reduction on blood pressure: A meta-analysis of randomized controlled trials. *Hypertension*, **38**(5), 1112–1117.

Zahr, N. M., Kaufman, K. L., & Harper, C. G. (2011). Clinical and pathological features of alcohol-related brain damage. *Nature Reviews Neurology*, 7, 284–294.

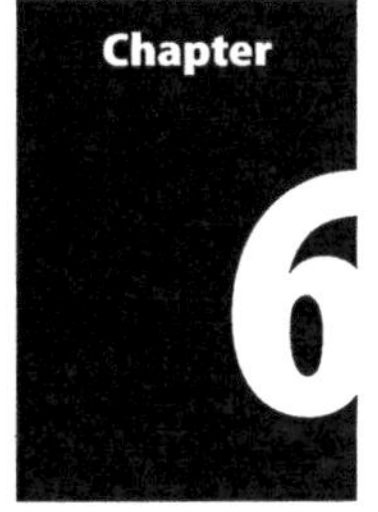

Chapter 6 Drinking problems and psychiatric disorders

Anyone working in the field of drinking problems must cultivate an awareness of the range of psychiatric disorders that may result from or lie behind the drinking. Very serious issues will otherwise be overlooked. Similarly, a lack of appreciation about the impact of alcohol and other substances on mental state may also result in substance misuse being ignored. Psychiatric disorders occur more commonly in individuals with drinking problems (and other substance use disorders [SUDs]) than in the general population. Although the term "dually diagnosed" is sometimes used to describe such individuals, they often have multiple problems; for example, alcohol and drug misuse, one or more psychiatric disorders, and physical health, behavioural, forensic, and social problems.

The aetiology of comorbidity is most likely to be multifactorial and due to an interaction between biological, psychosocial, environmental, and personality factors. Many psychiatric symptoms experienced by problem-drinking individuals are directly related to intoxication and/or withdrawal and will disappear with extended abstinence. At the same time, heavy alcohol consumption and dependence can also put individuals at increased risk for developing a psychiatric disorder (e.g., major depression) that persists even if abstinence is attained. In the same fashion, individuals with psychiatric disorders may be vulnerable to developing an alcohol or drug use disorder that has a life of its own. Drinking problems and psychiatric disorders may also co-occur independently. Comorbidity complicates treatment and prognosis and poses significant challenges to mental health services as well as primary care services. Clinicians are best able to meet these challenges when they focus on assessing the needs and problems of the patient rather than focusing solely on the diagnostic category(ies) into which they have been classified.

Clinical samples have higher prevalence rates of comorbidity than community samples because the presence of the comorbid disorder increases the likelihood of help-seeking. Indeed, comorbid individuals may seek help for a psychiatric symptom or disorder rather than their alcohol problems. They may not acknowledge or even realize that their alcohol consumption is contributing to their difficulties.

Epidemiology

The U.S. National Comorbidity Survey (Table 6.1) indicated that individuals with a lifetime history of an alcohol use disorder (AUD) have a higher risk of a mental health disorder and vice versa (Kessler, Crum, & Warner, 1997; Kessler et al., 1994). The 10-year follow-up of this study revealed that mood disorders and many anxiety disorders (panic, specific and social phobia, post-traumatic stress disorder [PTSD], separation anxiety) were predictive of developing subsequent substance dependence, with a particularly strong association with

Table 6.1. The U.S. National Co-morbidity Survey: The lifetime co-occurrence of psychiatric disorders with alcohol dependence versus those without

	Individuals with Alcohol Dependence			
	Men		*Women*	
Psychiatric Disorder	**(%)**	**OR**	**(%)**	**OR**
Anxiety	35.8	2.2	60.7	3.1
Mood	28.1	3.2	53.5	4.4
Drug dependence	29.5	9.8	34.7	15.8
Antisocial personality	16.9	8.3	7.8	17.0

Source: Kessler, Crum, & Warner (1997).

bipolar disorder (Swendsen et al., 2010). Notably, these psychiatric disorders had negligible to moderate impact on the risk of starting drinking or of "alcohol abuse" (in the nomenclature of the American Psychiatric Association's *Diagnostic and Statistical Manual of Mental Disorders* [DSM-IV]), but did increase the likelihood of a problem-drinking individual transitioning into alcohol dependence.

The evidence for lifetime comorbidity was stronger for alcohol dependence than for alcohol abuse, and comorbidity was more likely to occur in women than in men. The predominant comorbid disorders among men were other substance use disorders, conduct disorder, and antisocial personality disorder. Anxiety and affective disorders were the main contributors to comorbidity in women. The National Epidemiologic Survey on Alcohol Problems and Related Conditions (NESARC) in the United States found that, among individuals with AUDs (alcohol abuse and dependence) seeking treatment, 40.7 percent had at least one recurrent independent mood disorder and 33 percent had at least one current independent anxiety disorder (Grant et al., 2004). NESARC also revealed that transition from abuse to dependence occurs in 26.6 percent of individuals with alcohol abuse, mostly within about 3 years. Similar to the National Comorbidity Survey findings, NESARC data showed that a history of any mood, psychotic, or personality disorder showed an increased risk of transition to dependence on alcohol.

As the proportion of older people grows in the population, it becomes increasingly important to understand problem drinking and comorbidity among the elderly. Findings in younger adults may not generalize to older adults. For example, in NESARC participants aged 60 or older, substance use disorders did not predict incident mood or anxiety disorders, unlike for whole sample (Hasin & Kilcoyne, 2012). Researchers have less information on substance misuse and psychiatric disorders in late life than would be optimal. The National Comorbidity Survey, for instance, did not enroll older adults. Alcohol appears to be the main substance misused in mid to late life, with increasing use of prescribed opioids and benzodiazepines often co-occurring (Crome et al., 2011; Wu & Blazer, 2014).

There are gender differences in comorbidity patterns. Alcohol dependent women are at higher risk than alcohol dependent men for most externalizing disorders. On average,

Table 6.2. Prevalence of psychiatric disorder types among nondependent and nicotine-, alcohol-, and drug-dependent populations

	Nondependent population (%)	Nicotine-dependent population (%)	Alcohol-dependent population (%)	Drug-dependent population (%)
No disorder	87.5	77.0	69.4	52.9
Mixed anxiety disorder	6.2	10.2	9.9	16.3
Generalized anxiety disorder	2.4	4.1	5.3	7.3
Depression	1.2	3.7	7.3	9.1
Phobia	0.8	1.5	1.0	5.4
Panic disorder	0.5	1.5	2.7	2.5

Adapted from: Farrell et al. (2003).

alcohol dependence remits earlier in women despite lower treatment utilization than men (Khan et al., 2013).

Psychiatric comorbidity also affects whether individuals attempt to quit drinking and whether they succeed. In the NESARC study, about 10 percent of those with alcohol abuse and 18 percent with alcohol dependence tried to quit in a 3-year period (Chiappetta, García-Rodríguez, Jin, Secades-Villa, & Blanco, 2014). Of these individuals, about a third were successful. Quit attempts were more likely in those who were single, younger than 40 years, of low income, and who had a co-occurring psychiatric disorder and greater number of dependence symptoms. A greater severity of dependence, a greater number of psychiatric disorders, and a substance use disorder (including tobacco use disorder) decreased the likelihood of a quit attempt being successful.

Epidemiological studies conducted outside the United States generated results similar to NESARC and the National Comorbidity Survey. The British Psychiatric Morbidity Survey (Farrell et al., 2001) showed that individuals with nicotine, alcohol, and drug dependence had an increased risk of psychiatric morbidity compared with the nondependent population (Table 6.2). Most users of drug and alcohol services also experience mental health problems. In Australia, 18 percent of those with an AUD had an affective disorder, 15 percent had an anxiety disorder, and 17 percent had another drug use disorder (DUD). Looked at from the other direction, 16 percent of those with depression, 24 percent with PTSD, and 37 percent of those with a cannabis use disorder had an AUD (Burns, Teeson, & Lysnkey, 2001).

There are two broad categories of co-occurring psychiatric problems: (1) alcohol-induced disorders such as hallucinations, delirium, and delusions; and (2) common comorbid diagnoses such as depression, anxiety disorders, and the like. These will be discussed in turn. This section of the book should be considered a supplement to some of the material presented in Chapter 5 (e.g., regarding Wernicke–Korsakoff syndrome).

Alcohol-induced disorders

Transient hallucinatory experience

Transient hallucinatory experience deserves note for two reasons. First, it may herald the onset of delirium tremens (DTs) or alcoholic hallucinosis, and it can often give early warning of the likelihood of these much more serious illnesses. It may therefore be viewed as continuous with those states, rather than an altogether discrete clinical entity. Second, it is important to be aware that transient hallucinations may occur without the illness progressing to either of the major presentations. The diagnostician who is unfamiliar with these transient phenomena may be tempted to record incorrectly that the patient has "suffered from DTs" when this was not the case. Whether other drug use could have contributed should also be carefully assessed.

The essence of this condition is that the patient fleetingly and suddenly experiences any one of a variety of perceptual disturbances, often very much to their surprise and consternation, and with the episode then immediately over. These occurrences may be experienced during periods of continued, heavy, and chaotic dependent drinking or during withdrawal. There is no delirium or evidence of severe physiological disturbance as seen in DTs. Here are some examples of how patients described such experiences:

> I would be walking down the road and, ZOOM, a car would come up behind me and I'd jump on the pavement. Frightened out of my life. But it was all imagination.

> What used to happen was that I would turn around thinking someone had called my name.

The degree of insight is often characteristic; the patient immediately disconfirms the reality of the hallucination. A relatively stereotyped and limited kind of hallucinatory experience is also typical; for one patient, it is nearly always the car coming up from behind, for another a pigeon flying into the room. It is important to realize that some patients can experience such discomforting happenings for many months without progressing to a major disturbance. The meaning and significance of "continuity" will immediately become clear as we go on to discuss DTs and alcoholic hallucinosis.

Delirium tremens

DTs is a short-lived toxic confusional state that usually occurs as a result of reduced alcohol intake in alcohol dependent individuals with a long history of use (World Health Organization, 1992). It can produce a range of clinical pictures, but it is best viewed as a unitary syndrome with a continuum of severities and a variation in symptom clustering. The disturbance is often fluctuating, with the patient's condition worsening in the evening or when the room is unlit and shadowy. The classical triad of symptoms includes clouding of consciousness and confusion, vivid hallucinations affecting any sensory modality, and marked tremor. Delusions, agitation, sleeplessness, and autonomic arousal are frequently also present.

Symptoms of delirium usually occur from about 24–150 hours after the last drink although typically peaking between 72 and 96 hours. Prodromal symptoms are usually evident but may be overlooked. The onset is often at night with restlessness, insomnia and fear:

A 65-year-old widower was admitted to a general hospital via ambulance following a period of heavy drinking. On admission, he was written up for one dose of chlordiazepoxide (25 mg orally). A reducing dose was not commenced, even though the nursing and medical staff were aware that he had an alcohol problem. During the first 2 days of admission he was "pleasantly confused." On the third day, he went into the nursing office where he saw a nurse "organizing patients into groups." He suddenly realized that this meant everyone had to be evacuated because of a bomb scare. He left the ward in his pyjamas and bare feet and walked out of the hospital into a busy street, shouting that the hospital was in danger. He was duly found, returned, and reassured by nursing staff. Ten days later, he had a hazy recall of the event: "I knew it wasn't true, and yet I experienced a mounting and inexplicable fear and felt that I had to escape. Since then nothing extraordinary has happened."

Delirium

In delirium, the patient is more or less out of contact with reality and potentially disoriented as to person, place, and time. For instance, the patient may believe that they are cruising on a liner, mistake the nurse for a steward, and order a drink, but 5 minutes later, the patient knows that they are in a hospital and can correctly identify the people around them.

Hallucinations

Hallucinations are characteristically vivid, chaotic, and bizarre and occur in any sensory modality – the patient may see visions, hear things, smell gases, or feel animals crawling over them. The classical visual hallucinations are vivid and horrifying and typically include snakes, insects, rats, and other small animals that may appear to attack the patient as they lie in bed. They may also take a "microscopic" form (small furry men dancing on the floor), but any type of visual hallucination can occur. Patients often become completely preoccupied by and interact with the hallucinated objects. Thus, they brush away the spiders or argue with the little men.

Hallucinatory voices or bursts of music may be heard, or the threatening screams of animals. Hallucinations are often based on a ready tendency to illusional misrepresentation: the wrinkles in the bedclothes become snakes, patterns in the wallpaper become faces.

Tremor

As the illness develops, the patient becomes anxious and more fearful and develops tremor. At worst, the patient may shake so severely that the bed rattles, but, as with other symptoms, there can be a continuum of severity, and the tremor may not be very noticeable unless the patient is asked to stretch out their hands.

Fear

The patient may experience extremes of horror in reaction, for instance, to the snakes writhing all over their bed. But fearful reactions are not universal: on other occasions, the hallucinations may be enjoyable or entertaining, as if the patient is happily watching a private cinema show.

Paranoid delusions

The illness often has a degree of paranoid flavouring: enemies are blowing poisonous gas into the room, assassins lurk at the window, and there is a nameless conspiracy afoot. The mood can in fact be paranoid, with every happening and stimulus being misrepresented as it comes along, but the patient's mental state is too muddled for the delusional ideas to become systematized.

Occupational delusions or hallucinations

The barman, for instance, may believe that he is serving in his cocktail bar and pour out imaginary drinks. The bricklayer may be building an imaginary wall.

Restlessness and agitation

Partly as a consequence of the fearfulness of the hallucinatory experiences, the patient is often highly restless, clutching and pulling at the bedclothes, starting at any sound, or attempting to jump out of bed and run down the ward. This overactivity, when combined with a degree of weakness and unsteadiness, can put the patient seriously at risk of falls and other accidents.

Heightened suggestibility

The patient who is suffering from DTs can show a heightened susceptibility to suggestion, which occasionally becomes evident spontaneously but may only come out on testing. The older textbooks often mention such stories as the patient agreeing to deal from an imaginary pack of cards or "drinking" from a proffered empty glass.

Physical disturbances

Heavy sweating is typical. Appetite is usually lacking, the pulse is rapid, the blood pressure is likely to be raised, and the patient feverish. If the illness continues over many days, the picture gradually becomes that of dehydration, exhaustion, and collapse, with the possibility of a sudden and disastrously steep rise in temperature.

Aetiology and course

DTs is today generally viewed as essentially an alcohol withdrawal state, even though other factors, such as infection or trauma, sometimes play an ancillary role. The withdrawal state precipitating the attack may have been occasioned by admission to hospital, arrest and incarceration, or a self-determined effort to give up drinking. Often, though, there is no history of abrupt withdrawal, and the illness starts while the patient is still drinking, although there has probably been at least partial withdrawal. In some instances, the patient seems to have hovered on the brink of DTs for many preceding weeks, with much evidence of transient hallucinatory experience; in other instances, the illness has a more explosive onset. It is unusual for a patient to experience DTs without a history of at least several years of severe alcohol dependence and many years of excessive drinking, but an attack may occur even after 1 or 2 weeks if a previously abstinent patient rapidly reinstates dependence. Recurrent attacks are common once a patient has had one such episode.

The condition usually lasts for 3–5 days, with gradual resolution. On rare occasions, the illness drags on for some weeks, fluctuating between recovery and relapse. The possibility of severe physical complications has been mentioned, and, before the advent of antibiotics, intercurrent chest infection or pneumonia constituted serious risks. Reported mortality rates have varied from centre to centre and even with skilled care a degree of risk remains, with death occurring in 1–4 percent of hospitalized patients (Schuckit, 2014). Death is typically due to cardiovascular collapse, hypothermia, or intercurrent infection.

Possibilities of diagnostic confusion

DTs may seem so vivid and distinct as to make diagnostic mistakes unlikely. But there is always the possibility that an underlying condition, which is contributing to the picture, is being overlooked. Liver failure, pneumonia, and head injury should always be borne in mind. Confusion may also occur when the possibility of DTs is entirely overlooked, although in retrospect the diagnosis was plainly evident. This is often the case in the setting of a general hospital ward, where the patient is noted to be suffering from "confusion," to be "rambling a bit," or trying to get out of bed at night. In this situation, the condition may be put down to the nonspecific effects of infection, trauma, or an operation. The diagnosis is at times overlooked in the psychiatric hospital setting when it may be misdiagnosed as an "acute schizophrenic reaction"; for instance, when the acutely disturbed person with DTs has florid paranoid ideas, is found running up the street with a knife in their hand, and presents as an emergency admission from the police.

The following predict DTs during alcohol withdrawal: scores above 15 on the Clinical Institute Withdrawal Assessment for Alcohol Scale (CIWA)-Ar scale (see Chapter 11), particularly in association with cardiovascular disturbance (systolic blood pressure >150 mm Hg, pulse rate >100 beats per minute), recent withdrawal seizures (seen in 20 percent of individuals with delirium), prior withdrawal delirium or seizures, older age, recent misuse of other depressant agents, and concomitant medical problems (Schuckit, 2014).

In addition, patients may describe having had DTs but on closer questioning describe only "real bad shakes and sweats." It is therefore important to clarify their understanding of DTs.

The treatment of DTs is outlined in Chapter 11.

Alcohol-induced psychotic disorder

Alcohol-induced psychotic disorder, which includes alcoholic hallucinosis, is a comparatively rare disorder with auditory or visual hallucinations occurring either during or after a period of heavy alcohol consumption (Glass, 1989*a*, 1989*b*; Tsuang, Irwin, Smith, & Schuckit, 1994). The hallucinations are vivid, of acute onset, and typically occur in the setting of clear consciousness, which makes them different from DTs. They may be accompanied by misidentifications, delusions, ideas of reference, and an abnormal affect. Alcohol-induced psychotic disorder typically resolves over a period of weeks but can occasionally persist for months. DTs and other psychotic disorders (including those related to other psychoactive substances) must be ruled out before a diagnosis of alcohol-induced psychotic disorder can be made.

In alcohol-induced psychotic disorder, the auditory hallucinations may consist of unformed noises or snatches of music but usually take the form of voices. These voices may be talking to the patient directly, but more often they take the form of a running commentary about the patient. Sometimes there is only one voice, but often several engage in discussion, and the same voice may come back again on different occasions. The commentary may be favourable and friendly but is usually accusatory, threatening, or involves jealousy. Sometimes the voices command the patient to do things against their will, and this may result in acting-out behaviour or a suicide attempt. There is a lack of insight, and the voices are considered as real, but the patient will seldom elaborate any complex explanation as to the supposed mechanism by which the voices are reaching them. The voices may come and go or haunt the patient more or less incessantly.

Alcohol-induced psychotic disorder is almost certainly not a form of latent schizophrenia. Nevertheless, it may superficially resemble acute paranoid schizophrenia, and the differential diagnosis may be difficult. The delusions associated with alcohol-induced psychotic disorder are usually attempts to explain the hallucinations. There is no evidence of a complicated delusional system, thought disorder, incongruity of affect, or negative symptoms, and insight is regained as the voices diminish (Lishman, 1998).

Although these guidelines provide useful indications, in practice, it can still be difficult to make the distinction, and, in such circumstances, the sensible course of action is to admit the patient to the hospital, withdraw the patient from alcohol, and observe what happens. Remission may take place abruptly, but more often there is a slow fading of the symptoms. The voices become less persistent, do not make such an urgent demand on attention, and their reality begins to be doubted. Prognosis is generally good, but 10–20 percent may have a chronic schizophrenic-like course. The possibility that the illness will finally declare itself to be schizophrenia has, of course, also to be borne in mind. If symptoms have not ceased within a couple of months, the latter diagnosis becomes more likely, although it has been reported that alcohol-induced psychotic disorder may sometimes require up to 6 months for complete recovery. Some drug intoxications, including most notably amphetamine psychosis, can also result in a picture mimicking alcohol-induced psychotic disorder; with a presentation of this sort, it is always wise to carry out urine testing for drugs.

Alcoholic blackouts (alcohol-induced amnestic episodes)

The widely used but somewhat confusing lay term "alcoholic blackout" refers to transient memory loss that may be induced by intoxication (i.e., alcohol-related amnesia). There is no associated loss of consciousness. As described, the blackout may be related to a hyperglutamatergic state (see Chapter 2) and therefore may indicate the severity of impact that alcohol is having on brain function. Indeed, it may be thought of as the brain's equivalent of liver function tests. Clinicians should not enquire simply whether the patient has had a blackout and leave it at that. It is preferable to ask "Have you ever forgotten things you did while drinking?" Although such occurrences are reported in some two-thirds or more of alcohol dependent individuals, alcoholic memory blackouts are also relatively common in social drinkers after drinking too much, too fast. Approximately one-third of young men in the general population are likely to have experienced memory blackouts (Goodwin, Crane, & Guze, 1969*a*). Thus, although blackouts are an important warning sign of problem drinking, they are not necessarily pathognomonic of alcohol dependence.

Blackouts have been described as being of two types (Goodwin, Crane, & Guze, 1969*a*, 1969*b*). The en bloc variety is characterized by a dense and total amnesia with abrupt points of onset and recovery and with no subsequent recall of events for the amnesic period, either spontaneously or with prompting. This period may extend from 30 to 60 minutes up to as long as 2 or 3 days. In contrast, "fragmentary" blackouts or "greyouts" are patchy episodes of amnesia, with indistinct boundaries and islands of memory within these boundaries. They are often characterized by partial or complete subsequent recall and usually extend over a shorter period than the en bloc variety. In reality, alcoholic memory blackouts can occur with every degree of gradation, and although it is useful to recognize the two types, the experience of each patient has to be described separately.

Blackouts may begin to occur at a late stage in a career of excessive drinking or never at all. Once they start to be experienced with any frequency, they tend to recur, and a patient may often be able to identify the phase at which they "began to get bad blackouts." The reason for such varied susceptibility to the disorder is unknown, but blackouts are associated with an early onset of drinking, high peak levels of alcohol, and a history of head injury. Concurrent use of sedatives and hypnotics may increase the likelihood of amnesia. Blackouts are not predictive of long-term cognitive impairment.

During an alcoholic blackout, the individual can engage in any type of activity. To the observer, the drinker will not obviously be in an abnormal state of mind (other than being intoxicated), although a spouse or someone else who knows them well may claim to recognize subtle changes – for instance, "they get that glazed look." Patients sometimes report that during an alcohol blackout period they wandered away from home, later "waking up" in a strange place. Here is an example:

> When I came round I was sitting in a barber's chair having a shave. Hadn't a clue where I'd got to this time, terribly embarrassed, didn't like to ask. I had to go outside and look at the shop signs until I found the answer, and then to my amazement I discovered I was in this town 150 miles from home. To this day, I don't know how I got there. That was the worst experience of this kind, but time after time I woke up in strange places or found myself sitting on a train going to the coast.

Blackouts and their significance to the patient

One patient may mention blackouts only on direct questioning and appear untroubled about such experiences, whereas another patient may deem blackouts a leading reason for seeking help. Blackouts for that type of patient are often a matter of dread with, for instance, recurrent anguished fear that they may have hurt or killed someone while driving home; they do not remember getting their car into the garage the previous night, and they go out in the morning fearfully to check the paint work.

Alcohol-related brain damage and cognitive impairment

The question often arises as to whether the patient with a drinking problem is suffering from "brain damage" or cognitive impairment. In some individuals, it is immediately apparent that they are having difficulty giving accurate information about themselves and their drinking history. It is then important to determine if any impairment is due to Wernicke's encephalopathy, which is a medical emergency requiring immediate treatment, or is due instead to acute effects of alcohol consumption:

> A 53-year-old man comes into a drop-in session at the local alcohol treatment centre on and off over a number of weeks. Although he sees his drinking as "a bit heavy," he is not particularly interested in stopping. Nevertheless, his support worker helps him make some reductions in his drinking although it is obvious that his main motivation for attending is to get help with filling in application forms for better-quality housing. Over the weeks, his support worker concludes that the man has poor reading and writing skills and attributed him forgetting their previous conversations to his current drinking. However, on one occasion, the man attended confused, unsteady on his feet, and not smelling of alcohol. A medical assessment confirmed Wernicke's encephalopathy, and a medical admission was arranged for treatment with intravenous thiamine.

A familiar scenario, however, is that of alcohol-related brain damage (ARBD) and is discussed more fully in Chapter 5 in relation to the physical damages that can result from drinking. Much the same sort of picture is seen when the patient is developing a dementia for any other reason (presenile dementia, for instance, or senile or multi-infarct dementia). The patient with ARBD will typically give a history of many years of heavy drinking with ultimate development of brain damage. With dementia due to other causes, the sequence of events is the other way round: the patient develops dementia and, as a result of the ensuing disinhibition and personality deterioration, becomes involved in drinking.

The fact that brain damage can be a cause as well as a consequence of drinking needs to be written into any diagnostic checklist. In addition to brain damage due to degenerative processes such as those already mentioned, the significance of a history of brain injury deserve particular attention. Instances occur when personality change as a sequel to head injury is disproportionate to any fall-off in intellectual functioning, and this type of personality change may, for instance, result in drinking problems as a late sequel of a road accident. The following brief case extracts show some of the many possible organic relationships that should be on that checklist:

> A 48-year-old career civil servant of previously unblemished record suffered a subarachnoid haemorrhage (a bleed into the space around the brain). The leaking blood vessel was operated on, and she felt she had "recovered completely." But she had, in fact, sustained a degree of brain damage. Work habits, which had for a lifetime been almost overmeticulous, now deteriorated, and she was found to be drinking secretly in the office.

> A divorced woman of 60 presented with alcohol dependence, seemingly of recent onset. Over the past few months, friends had also noticed that she seemed increasingly unhappy and irritable but put this down to her son and family moving away. They realized something was wrong when, on a night out, she acted out-of-character by being very flirtatious with the waiter and attempted to grab him. She was found to have a brain tumour.

Some of these case histories illustrate only rather rare associations, and the precise part that brain damage played in the aetiology of the drinking is in some instances difficult to establish. However, the general picture, which is being built up by listing these diverse cases, is valid and important. Some associations between brain damage and alcohol dependence are relatively common (personality deterioration following head injury, for example), whereas others, such as tumour, are rare; the general message has to be stressed that no diagnostic assessment is complete without thinking about the possible significance of brain involvement. Alcohol dependence can also supervene as a complication of learning disability of any origin.

Whatever the underlying brain syndrome associated with alcohol dependence, the clinical features can be grouped under a number of headings. There are, of course, first the primary symptoms of the brain damage itself. Features of the drinking problem will also stand in their own right, but it is the interaction of the underlying brain damage and the drinking that gives these cases their colouring. Personal and social deterioration may seem to be disproportionate to the drinking or suddenly to have accelerated. Drunken behaviour when there is underlying brain damage often appears to be particularly heedless of consequences or antisocial. There may be increasing episodes of violence, or the patient sets their lodgings on fire. There is also an increased sensitivity to alcohol; the patient gets drunk on less drink, and, with relatively little alcohol, becomes disinhibited or begins to fall about.

Given proper alertness to the possibility of such underlying problems, what, then, are the practical implications? If involvement of an underlying brain condition is in any way suspected, appropriate neurological and psychological investigations need to be carried out with a sober patient, which may require hospital admission. The sad fact is that most of the possibly relevant brain conditions are going to prove more diagnosable than treatable. Even so, an accurate diagnostic formulation is the necessary basis for working out what is best to be done. If, for instance, an individual with alcohol dependence is severely cognitively impaired, the only kind and safe policy may be to propose care in a supportive residential community. If there is milder impairment, the patient will be able to keep going outside an institution, but they may be more likely to drink alcohol, and further troubles are probably to be expected. The continuing treatment plan must be set up to meet these sorts of eventualities and be designed to support the family in what may well be a difficult situation. The emphasis may sometimes have to be placed on directive intervention, such as ensuring that money is properly handled or that local pub owners will not serve the person drinks. But, even here, there is no cause for absolute pessimism because sometimes a patient with significant cognitive impairment will be able to stop drinking, the progression of such damage will be arrested, and the patient's behaviour will improve.

Comorbid psychiatric disorders

A number of comorbid disorders are considered here: depressive disorder, suicide, bipolar disorder, anxiety disorder, PTSD, personality disorder, eating disorders, attention deficit hyperactivity disorder (ADHD), and psychosis. In this section, the emphasis will be on clinical presentation; treatment will be described in Chapter 13. Alcohol services should be in a position to assess psychiatric comorbidity, particularly mood and anxiety, and provide or signpost individuals to appropriate treatment depending on their severity. Specialist alcohol services will usually be in a position to offer treatment or to work in a coordinated way with other specialist services. Clinicians should be mindful that many studies and trials of alcohol dependence do not include patients with comorbidity, and evidence from such studies may not adequately inform the management of dually diagnosed patients (Humphreys, Weingardt, Horst, Joshi, & Finney, 2005).

Depression

Depression, or at least depressive symptoms, are common among individuals with drinking problems and may be the decisive factor in seeking treatment. However, the nature of the relationship between the two is still poorly understood. What seems on the surface to be a simple association is in fact extremely complex. Part of the problem is a lack of clarity in terminology. The word "depression" has a variety of meanings, and a distinction has to be made between the experience of feeling depressed and depressive illness.

Depression as a psychiatric illness must be distinguished from feelings of sadness and unhappiness that can occur as a normal reaction to adversity. The essential feature of a depressive episode is a period of at least 2 weeks during which there is depressed mood and loss of interest or pleasure in nearly all activities. The mood disturbance is often worse at a particular time of day, usually the morning. Loss of energy, fatigue, and diminished activity are common, as is marked tiredness after slight effort. Other symptoms include reduced concentration and attention, reduced self-esteem and self-confidence, ideas of guilt and unworthiness, bleak and pessimistic views of the future, disturbed sleep and early-morning wakening, diminished appetite and weight loss, and ideas of self-harm and suicide (World Health Organization, 1992). Sexual interest is reduced or lost. Somatic complaints, rather than feelings of sadness, may be emphasized, and the patient believes that they are physically ill. There is often increased irritability, an impaired ability to think or make decisions, and poor concentration. The patient may be agitated or slowed. Psychotic symptoms such as delusions, hallucinations, or depressive stupor can occur in a severe depressive episode.

Depressive illness exists in degrees, and there are many variations in which symptoms cluster and present. No one description can do justice to the true variety of presentations. The picture will be influenced by culture and the patient's age and personality. Many attempts have been made to typologize this disorder – endogenous versus reactive, "neurotic depression" versus true depressive illness, and so on. Current diagnostic classification is set out in the International Classification of Disease (ICD) and DSM manuals. A distinction is made between unipolar affective disorder and bipolar affective disorder, with the latter characterized by repeated episodes in which the patient's mood and activity levels are significantly disturbed, sometimes in terms of elevation of mood (elation) and increased energy and activity (mania or hypomania) and at other times by episodes of depression.

Deciding whether a person is just miserable or, on the other hand, ill with depression can be extraordinarily difficult when the person is drinking. Depressive illness is often overdiagnosed in problem drinkers, with consequent needless prescribing of medications; on other occasions, the diagnosis may be overlooked. This is an instance when correct diagnosis will speak very importantly to appropriate management. If the patient is suffering from nonspecific unhappiness rather than a depressive illness, that aspect of their situation may require skilled help, but not the same type of help as would be indicated for undoubted depressive illness. A picture of drinking problems together with a complaint of depression is illustrated by the following case abstract:

> A divorced woman aged 35 had been drinking excessively for 3 or 4 years. Concerned about her well-being, the pastor of her church visited the woman and discovered that the house was in a terrible state and the teenage children appeared to have been mostly left to fend for themselves. The woman herself was disheveled, obviously rather drunk, and declaring in a maudlin fashion that she was no good and that the family might as well be rid of her. The pastor persuaded the woman to allow him to drive her to the emergency psychiatric services unit, where they met together with a psychiatric resident.

How should the psychiatric resident respond to this situation? Quite certainly, an entirely inadequate course of action would be simply to write a prescription for antidepressant drugs and let the patient take them whilst still drinking. Treatment cannot be intelligently and usefully started until it is known what must be treated. The obverse approach, and one as misguided as the ill-thought-out use of pharmacotherapy, is to assume that all problem drinkers can be a bit morose at times and to dismiss this woman's complaint as "just the alcoholic miseries" – later perhaps to hear that she killed herself.

How, in practice, does the clinician decide whether such a patient is suffering from a depressive illness? Assessment of the history is very important – a history of depressive illness, an event such as childbirth or bereavement that might have precipitated the illness, or a sense of some more or less demarcated point where "things changed" and the patient knew that, whatever the previous ups and downs of mood, something was now being experienced that was fixed and of different degree. A family history of depression can also be an important indicator of potential vulnerability. Information on familial and personal history is useful in diagnosis because present behaviour and mental state may not in themselves be dispositive. Many problem drinkers will, when drinking, show emotional lability, will cry easily, and will talk of the hopelessness of their lives. To leap to an immediate diagnosis of depressive illness in all such instances would result in a great deal of overdiagnosis. The dilemma can be very real, and even experienced clinical judgment may be unable to resolve this diagnostic question while that patient is intoxicated. The patient's account may be inconsistent, it may seem to be overdramatized, the immediate life situation may be distressingly fraught and chaotic, but it is still unclear whether or not behind this drinking lies a depressive illness.

In such circumstances, the sensible rule is to admit that diagnosis cannot be made in the presence of drinking. Stopping drinking is the prerequisite to a resolution of the diagnostic difficulty. In most individuals, depressive symptoms resolve following 2–3 weeks of abstinence. Alternatively, it may become very apparent that a classical depressive illness now stands out as certainly as a rock left by the tide. Sometimes, however, even after a period of in-patient observation and continued sobriety, it may be difficult to know whether what is emerging is a depressive illness or a personality chronically prone to unhappy feelings and explosive declarations of misery. The ultimate resolution of the diagnostic problem might, for instance, be that the woman described in the case study had always been a rather unhappy and insecure person and that, in this setting, she had gradually started to drink more and had been drinking heavily for 5 or more years; but, against all this background, she had undoubtedly a year previously developed a postpartum depressive illness that had been untreated. The unravelling of such a story may require a lot of time, but arriving at a proper understanding is no optional extra if the depressed drinker is to be effectively treated.

The relationship of drinking problems and depression

In many cases, depression is secondary to the alcohol problem. However, a proportion of problem drinkers have an independent depressive disorder that may predispose them to the development of an alcohol problem or exacerbate it once it has developed. Depression more commonly predates alcohol problems in women than in men (Helzer & Pryzbeck, 1988). The relationship may also vary with age and sex; for instance, adolescent girls are at greater risk of depression than are boys, which may be why some studies find association with drinking problems in females but not males (Boden & Fergusson, 2011). The association with major depressive disorder is stronger with alcohol dependence than abuse (Pacek, Martins, & Crum, 2013). Other predisposing factors for depression in people with drinking problems include a history of anxiety, other drug misuse, and previous suicide attempts (Roy et al., 1991). A history of recent, particularly negative, life events and a family history of depression appear to increase risk factors for secondary depression in male alcoholics (Roy, 1996).

Depressive symptoms are common during alcohol withdrawal, particularly following a period of heavy consumption. Clinically significant levels of depression are found among in-patients with drinking problems during the early stages of admission and alcohol withdrawal, but, in most people, these symptoms improve after a few weeks of abstinence. However, depressive symptoms may persist or may even emerge during abstinence, and the astute clinician should always be on the lookout for this. Long-term follow-up studies suggest that depressive symptoms usually decline with continued abstinence.

In the clinical situation, it may be helpful to differentiate between alcohol-induced depressive syndromes and independent depressive episodes. Major depressive episodes occurring during a period of active alcohol dependence are considered to be alcohol-induced. Independent major depression may be defined as an episode that occurred either before the onset of alcohol dependence or during a period of 3 or more months of abstinence. However, labelling either depression or problem drinking as "primary" and the other "secondary" should not result in either receiving less attention because both need treatment (see Chapter 13). It should also not be a reason for either a psychiatric or alcohol treatment service not to accept a referral; instead, the referred service must make further enquiries and possibly offer an assessment; joint working is optimal.

Depression and drinking problems: the practical importance of the diagnostic question

There are several reasons to determine whether a patient with a drinking problem is also suffering from a depressive illness. If such an illness exists, it of course deserves treatment (e.g., with cognitive behavioural therapy [CBT] or an antidepressant medication). If co-occurring depression is untreated, attempts to treat the drinking problem will be grossly handicapped. A depressed patient may find it extremely difficult to stop drinking, and untreated depression can on occasion persist for 2 or 3 years, or even longer, perhaps with partial remissions and further relapses making the time course even more blurred and extended. Another important reason for taking the diagnostic question extremely seriously is the issue of suicidal risk (see later discussion). Problem drinkers who are not suffering from depressive illness may take their own lives, but the risk is certainly enhanced if this illness is present.

Knowledge of a depressive illness has a bearing on long-term management, and this must be openly discussed with the patient. Once someone has suffered from one such illness, they are at some risk of developing depression again at some point. If they can recognize early signs and seek appropriate help, significant suffering may be averted. An episode of depression is not an uncommon cause of relapse into drinking after a long period of sobriety. Paradoxically, the development of an underlying depression may be the reason for a drinker to eventually seek help. It may be an expression of their depressive illness when they say they "can't go on any longer," start to blame themselves rather than others for their drinking or make the suicidal gesture that gets them into hospital.

> A 35-year-old woman who worked mainly from home with her catering business was found by her partner, who arrived home early, to have taken an overdose. Her family history showed a heavy loading both with depressive illness and alcohol dependence, and she undoubtedly was suffering from both problems. She accepted that she had to stop drinking and responded well to relapse prevention medication alongside an antidepressant and CBT.

Summing the matter up, an awareness of the significance of depressive illness is so essential to working with problem drinkers that every clinician should develop a good understanding of depression and how best to treat it. Clearly, it is important to assess the severity of depression and any suicidal ideation and to manage them accordingly. However, for many, their depression will improve with reduced drinking or abstinence. Therefore, the therapeutic priority is to aid and persuade those patients to stop drinking (offering perhaps immediate admission to achieve this purpose). Their depression should be monitored throughout and treated accordingly. It is generally messy and ineffective to try to treat a depressive illness without supporting the patient to change their problem drinking at the same time.

Suicide and deliberate self-harm

Alcohol consumption precedes or is part of an episode of deliberate self-harm in about half of individuals who then present to a hospital (Hawton et al., 2007). The lifetime risk of suicide in alcoholics was previously estimated to be 15 percent (Murphy & Wetzel, 1990), but this figure was challenged by a meta-analysis of mortality studies that calculated a lifetime risk of 7 percent (Inskip, Harris, & Barraclough, 1998). When national suicide rates are taken into account, lifetime risk is somewhere between 2.5 and 7 percent (Jenkins, 2007). A 25-year follow-up study of almost 50,000 Swedish male conscripts born in 1950 and 1951 showed that those who had abused alcohol had a highly elevated risk of suicide attempts (odds ratio of 27.1) and of completed suicide (odds ratio of 4.7) (Rossow, Romelsjö, & Leifman, 1999). The odds ratios remained elevated when the data were adjusted for psychiatric comorbidity (8.8 and 2.4, respectively). Intoxication was the main component in nonfatal suicide behaviour. The role of hazardous and harmful alcohol use in suicidal behaviour, particularly in male adolescents and young men, has been highlighted in a number of other studies (Fombonne, 1998; Pirkola et al., 1999; Vassilas & Morgan, 1997).

Stressful life events are key contributors to suicide or deliberate self-harm in individuals with alcohol problems. Other factors include isolation; lack of social support; unemployment; comorbid disorders such as anxiety, depression, and personality disorder; and medical problems. Close attention to these factors may help in the assessment of suicidal risk in such individuals when they present to emergency services and to other healthcare professionals. Suicidal ideation should be taken seriously, their drinking and comorbid disorders assessed carefully, and appropriate treatment instituted (Brady, 2006; Pirkola, Suominen, & Isometsa, 2004).

Bipolar disorder

Bipolar disorder is a chronic illness involving severe fluctuations in mood much greater than the "ups and downs" that everyone experiences. Symptoms of mania include feeling "high," elation, irritability, distractability, flight of ideas, having enormous energy with little need for sleep, impulsive behaviour, and unrealistic belief in ability (e.g., thinking they can fly). In a depressive state, individuals describe being tired, losing interest in activities, not experiencing pleasure, and having suicidal thoughts. Bipolar I disorder is characterized by manic and depressive episodes, whereas in bipolar II disorder, depression occurs with hypomania. Hypomania describes elated states without significant functional impairment, whereas such an adverse impact is always seen in mania. Occasionally, the hypomanic patient finds that alcohol can ameliorate unpleasant elements in their feelings: accompanying the basic elevation of mood, the hypomanic state may be characterized by a considerable admixture of anxiety, irritability, and suspiciousness.

The frequency of episodes in bipolar disorder may vary between individuals but generally last for a few weeks, with periods of stability in between. In some however, the fluctuations in mood are more rapid such that at least four distinct mood episodes such as major depression, manic, hypomanic, or mixed states occur within 12 months. Mixed affective illnesses exist where the patient is both excited and tearful, with a confusing presentation that moves within minutes from elation to depression. Such "rapid cycling" is more commonly seen in those who abuse alcohol or illicit substances (Frye & Salloum, 2006). If a patient presents with such a pattern, alcohol misuse should be investigated.

In bipolar disorder, as many as 45 percent may also have an AUD (Farren, Hill, & Weiss, 2012). The odds ratio for AUD in bipolar I disorder (3.5) is higher than for bipolar II disorder (2.6). Mania in particular is highly associated with AUD (see Table 6.1). Patients with repeated hypomanic or manic episodes may give the appearance of "bout drinking." During an attack, they are likely to lose their social judgment and to spend large sums of money and live things up, and this general disinhibition, as well as the more specific seeking of relief from unpleasant feelings, may contribute to their drinking. The onset of bipolar disorder comorbid with alcoholism tends to be earlier than the onset of either disorder alone (i.e., early 20s compared with mid to late 20s). Not surprisingly, the course of bipolar disorder in the presence of alcoholism is worse than when it is not present, and treatment response to lithium is also reduced.

A 40-year-old lawyer was persuaded by his colleagues to seek help because they thought his excessive drinking was making him unpredictable and bad-tempered. At interview, it became clear that he was developing a manic swing of a bipolar illness. His generally heavy background drinking was apt to go out of control during this kind of episode. With treatment for his bipolar disorder instituted and his own decision that drinking was "best cut out," he returned to practice.

A more difficult diagnostic problem arises when there is a suspicion that the patient's mood may phasically become slightly elevated but not approaching a hypomanic illness in severity. This slight elevation and disinhibition may appear sufficient to spark off some weeks of drinking, and, on occasion, this is a plausible explanation of "periodic drinking." What is being discussed here is a mood disturbance, *cyclothymia*, which occurs when individuals have episodes of hypomania and mild depression for at least 2 years that do not meet the threshold for bipolar disorder. Alternatively, it may be a character trait (cyclothymic personality), but there is no absolute demarcation between this sort of state and hypomania. In turn, hypomania merges with mania, with the latter term indicating a state of appalling overexcitement or the traditional picture of "raving madness." A patient with fully developed mania is far too disordered to be other than rapidly admitted to a hospital, and drinking as a complication of this illness needs immediate consideration if medication is required for detoxification and then later for relapse prevention.

Anxiety

Symptoms of anxiety are particularly prominent after a bout of heavy drinking and during alcohol withdrawal. Alcohol withdrawal symptoms can mimic anxiety and panic disorder, probably due to a common dysregulation in the GABA-ergic system. Individuals with alcohol dependence and anxiety disorder have been found to experience more severe alcohol withdrawal symptoms than a non-anxious control group, even though the two groups had similar drinking histories (Johnston, Thevos, Randall, & Anton, 1991). Anxiety symptoms typically diminish in the early stages of abstinence and continue to improve with prolonged abstinence.

This case example illustrates one kind of possible clinical relationship between alcohol and anxiety:

> A woman, aged 53, was admitted to the hospital with a long history of drinking. She worked as an office cleaner, so rose early. She would have a drink at 5 o'clock before leaving the house and would then put a couple of bottles of wine into her bag. Information from her case notes revealed that she had first attended the clinic many years previously. Her presenting complaint then was agoraphobia and difficulty in leaving her house. Careful questioning revealed that phobic anxiety symptoms still very much persisted, although alcohol dependence had now developed as a problem in its own right.

As with depression, the ideal clinical approach when a problem drinker appears to be suffering from an anxiety state is to take a full comprehensive history to ascertain the relationship between the drinking and anxiety. It is key to make a correct diagnosis or diagnoses in order to inform appropriate treatment. It is difficult to assess the true severity or fixedness of anxiety symptoms until the patient has been completely off alcohol for about 4 weeks, and sometimes a longer period of observation is required. At that point, seemingly rather severe anxiety symptoms may fade away following detoxification, and, in that event, there is no anxiety to be treated. The symptoms were part of the general "bad nerves" related to alcohol dependence.

If, however, severe anxiety symptoms persist, an effort must be made to treat them. Like depression, anxiety often diminishes with reduction/cessation of drinking, so this must be encouraged. However, in some cases, concurrent treatment of the anxiety disorder will be required (e.g., exposure therapy or medication). The response is often excellent provided that the patient can maintain abstinence and cooperate with treatment, that the background level of anxiety is not too high, and that the phobic situations are not too universal. It would be optimistic to suppose that CBT is a panacea because such favourable conditions do not always exist.

> John was a 41-year-old divorced teacher who presented to the in-patient unit for treatment. He had been alcohol dependent for about 15 years but had never sought any specialist alcohol treatment. However, he had been receiving treatment for anxiety and depression for about 20 years, having first presented to psychiatric services following an overdose. During his admission, he successfully completed a medically assisted withdrawal from alcohol and then had a full psychiatric assessment. This revealed social anxiety and lack of confidence, difficulties relating to others, chronic depressive features, and feelings of inadequacy, all of which had been present since childhood.
>
> Following discharge from the hospital, he attended a 12-step day programme and had 16 sessions of CBT with a clinical psychologist. He continued to visit his psychiatrist, who helped to monitor progress and liaised with the psychologist and general practitioner. John took to the cognitive model very well and found it quite revelatory in terms of his ability to focus on and identify aspects of his difficulties of which he had not previously been aware. After seven sessions, he was less depressed and more optimistic but continued to experience significant social anxiety and still felt "socially inadequate." However, after a further nine sessions (and 6 months later) there had been an improvement in his anxiety symptoms, which were now within the normal range. It was clear that he had used alcohol to cope with his social anxiety and feeling of social inadequacy. By this time, he was back at work and feeling satisfied with the changes that he had been able to achieve. In the early days of abstinence, he attended Alcoholics Anonymous (AA) nightly. He concluded the CBT with the psychologist. A year later, he was still abstinent and attending AA twice a week.

Post-traumatic stress disorder

PTSD is an anxiety disorder that develops following exposure to an extremely traumatic stressor considered to be exceptionally threatening or catastrophic in nature. Current and former members of the military with combat experience are a particular group of alcohol abusing patients who often have co-occurring PTSD. Characteristic symptoms include persistent re-experiencing of the traumatic event, persistent avoidance of stimuli associated with the trauma, numbing of general responsiveness, and persistent symptoms of hyperarousal. PTSD may exist with major depressive disorder and may present as a combination of the listed symptoms and typical grief. Surveys have revealed that around a third of individuals with PTSD also had a diagnosis of alcohol dependence during the lifetime, with increasing PTSD severity associated with greater likelihood of alcohol problems (Blanco, Xu, Brady, Pérez-Fuentes, Okuda, & Wang, 2013; Kessler et al., 1997). In about 50 percent of cases, alcohol dependence began in the same year or after PTSD was diagnosed. Whatever the order of onset, each disorder makes more challenging the treatment of the other.

Several hypotheses have been proposed to explain the link between PTSD and alcohol misuse, including the involvement of the stress system in both disorders. Early substance misuse may occur in the context of other "high-risk" behaviours that increase the likelihood of exposure to potentially traumatizing events and hence the likelihood of developing PTSD. Additionally, individuals who begin using alcohol at an early age may also be susceptible to the development of PTSD following traumatic exposure because they have historically relied on alcohol as a way of combatting stress and have failed to develop more effective stress reduction strategies. In the clinical setting, it is helpful to differentiate between experiences of childhood and adult trauma and to assess how these experiences have affected the individual.

The association between PTSD and alcohol misuse or dependence is particularly strong in individuals who have experienced childhood physical and sexual abuse (most commonly, but not entirely, females). Early experiences of physical and sexual abuse put individuals at a greater risk of developing PTSD symptoms following traumatic events in adulthood (Breslau, Chilcoat, Kessler, & Davis, 1999). PTSD and alcohol dependence are associated with higher prevalence of childhood trauma, earlier onset of alcohol dependence, lower socioeconomic status, and poorer physical health compared with alcohol dependence only (Blanco et al., 2013).

In an ideal world, individuals with alcohol dependence and PTSD should be enabled to tackle both problems simultaneously. As with other psychiatric comorbidities, evidence on how to do this or which condition should be treated first is limited. Clearly, treatment for PTSD should ideally not be so traumatic as to escalate or cause relapse to heavy drinking, as illustrated in the following case example:

> A 36-year-old man was referred to a specialist PTSD clinic. He had a long history of heavy drinking that developed into alcohol dependence after a bus accident that caused him to develop PTSD followed by depression. He had made several attempts to overcome his PTSD with counselling, but each time he found himself drinking more alcohol to cope with the memories of the accident. With support from his wife, he managed to reduce his drinking to a low level and was motivated to engage in treatment for his PTSD. Unfortunately, he relapsed to dependent drinking after only four treatment sessions, during which he had been "exposed" to the traumatic memories and encouraged to relive them as

vividly as possible. His wife felt that she had to move out because he was violent to her while intoxicated, and she worried for her own and the children's safety. There followed a number of episodes where he engaged with the community alcohol team and underwent several alcohol detoxes but was unable to sustain any substantial period of abstinence. Over the next few years, he spent some time being cared for in psychiatric wards but rarely stayed long and never received any services directed at his alcohol problem. It was hard to find an addiction treatment unit that would accept his medication for PTSD. Several years later, he remained in and out contact with out-patient services with various approaches including motivational enhancement therapy, CBT, and pharmacotherapy for alcohol dependence, PTSD, and depression not resulting in sustained robust improvements in his drinking, depression, and PTSD. He now lives on his own, continues to drink, and has only intermittent contact with his children. Although his wife remains supportive, she still lives with her parents.

Treatment of comorbid AUD and PTSD is more fully described in Chapter 13.

Personality disorder

It is impossible to work with drinking problems without becoming aware of the relevance of personality to an understanding of the genesis of drinking and the treatment of excessive drinking and dependence. Patients with drinking problems are sometimes and to various degrees angry, unhappy, nonconformist, rule-breaking, aggressive, and handicapped in their ability to deal with social demands and expectations. It can be difficult to determine how much such seeming disturbances are cause and how much are the consequences of excessive drinking. Personality disturbance can make treatment difficult and has to be dealt with clinically as a significant issue.

Studies in population and clinical settings show a higher prevalence of personality disorder among people with AUDs (and drug use disorders) than among the general population, with antisocial and borderline personality disorder being particularly prominent. Borderline personality traits have been shown to predict later alcohol use problems (Stepp, Trull, & Sher, 2005). Antisocial, borderline, and schizotypal personality disorders consistently predict a persistent course of alcohol, nicotine, and cannabis use disorders (Hasin & Kilcoyne, 2012). Specialist alcohol services are accustomed to dealing with people with personality disorder, especially antisocial and borderline personality disorder.

Attention deficit hyperactivity disorder

ADHD is an early-onset neurobehavioural disorder characterized by symptoms of inattention, hyperactivity, and impulsivity; it affects between 4 and 7 percent of children (Spencer, Biederman, & Mick, 2007). Children with the disorder typically have trouble concentrating and staying still, and this can lead to problems at school. Diagnosis of ADHD in an adult requires childhood onset of these symptoms and is evidenced by history of limited life, academic, and occupational achievements. However, such symptoms and difficulties are also seen in foetal alcohol spectrum disorder, and this diagnosis should also be carefully considered.

Individuals with ADHD can present to alcohol treatment services as adolescents or adults. Several studies have shown a high incidence of AUDs (33–44 percent) in adults with ADHD and, other psychiatric disorder are also often seen, such as depressive or anxiety disorders (Spencer et al., 2007). It is worth bearing this diagnosis in mind when seeing patients with multiple comorbidities, particularly if they are using stimulants. In addition, adolescents and adults with ADHD are at increased risk for tobacco dependence. On the other hand, early diagnosis and treatment of the ADHD may help to reduce the onset of other addictions (Ohlmeier et al., 2007).

Psychosis and schizophrenia

Prevalence studies suggest that approximately 40–50 percent of schizophrenia patients have a lifetime history of SUDs (Menezes et al., 1996; Weaver et al., 2001). With a prevalence rate of greater than 80 percent, tobacco smoking is the most common drug use behaviour of patients with schizophrenia. Lifetime prevalence of AUDs is about 20 percent in schizophrenia (Duke, Pantelis, & Barnes, 1994) and 32 percent in psychosis (Menezes et al., 1996). Alcohol use may be an added risk factor for the development of tardive dyskinesia in some patients with schizophrenia (Duke et al., 1994).

It is not uncommon for clinicians to focus on their psychotic patient's illicit drug use, particularly cannabis, but give alcohol misuse little attention. For comparison, the lifetime prevalence is 27 percent for cannabis use disorders. The remaining illicit drugs, such as psychostimulants like cocaine, amphetamine, and methamphetamine, are generally less commonly used, although rates may be high in particular environments.

There are several theories as to why patients with schizophrenia use illicit psychoactive substances, and, in any one individual, there will be a number of different contributions. Using substances to attenuate or cope better with either their psychiatric symptoms or the side effects of antipsychotic medication has been a popular explanatory hypothesis among psychiatrists and psychodynamically oriented psychologists. However, this theory has had limited empirical support over the years (Lembke, 2012) and indeed seems even less compelling today when one considers that newer antipsychotics incur fewer side effects and improved symptom control. An alternative view is to see that dysregulation in the dopaminergic system underpins vulnerability to both psychosis and substance misuse. This is supported by some preclinical evidence that drug use can precede schizophrenia and that patients with schizophrenia tend to overvalue the positive consequences of drug use and undervalue its negative consequences (Thoma & Daum, 2013). It also has to be remembered that people with schizophrenia may use substances for the same reasons as those without schizophrenia (e.g., pleasure, relaxation).

Alcohol consumption is a risk factor for violence in individuals with schizophrenia (Fazel et al., 2009). Treatment should minimize this risk by reducing alcohol consumption.

Eating disorders and obesity

The most common disorders of body weight that result from excessive drinking are obesity due to the high caloric content of alcohol and the loss of weight and general malnutrition that are consequences of the dietary neglect that frequently accompanies heavy drinking. It is not an uncommon clinical scenario to see individuals abusing alcohol and engaging in altered eating patterns (such as bingeing on food) and in deliberate self-harm (such as cutting for emotional regulation). As one behaviour is brought under control, another may increase in intensity, thus providing a challenge to the clinician.

About half of patients with an eating disorder misuse alcohol or other drugs, and, in those with a SUD, about a third have an eating disorder (Gregorowski, Seedat, &

Jordaan, 2013). The association between AUDs is stronger with binge eating and bulimia nervosa, particularly purging-type, rather than anorexia nervosa. The association between drinking problems and eating disorders may be due to a common dysregulation in impulse control or to an attempt to moderate mood or distress. Comorbid alcohol abuse with eating disorders increases the number of complications and challenges as well as risk of mortality in anorexia nervosa (Franko et al., 2013). Individuals with eating disorders and AUDs may also have a predisposition toward other "impulse" disorders such as self-harm and misuse of illicit or prescribed drugs.

There is increasing interest in whether substance dependence has similarities to obesity in that being overweight results from excessive consumption and altered responding to food rewards. Similarities of seeking and consuming a rewarding substance exist across sugar and alcohol/drugs (Volkow, Wang, Tomasi, & Baler, 2013).

Psychiatric disorders: the general implications

Many types of psychiatric disorder can be associated with excessive drinking and in a range of ways. This reality must not be interpreted as meaning that only the psychiatrist can treat the problem drinker. Neither does the fact that psychiatric treatment or admission to a psychiatric hospital may be indicated for some of these patients mean that the treatment of alcohol problems is a psychiatric preserve. However, what must be evident is that psychiatry may quite often have a part to play and that a working liaison with psychiatric services should be available to clinicians engaged in treating drinking problems. An awareness of this psychiatric dimension is vital, regardless of the clinician's professional discipline.

References

Blanco, C., Xu, Y., Brady, K., Pérez-Fuentes, G., Okuda, M., & Wang, S. (2013). Comorbidity of posttraumatic stress disorder with alcohol dependence among US adults: Results from National Epidemiological Survey on Alcohol and Related Conditions. *Drug and Alcohol Dependence*, **132**, 630–638.

Boden, J. M., & Fergusson, D. M. (2011). Alcohol and depression. *Addiction*, **106**, 906–14.

Brady, J. (2006). The association between alcohol misuse and suicidal behaviour. *Alcohol and Alcoholism*, **41**, 473–478.

Breslau, N., Chilcoat, H. D., Kessley, R. C., & Davis, G. C. (1999). Previous exposure to trauma: Results from the Detroit Area Survey of Trauma. *American Journal of Psychiatry*, **156**, 902–907.

Burns, L., Teesson, M., & Lynskey, M. (2001). *The epidemiology of comorbidity between alcohol use disorders and mental disorders in Australia: Findings from the National Survey of Mental Health & Well-Being* (Technical Report 118). Sydney, Australia: National Drug and Alcohol Research Centre.

Chiappetta, V., García-Rodríguez, O., Jin, C. J., Secades-Villa, & R., Blanco, C. (2014). Predictors of quit attempts and successful quit attempts among individuals with alcohol use disorders in a nationally representative sample. *Drug and Alcohol Dependence*, **141**, 138–144.

Crome, I., Brown, A., Dar, K., Harris, L., Janikiewicz, S., Rao, T., … Tarbuck, A. (2011). *Our invisible addicts: First report of the Older Persons' Substance Misuse Working Group of the Royal College of Psychiatrists*. London: Royal College of Psychiatrists.

Duke, P., Pantelis, C., & Barnes, T. R. E. (1994). South Westminster Schizophrenia Survey. Alcohol use and its relationship to symptoms, tardive dyskinesia and illness onset. *British Journal of Psychiatry*, **164**, 630–636.

Farrell, M., Howes, S., Bebbington, P., Brugha, T., Jenkins, R., Lewis, G., … Meltzer, H. (2001). Nicotine, alcohol and drug dependence, and psychiatry morbidity – results of a national household survey. *British Journal of Psychiatry*, **179**, 432–437.

Farren, C. K., Hill, K. P., & Weiss, R. D. (2012). Bipolar disorder and alcohol use disorder: A review. *Current Psychiatry Reports*, **14**, 659–666.

Fazel, S., Långström, N., Hjern, A., Grann, M., & Lichtenstein, P. (2009). Schizophrenia, substance abuse and violent crime. *Journal of the American Medical Association*, **301**, 2016–2023.

Fombonne, E. (1998). Suicidal behaviours in vulnerable adolescents. *British Journal of Psychiatry*, **173**, 154–159.

Franko, D. L., Keshaviah, A., Eddy, K. T., Krishna, M., Davis, M. C., Keel, P. K., & Herzog, D. B. (2013). A longitudinal investigation of mortality in anorexia nervosa and bulimia nervosa. *American Journal of Psychiatry*, **170**(8), 917–925.

Frye, M. A., & Salloum, I. M. (2006). Bipolar disorder and comorbid alcoholism: Prevalence rate and treatment considerations. *Bipolar Disorder*, **8**(6), 677–685.

Glass, I. (1989a). Alcoholic hallucinosis: A psychiatric enigma – I. The development of an idea. *British Journal of Addiction*, **84**, 29–41.

Glass, I. (1989b). Alcoholic hallucinosis: A psychiatric enigma – 2. Follow-up studies. *British Journal of Addiction*, **84**, 151–164.

Goodwin, D. W., Crane, B. J., & Guze, S. B. (1969a). Phenomenological aspects of the alcoholic "blackout." *British Journal of Psychiatry*, **115**, 1033–1038.

Goodwin, D. W., Crane, B. J., & Guze, S. B. (1969b). Alcoholic "blackouts": A review and clinical study of 100 alcoholics. *American Journal of Psychiatry*, **126**, 191–198.

Grant, B. F., Stinson, F. S., Dawson, D. A., Chuo, S. P., Dufour, M. C., Compton, W., … Kaplan, K. (2004). Prevalence and co-occurrence of substance use disorders and independent mood and anxiety disorders: Results from the National Epidemiologic Survey on Alcohol and Related Conditions. *Archives of General Psychiatry*, **61**, 807–816.

Gregorowski, C., Seedat, S., & Jordaan, G. P. (2013). A clinical approach to the assessment and management of co-morbid eating disorders and substance use disorders. *BMC Psychiatry*, **13**, 289.

Hasin, D., & Kilcoyne, B. (2012). Comorbidity of psychiatric and substance use disorders in the United States: Current issues and findings from the NESARC. *Current Opinion in Psychiatry*, **25**(3), 165.

Hawton, K., Bergen, H., Casey, D., Simkin, S., Palmer, B., Cooper, J., … Owens, D. (2007). Self-harm in England: A tale of three cities. Multicentre study of self-harm. *Social Psychiatry and Psychiatric Epidemiology*, **42**, 513–521.

Helzer, J. E., & Pryzbeck, T. R. (1988). The co-occurrence of alcoholism with other psychiatric disorders in the general population and its impact on treatment. *Journal of Studies on Alcohol*, **49**, 219–224.

Humphreys, K., Weingardt, K. R., Horst, D., Joshi, A. A., & Finney, J. W. (2005). Prevalence and predictors of research participant eligibility criteria in alcohol treatment outcome studies, 1970–98. *Addiction*, **100**, 1249–1257.

Inskip, H. M., Harris, E. C., & Barraclough, B. (1998). Lifetime risk of suicide for affective disorder, alcoholism and schizophrenia. *British Journal of Psychiatry*, **172**, 35–37.

Jenkins, R. (2007). Substance use and suicidal behaviour. *Psychiatry*, **6**, 19–22.

Johnston, A. L., Thevos, A. K., Randall, C. L., & Anton, R. F. (1991). Increased severity of alcohol withdrawal in in-patient alcoholics with a co-existing anxiety diagnosis. *British Journal of Addiction*, **86**, 719–725.

Kessler, R. C., Crum, R. M., & Warner, L. A. (1997). Lifetime co-occurrence of DSM-III-R alcohol abuse and dependence with other psychiatric disorders in the National Comorbidity Study. *Archives of General Psychiatry*, **54**, 313–321.

Kessler, R. C., McGonagle, K. A., Zhad, S., Nelson, C. B., Hughes, M., Eshleman, S., … Kendler, K. S. (1994). Lifetime and 12-month prevalence of DSM-III psychiatric disorders in the United States: Results from the National Comorbidity Survey. *Archives of General Psychiatry*, **51**, 8–19.

Khan, S., Okuda, M., Hasin, D. S., Secades-Villa, R., Keyes, K., Lin, K. H., … Blanco, C. (2013). Gender differences in lifetime alcohol dependence: Results from the national epidemiologic survey on alcohol and related conditions. *Alcoholism: Clinical and Experimental Research*, **37**, 1696–1705.

Lembke, A. (2012). Time to abandon the self-medication hypothesis in patients with psychiatric disorders. *American Journal of Drug and Alcohol Abuse*, **38**, 524–529.

Lishman, W. A. (1998). *Organic psychiatry* (3rd ed.). Oxford: Blackwell Scientific.

Menezes, P., Johnson, S., Thornicroft, G., Marshall, J., Prosser, D., Bebbington, P., & Kuipers, E. (1996). Drug and alcohol problems among individuals with severe mental illness in South London. *British Journal of Psychiatry*, **168**, 612–619.

Murphy, G. G., & Wetzel, R. D. (1990). The lifetime risk of suicide in alcoholism. *Archives of General Psychiatry*, **47**, 383–392.

Ohlmeier, M. D., Peters, K., Kordon, A., Seifert, J., Wildt, B. T., Wiese, B., ... Schneider, U. (2007). Nicotine and alcohol dependence in patients with comorbid attention-deficit/hyperactivity disorder (ADHD). *Alcohol and Alcoholism*, **42**, 539–543.

Pacek, L. R., Martins, S. S., & Crum, R. M. (2013). The bidirectional relationships between alcohol, cannabis, co-occurring alcohol and cannabis use disorders with major depressive disorder: Results from a national sample. *Journal of Affective Disorders*, **148**, 188–195.

Pirkola, S., Marttunen, M. J., Henriksson, M. M., Isometsa, E. T., Heikkinen, M. E., & Lönnqvist, J. K. (1999). Alcohol-related problems among adolescent suicides in Finland. *Alcohol and Alcoholism*, **34**, 320–329.

Pirkola, S. P., Suominen, K., & Isometsa, E. T. (2004). Suicide in alcohol-dependent individuals: Epidemiology and management. *CNS Drugs*, **18**, 423–436.

Rossow, I., Romelsjö, A., & Leifman, H. (1999). Alcohol abuse and suicidal behaviour in young and middle-aged men: Differentiating between attempted and completed suicide. *Addiction*, **94**, 1199–1207.

Roy, A. (1996). Aetiology of secondary depression in male alcoholics. *British Journal of Psychiatry*, **169**, 753–757.

Roy, A., DeJong, J., Lamparski, D., George, T., & Linnoila, M. (1991). Depression among alcoholics. *Archives of General Psychiatry*, **48**, 428–432.

Schuckit, M. A. (2014). Recognition and management of withdrawal delirium (delirium tremens). *New England Journal of Medicine*, **371**(22), 2109–2113.

Spencer, T. J., Biederman, J., & Mick, E. (2007). Attention-deficit/hyperactivity disorder: Diagnosis, lifespan, comorbidities and neurobiology. *Journal of Pediatric Psychology*, **32**, 631–642.

Stepp, S. D., Trull, T. J., & Sher, K. J. (2005). Borderline personality features predict alcohol use problems. *Journal of Personality Disorders*, **19**, 711–722.

Swendsen, J., Conway, K. P., Degenhardt, L., Glantz, M., Jin, R., Merikangas, K. R., ... Kessler, R. C. (2010). Mental disorders as risk factors for substance use, abuse and dependence: Results from the 10-year follow-up of the National Comorbidity Survey. *Addiction*, **105**, 1117–1128.

Thoma, P., & Daum, I. (2013). Comorbid substance use disorder in schizophrenia: A selective overview of neurobiological and cognitive underpinnings. *Psychiatry and Clinical Neurosciences*, **67**(6), 367–383.

Tsuang, J. W., Irwin, M. R., Smith, T. L., & Schuckit, M. A. (1994). Characteristics of men with alcoholic hallucinosis. *Addiction*, **89**, 73–78.

Vassilas, C. A., & Morgan, H. G. (1997). Suicide in Avon. Life stress, alcohol misuse and use of services. *British Journal of Psychiatry*, **170**, 453–455.

Volkow, N. D., Wang, G. J., Tomasi, D., & Baler, R. D. (2013). The addictive dimensionality of obesity. *Biological Psychiatry*, **73**(9), 811–818.

Weaver, T., Rutter, D., Madden, P., Ward, J., Stimson, G., & Renton, A. (2001). Results of a screening survey for co-morbid substance misuse amongst patients in treatment for psychotic disorders: Prevalence and service needs in an inner London borough. *Social Psychiatry and Psychiatric Epidemiology*, **36**, 399–406.

World Health Organization. (1992). *The ICD-10 classification of mental and behavioural disorders*. Geneva: Author.

Wu, L. T., & Blazer, D. G. (2014). Substance use disorders and psychiatric comorbidity in mid and later life: A review. *International Journal of Epidemiology*, **43**(2) 304–317.

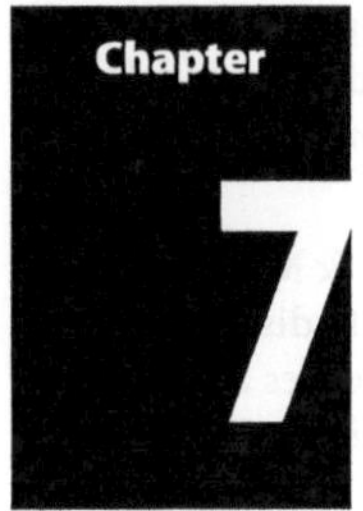

Alcohol and other drug problems

Alcohol is a drug (see Chapter 2) that is often used with other drugs, ranging from simple combinations, such as alcohol and nicotine at one end of the spectrum, to multiple combinations at the other end. Drugs may be used concurrently with alcohol, as a substitute for it, or in response to withdrawal from it. It is important to clarify how and why they may be used together (e.g., to heighten positive experiences or minimize negative ones). In the clinical situation, one may see alcohol dependent patients who report that they have been abstinent from alcohol for some considerable time, but this "abstinence" has been achieved by substituting another drug such as benzodiazepines or cannabis, or both. The patterns of relationship that can exist between the uses of different types of drugs are myriad, and the following case extract illustrates one variation on this theme:

> The patient was a successful businessman, aged 35. His working day was lived at a fast pace, and most evenings were spent entertaining business associates in restaurants and nightclubs. He and his guests would get through a lot of alcohol, drinking on average a couple of bottles of wine each as well as "a few" double vodkas. Although he said he might not be as sharp as he would like, rarely did he become, in his terms, "pretty incoherent." However, he was beginning to feel "dreadful, sick, sweaty" on most mornings, and occasionally he would be unable to remember how he had reached his bed. Cocaine then began to be available in his social circle, and, before long, he discovered that this drug appeared to provide an antidote to some of the unwanted effects of alcohol. For instance, if he snorted (sniffed) cocaine a few times during the evening, "it lifted me up, I could go on drinking, it stopped me from passing out with the alcohol." He also found that a line or two of cocaine helped to alleviate the unpleasant early-morning symptoms caused by the previous night's drinking. Within a few months, he progressed from snorting to smoking crack cocaine, and his cocaine use rapidly and disastrously went out of control. His problem came to attention when he was arrested for possession of cocaine. Seen by a doctor at the request of his solicitor this man said: "OK, I'm addicted to cocaine but alcohol is not a problem."

This patient's history illustrates how another drug often lies behind the immediately presenting drug. It would be unprofitable in such circumstances to debate whether alcohol or cocaine was the "real" problem. This man's problem was his tendency to misuse substances. Both the alcohol and cocaine aspects of his history have to be taken seriously, but what the patient himself and those who are seeking to help him need to realize is that dependence can often resemble the many headed Hydra of mythology: one head can be lopped off and two grow in its place. With such a patient, unless there is a focus on the central issue of his tendency to develop dependence on substances, the story will all too

Table 7.1. Alcohol and other drug problems: key issues

- Polydrug use is common and indeed normative in many treatment settings.
- The majority of individuals dependent on illicit drugs have a co-occurring drinking problem.
- The majority of individuals diagnosed with alcohol dependence do not have a co-occurring illicit drug problem.
- Nicotine is the most common other drug used by people with drinking problems.
- Polydrug use is associated with significant physical and psychosocial morbidity.
- Clinicians and treatment services need the skills to meet mixed problems.

probably progress in terms of a further switching or mixing of different substances – in terms perhaps of tranquillizers or sleeping tablets then being added to alcohol.

This chapter describes some of the more frequently encountered connections between alcohol and other drug use (Table 7.1). It also considers the general implications both for prevention and for clinical practice that stem from the realization that alcohol and other drug problems potentially constitute one continuous domain rather than two distinct problem areas. Services may be set up or commissioned to manage alcohol problems without necessarily being skilled in or expected to deal with an individual's use of other substances. However, given the prevalence of polydrug use, all services should be able to manage *all* drug misuse or at least refer to and work collaboratively with another service.

Polydrug use

Polydrug use has become increasingly the norm over recent decades, even without including tobacco smoking. It occurs in the general population and is not confined to individuals heavily involved in the "drug scene" or in contact with treatment services. It has been accentuated by the rising availability of prescribed, abusable drugs, most notably opioids and benzodiazepines. Many factors are implicated in the initiation and perpetuation of other drug use in people who have drinking problems, and these can be considered under general headings such as psychological, socioeconomic, pharmacological, and genetic–environmental. Such factors do not occur in isolation but are often multiple and interrelated.

Polydrug use has been defined by the World Health Organization (1994) as the consumption of more than one psychoactive drug or drug class at the same time (concurrent use) or in succession (sequential use). Various patterns may exist for any given alcohol–drug combination. Assessment should tease out the relationship between alcohol and other drug use and how it may change during treatment. The interaction of alcohol with other drugs involves multiple risks of which patients should be made aware, most notably the potential for fatal respiratory depression from combined opioid and alcohol use (or heroin, alcohol, and benzodiazepines).

Polydrug use serves a number of purposes (Leri, Bruneau, & Stewart, 2003). Some drugs can enhance the effect of others, counteract or attenuate negative effects, or can be used as a substitute for another drug when it is not available. For instance, alcohol can enhance the effects of stimulants such as cocaine and amphetamines, and also the effects of benzodiazepines and volatile solvents. Alcohol can also reduce the jittery feelings associated with stimulant use and moderate the symptoms of the withdrawal phase or "crash." A heroin user may substitute with alcohol, cannabis, or benzodiazepines, either alone or in combination, to tide them over until heroin is again available. Thus, combinations and patterns of polydrug use vary according to the characteristics of users, the availability of drugs, peer influence and fashion, the context of drug use, and prescribing practices (European Monitoring Centre for Drugs and Drug Addiction, 2009). Consuming several drugs is not necessarily done in a haphazard fashion. Users make take drugs in a particular order and at particular relative doses specifically to achieve a desired effect. Aside from each drug interacting with the brain's chemistry to produce its effects, such polydrug use may also affect the pharmacokinetic properties of other drugs (e.g., augmenting plasma concentrations; Barrett, Darredeau, & Pihl, 2006). Although particular combinations may be seen quite commonly, some groups of patients (e.g., addicted healthcare professionals) may use rarer combinations because of their privileged access to a wide range of drugs.

Polydrug use can lead to significant medical, neuropsychological, and psychosocial complications, and thus it has a significant impact on public health. It is associated with increased risk-taking behaviours in multiple domains, thus increasing the risk of negative outcomes ranging from road traffic accidents to contracting and transmitting HIV, hepatitis, and other sexually transmitted infections. For instance, in UK HIV services, illicit drug use is associated with problem drinking and risky sexual practices (Daskalopoulou et al., 2014). Heavy drinking in former or current illicit drug users is common and is associated with a range of adverse health consequences. This is particularly true for those who are hepatitis C positive, in whom drinking may prevent the individual from being allowed to start treatment and may also increase damage to the liver. Most drug-related attendances to Emergency Rooms involve polydrug use, in particular the combination of alcohol and prescription drugs (McCabe, Cranford, & Boyd, 2006). Polydrug users are more likely to have psychiatric comorbidity (see Chapter 6).

In developed Western countries, alcohol and nicotine is the most common polydrug combination, followed by the addition of cannabis. This is particularly seen in younger people. For instance, in Kelly and colleagues' (2014) recent survey of 18- to 29-year-old Australian drinkers, the majority used alcohol only (51 percent), and 37 percent also smoked tobacco but had no other drug use. The remainder used alcohol, tobacco, and also illicit drugs. Kelly et al. noted that this profile had not changed substantially in the past half-decade. In South London residents over the age of 16, similar findings have been reported, with alcohol, cigarettes, and cannabis associated with the highest probability of polydrug use (Carter et al., 2013). A UK-wide study also reported that hazardous alcohol use and tobacco use were strongly associated with illicit polydrug use and that polydrug use was associated with adverse mental health outcomes, including suicide attempts (Smith, Farrell, Bunting, Houston, & Shevlin, 2011).

Similar patterns of polydrug use have been described in the United States. In addition to the use of alcohol, the use of cannabis and tobacco before the age of 16 was associated with problematic use of substances, including misuse of prescription drugs (Moss, Chen, & Yi, 2014). Another survey of adults revealed that about 10 percent of current drinkers also used cannabis in the past 12 months, with 7 percent using them together; tobacco use was not assessed (Midanik, Tam, & Weisner, 2007). Using alcohol and cannabis together was strongly associated with depression, alcohol dependence, and adverse social consequences. Interestingly, using both substances in the past 12 months but not at the same time was only associated with depression. This emphasizes that the impact of concurrent use may differ from sequential use due to drug interactions, an area that receives little research attention. After cannabis, the next most common group of drugs used were prescription painkillers, followed by illicit drugs such as cocaine. Other U.S. studies have reported the most common two-drug combinations are alcohol with either cocaine, cannabis, opiates, or sedatives (Kedia, Sell, & Relyea, 2007; Martin et al., 1996; Staines et al., 2001; Substance Abuse and Mental Health Services Administration, 2002).

These studies also illustrate that although cannabis has often been seen as the "gateway drug" (i.e., its use leads to further illicit drug use, such as heroin or cocaine), in fact use of tobacco or alcohol generally precedes cannabis use.

Many other drugs are used in combination with alcohol, including over-the-counter (OTC) medicines like paracetamol (acetaminophen) and the nonsteroidal anti-inflammatory drug (NSAID) ibuprofen. NSAIDs are associated with gastritis (inflammation of the stomach lining), as is alcohol, so this combination may result in indigestion/reflux and ultimately an ulcer and bleeding. Analgesics may help to relieve headache, musculoskeletal pain, or pain associated with pancreatitis or gout, but, after a time, simple aspirin and paracetamol/acetaminophen may not afford adequate pain relief, leading the drinker to progress to stronger analgesics, such as codeine or dihydrocodeine. High doses of analgesics can lead to both liver and renal problems, so the clinician should try to intervene before the patient – who may already have a compromised liver – ends up in intensive care with liver and renal failure.

Drinkers with chronic pancreatitis typically experience severe incapacitating pain and often seek opiate analgesia from their family doctor or hospital specialist. If these drinkers are economical with the truth or do not realize that their painkillers are opiate drugs, subsequent doctors may be unaware that they are obtaining such prescriptions for opioids. There is a real risk that when individuals with chronic pancreatitis or other chronic pain syndromes finally manage to become abstinent, they find that they are dependent on opioids.

Many drinkers complain of nonspecific pain in their joints, arms, and legs. It is important to take a history because the pain may have its origin in injuries sustained while intoxicated (e.g., due to a fist fight, a tumble down a flight of stairs, a violent alcohol withdrawal seizure, or an automobile accident). These patients may have little memory of the episode, relating, for instance, how "I woke up in intensive care with a mangled shoulder/leg/arm." The perceived pain from such injuries can be compounded by long periods of self-neglect, poor diet, and lack of exercise, and also from alcohol-induced myopathy.

Prescription drugs are increasingly also available without a prescription via the Internet and are typically used in a manner not intended by a prescribing doctor. They are also widely stolen out of medicine cabinets or begged from friends and family. Problem or dependent drinkers often use OTC or prescribed drugs to obtain relief from chronic conditions such as insomnia, pain, and perceived stress.

Adolescents and polydrug use

As described previously, early use of drugs including nicotine and alcohol is associated with increased likelihood of use of additional drugs. Use of drugs in the young also raises concern about impact on the developing brain. In adolescence, the reward and motivation system develops early and is active, whereas the frontal lobes that control such behaviour do not fully mature until the early-to-mid 20s. The developing brain appears much more sensitive to the effects of drugs, and exposure during this age may lead to long-lasting changes in the brain's connections.

The initiation of substance use in adolescents is heavily determined by environmental factors such as availability, price, social situation, peer group usage, and fashion (Han, McGue, & Iacono, 1999). Adolescents are prone to risk-taking behaviour. In moderation, this is part of healthy development. Indeed, adolescents who experiment a little are usually better adjusted as adults than are those who abstain completely. However, adolescent substance use is a powerful predictor of substance use disorders in adulthood (Grant & Dawson, 1997), and those with psychological traits such as impulsivity, alienation, and distress may be more vulnerable. Rates of tobacco, alcohol, and illicit drug use increase in the teenage years. Young people using one or more of these substances, especially alcohol, are more likely to use other substances subsequently. Teenagers with heavier drinking and smoking patterns are at greater risk of later drug use and dependence. Religious influences may help to attenuate the influence of substance use risk factors (Humphreys & Gifford, 2006). Drug fashions come and go, but alcohol is almost always implicated in the shifting picture of multiple substance use.

Recreational polydrug use is common in younger people in dance-club settings (the "clubbing scene"), and the drugs used here are typically alcohol, cannabis, and stimulants (including "legal highs") (European Monitoring Centre for Drugs and Drug Addiction, 2009; see later discussion). In young people, cocaine use is prevalent, particularly in the Republic of Ireland and the United Kingdom, and, therefore, its use with alcohol should be assessed. One survey of Irish adolescents revealed that cocaine was often first used whilst intoxicated with alcohol (Apantaku-Olajide, Darker, & Smyth, 2013). This is consistent with evidence from other surveys and emphasizes the importance of targeting adolescent alcohol drinking.

Older adults and polydrug use

The challenge of managing polydrug use in an increasingly elderly population is only beginning to be realized. Referred to as "invisible addicts" in a recent report, it was emphasized that mortality rates linked to drug and alcohol use are higher in older compared with younger people (Crome et al., 2011). There are also high rates of mental health problems in older people including, in particular, cognitive disorders. In this population, prescribed medication for a range of physical health problems is the norm. In addition, individuals may buy OTC medications as well as use a combination of licit and illicit substances. Such polypharmacy creates increased risk and a clinical challenge. Careful assessment is required to assess all possible licit, illicit, prescribed, and OTC drug use, and gentle but persistent questioning may be required.

The reasons underpinning starting substance misuse in later life are likely to include loss of a job, bereavement (e.g., of a spouse), retirement, or medical problems. Prognosis is generally better than for those with an earlier onset, but careful assessment is advisable before concluding that a late-life problem is truly new versus being an exacerbation of a long-standing but milder problem or one that can no longer be hidden (e.g., daytime drinking no longer being concealable from a spouse once the person has retired).

Specific drugs used by patients with drinking problems

The evidence base on the use of alcohol in combination with other drugs is better developed for epidemiologic research than for treatment research because substance use disorder treatment studies often focus on patients who have difficulties with only one substance

(Connor, Gullo, White, & Kelly, 2014; Humphreys, Blodgett, & Roberts, 2015). The next section thus puts more weight on the former, although some comments regarding treatment management are also offered. A more extended discussion of treatment strategies in presented in Chapter 13.

Alcohol and nicotine

As described, alcohol use and tobacco smoking is the most common substance use combination. Several psychological and neuropharmacological models have been proposed to explain the association between alcohol use disorders (AUDs) and tobacco smoking. Clinical and preclinical models have shown that use of either alcohol or nicotine may increase use of the other, and each can act as a conditioned cue for the other substance (McKee & Weinberger, 2013). Nicotinic receptors are key modulators of the dopaminergic reward mesolimbic system, and it has been suggested that the synergistic effects of alcohol and nicotine are due to their combined effect on this system. There may also be a common genetic vulnerability (Daeppen et al., 2000; Madden & Heath, 2002).

In general population epidemiological surveys, about 50 percent of alcohol dependent individuals smoke versus more than 80 percent in treatment populations (Kalman et al., 2011; McKee & Weinberger, 2013). Among smokers, alcohol dependence is 10 times more common than in nonsmokers. Nicotine dependence is associated with a greater severity of alcohol dependence and alcohol-related problems. Alcohol dependent individuals who smoke have high rates of tobacco-related disease, and they are more likely to die from tobacco-related disease than from their alcohol dependence. Some disorders are more common in those problem drinkers who also smoke, such as head and neck cancers, cirrhosis, and pancreatitis (Pelucchi et al., 2006). In addition, both alcohol and nicotine dependence are associated with mood and anxiety disorders (Le Strat, Ramoz, & Gorwood, 2010).

As described, cigarette use is strongly associated with alcohol and other drug use in adolescents. Such adolescents have an increased risk of having difficulties at school, delinquency, and use of other drugs (Myers & Kelly, 2006). Young adults who smoke are also more likely to report binge drinking (McKee & Weinberger, 2013). Young people who are treated for alcohol and other drug use are typically heavy smokers, and smoking tends to persist after treatment.

There is a wealth of evidence and guidelines about stopping tobacco smoking (e.g., Fiore et al., 2009; Lingford-Hughes, Welch, Peters, Nutt, & BAP Group, 2012; NICE, 2013) but little for comorbid alcohol use and tobacco smoking. In part, the problem stems from tobacco cessation researchers having the disappointing habit of excluding patients with drinking problems from clinical trials (Lembke & Humphreys, 2015), which leaves clinicians in the dark about how to handle this common comorbidity.

Many people take the approach of "one vice at a time" when thinking about dealing with their tobacco smoking and problem drinking. However, given that use of one drug can increase the use of the other and that use of either drug can trigger relapse among individuals who have stopped using the other, is it better to give both up simultaneously? Alcohol dependent individuals are open to advice on smoking (Harris et al., 2000). In discussing what approach to take with a patient, clinicians should explore how they smoke and drink; for example, always together? Or, if the patient cannot drink, do they smoke more? Given the adverse health consequences, all patients who smoke should receive advice about quitting smoking or at least reducing. There are reports of increased smoking to compensate for not drinking, so this should be monitored. A meta-analysis of concurrent tobacco and alcohol treatment compared with alcohol-only treatment reported higher abstinence rates from alcohol with concurrent treatments (Prochaska, Delucchi, & Hall, 2004). Smoking cessation interventions have been reported to result in low quit rates in alcohol dependent individuals. However, these trials were primarily done prior to widespread smoke-free policies. In-patient units are now smoke-free, and nicotine replacement therapy (NRT) can be offered during the course of the medically assisted withdrawal programme and thereafter. The spread of smoke-free policies in places where people drink (e.g., pubs, restaurants) may have contributed to a reduction in the onset of alcohol abuse in the population and reduced drinking by heavy drinkers (McKee & Weinberger, 2013).

The use of e-cigarettes containing nicotine (they can also be used to consume cannabis) is increasing, both by those using it as a substitute for smoking when in smoke-free areas and by those trying to quit. Because e-cigarettes are seen as safe, some may start to use them who otherwise would not have started tobacco smoking, including adolescents. The debate about regulations that should be in place for e-cigarettes is under way. The relationship between e-cigarettes and alcohol abuse is not yet clear.

Whilst counselling with or without NRT is the most common approach to quit or reduce tobacco smoking, there are other medications available. These all have been shown to be effective (Lingford-Hughes et al., 2012; NICE, 2013). Bupropion, an atypical antidepressant that is licensed as an aid for smoking cessation, has been shown to be effective in a few small studies, including those enrolling individuals with a history of major depression and alcoholism (Hayford et al., 1999) and recently abstinent alcohol dependent individuals (Karam-Hage, Strobbe, Robinson, & Brower, 2011). Adding bupropion to a nicotine patch did not improve smoking outcomes in abstinent alcohol dependent individuals (Kalman et al., 2011) compared with nicotine patch alone. Varenicline is another medication shown to be effective in smoking cessation (Lingford-Hughes et al., 2012; NICE, 2013). It is a partial agonist at the alpha$_4$beta$_2$ nicotinic receptor that modulates the mesolimbic dopaminergic reward pathway as well as processes involved in memory and learning. Varenicline has also been investigated as a treatment for alcoholism and could therefore have particular utility in comorbid alcohol and nicotine dependence (Nocente et al., 2013).

Alcohol and stimulants

The combination of alcohol and a stimulant such as cocaine, amphetamine, methamphetamine, or ecstasy is a not uncommon pattern of polydrug use. For instance, cocaine use in heavy drinkers increases the risk of developing alcohol dependence fourfold, with more frequent cocaine use associated with more rapid progression (Rubio et al., 2008). Greater alcohol use and greater levels of psychological problems are seen in those who are alcohol dependent and use cocaine (Heil, Badger, & Higgins, 2001). Similarly, in young people, it has been reported that alcohol is used in greater quantities with cocaine than when it is used alone (Barrett et al., 2006). Binge drinking in young people is associated with stimulant intoxication, where the stimulant could be cocaine, ecstasy, amphetamine, or methamphetamine (McKetin, Chalmers, Sunderland, & Bright, 2014).

Cocaine may be taken by different routes, such as snorting it in powder form, injecting liquefied cocaine, or smoking "crack cocaine." Generally, the use of crack cocaine is associated with a higher degree of physical dependence on the drug. Those who smoke crack cocaine and drink alcohol tend to be older with lower education and employment levels compared with those who snort cocaine and drink alcohol (Gossop, Manning, & Ridge, 2006). Improving sociability has been cited as a motivation for concurrent alcohol drinking and snorting cocaine but not for smoking crack cocaine (Martin, Macdonald, Pakula, & Roth, 2014).

Whereas much concurrent use may be unplanned, alcohol and stimulants may be used together intentionally for a variety of differing reasons. Consuming alcohol during a cocaine binge may prolong the euphoriant effects of cocaine, diminish the unpleasant experiences associated with cocaine use (e.g., agitation and paranoia), provide sedation, and ameliorate the dysphoria associated with withdrawal and early abstinence from cocaine (the "crash"). Alternatively, cocaine or other stimulants such as amphetamine appear to attenuate the intoxicating and sedative effects of alcohol, thus allowing drinkers to drink more alcohol and tolerate these considerable quantities without becoming obviously intoxicated. The Friday night drinking session can be extended over a weekend and only comes to an end on Sunday night as the working week looms nearer. Once regular cocaine and alcohol use is established, it may be difficult to give up one substance without giving up the other because alcohol can become a powerful conditioned cue for cocaine.

Cocaethylene, a pharmacologically active metabolite, is formed when cocaine and alcohol are taken together. It enhances and extends cocaine-induced euphoria and also increases heart rate and blood pressure. Cocaethylene is formed in the liver and, not surprisingly, greater levels are formed from taking cocaine orally compared with routes with less hepatic involvement (i.e., injecting or smoking; Herbst et al., 2011).

For many patients, treatment of the cocaine problem leads to an improvement in the alcohol problem. However, the presence of alcohol problems and dependence in treated cocaine users is associated with more severe dependence, poorer retention in treatment, and a poorer outcome compared with either disorder alone (Brady et al., 1995; Carroll, Power, Bryant, & Rounsaville, 1993; Carroll, Rounsaville, & Bryant, 1993). Because no medication has been robustly shown to treat cocaine addiction, psychosocial interventions such as contingency management are the mainstay of treatment (Lingford-Hughes et al., 2012). There is limited evidence to guide what might be the best course of treatment for comorbid alcohol and cocaine misuse. Treatment with disulfiram for 12 weeks was reported to be associated with better treatment retention and abstinence, particularly when combined with "active" out-patient psychotherapy (cognitive behavioural coping skills and therapy) and 12-step facilitation (Carroll et al., 1998, 2000; Lingford-Hughes et al., 2012). Disulfiram in combination with naltrexone has been shown to be more likely to result in abstinence from cocaine and alcohol, although the difference was not statistically different from either drug alone in this trial, and adherence was low (Pettinati et al., 2008).

Alcohol and cannabis

Cannabis is the most commonly used drug worldwide after alcohol and nicotine. As its legal status and availability changes in some parts of the world, it will be interesting to see how cannabis use alters in response. The main intoxicating effects of cannabis are due to delta-tetrahydrocannabinol (THC). "Skunk" and butane hash oil are particular forms of cannabis with higher THC levels. Simultaneous use of alcohol and cannabis is common in adolescents, and this may have detrimental effects on brain development including predisposition to more severe cannabis- or alcohol-dependence symptoms. Alcohol and cannabis may alter each other's absorption, although evidence is mixed on whether the combined impact on impairment (e.g., driving ability) is multiplicative or additive (Hartman et al., 2015; National Highway Traffic Safety Administration, 1999). Simultaneous use can sometimes be unpleasant, with individuals experiencing nausea, vomiting, dizziness, and sweating. This most likely occurs because alcohol speeds up the absorption of THC, leading to a stronger cannabis effect. Alcohol and cannabis are often used when "coming down" from ecstasy.

A number of synthetic cannabis-like compounds are available as "legal highs" via the Internet or through "head shops" (see the section on novel psychoactive substances). Often containing the name "spice," some of these products appear quite potent and may have more than cannabis-like compounds in them. As with stimulants, psychosocial approaches are the mainstay of treatment of cannabis misuse. Cognitive-behavioural, motivational enhancement, and contingency management approaches can all be helpful for reducing use (Babor, 2004).

Alcohol and opioids

Alcohol and opioids can engage in a complex dance in the lives of those who use both simultaneously or at different times of life, as this case extract illustrates:

> A 34-year-old unemployed man was referred for assessment of his heavy drinking and depression. He had experienced extreme emotional deprivation in childhood and had been in care. At 14, he began to drink beer and smoke cannabis "for comfort." His daily alcohol consumption gradually increased to 3–4 cans of strong lager, and he began to experiment with mixing it with opioid medications that he stole from his parents' and friends' medicine cabinets. He first smoked heroin in his early 20s and very soon switched to intravenous use, sharing needles. He experienced multiple alcohol-opioid overdoses in his late 20s, including one that was nearly fatal. When he was 30, he entered a residential rehabilitation unit and gave up all illicit drug use. However, his alcohol consumption escalated, and, 4 years later, at the time of referral, his drinking was out of control. He was also experiencing a marked craving for heroin and was worried that he would begin using it again.

Problematic use of alcohol is a common problem in opioid users. Alcohol consumption typically precedes first use of heroin in the early career of heroin addicts, but levels of alcohol use tend to drop off when regular opioid use is established. Alcohol problems may substitute for opioids when heroin users attempt to detoxify on their own or enter a treatment programme, or during prolonged periods of abstinence. A seemingly promising recovery from a drug problem can be brought down by alcohol if, for example, a patient on methadone maintenance overdoses due to a drinking binge. Relative to those patients whose dependence is confined to opioids, opioid-dependent patients who go on to develop alcohol problems are more likely to have had disruptive childhoods, more legal problems and polydrug use, more problems with social functioning, and higher rates of psychiatric disorders.

Concomitant use of alcohol and opioids heightens risk of overdose. This risk is even more pronounced if the individual also uses benzodiazepines. Many "opioid overdoses" are in fact alcohol-opioid overdose, benzodiazepine-opioid overdoses, or benzodiazepine-alcohol-opioid overdoses (Darke, Degenhardt, & Mattick, 2007).

Treatment of opiate dependence generally involves use of opiate substitute medication, most commonly methadone or buprenorphine (with or without naloxone). Both medications reduce the intoxicating effect of opioids, and some addicts may respond by looking for another intoxicating substance. Up to a third of individuals in methadone maintenance programmes are alcohol dependent, in addition to a similar proportion drinking in a hazardous or harmful manner (Otomanelli, 1999; Srivastava, Kahan, & Ross, 2008). In methadone maintenance programmes, alcohol misuse is commonly associated with poorer outcomes, nonadherence with methadone, and greater physical and mental health complications (Roux et al., 2014; Srivastava et al., 2008). Although the majority of studies do not show an increase in alcohol consumption during methadone maintenance, many trials do not show a reduction either (Srivastava et al., 2008). Relative to methadone, buprenorphine may currently be used clinically to treat less complex opiate-addicted individuals, which may be the reason that alcohol dependence has been reported not to affect the outcome of buprenorphine maintenance (Dreifuss et al., 2013). Treating alcohol and opiate comorbidity is challenging, with thorough initial assessment of both substances used and early intervention critical. Despite how commonly this comorbidity is encountered and its significant associated harms, there is limited evidence available to guide treatment. It is also not uncommon for opiate substitution programmes to have insufficiently developed strategies to deal with alcohol misuse compared with illicit heroin use.

Alcohol and benzodiazepines

Benzodiazepines were introduced to clinical practice in 1960 and soon became widely used in the treatment of anxiety and insomnia. They are also accepted as the treatment of choice for medically assisted alcohol detoxification (see Chapter 11). A wide variety of benzodiazepines have been marketed, and Table 7.2 lists the commoner substances, giving both their official and trade names. Whereas the anxiolytic or sedative effects of different benzodiazepines may not differ substantially, important differences exist in relation to the duration of action either of the drug itself or of its active metabolite. Lorazepam, oxazepam, and temazepam are all relatively short-acting; chlordiazepoxide and diazepam are long-acting, whereas the other benzodiazepines listed in Table 7.2 produce an action of intermediate duration. It must also be remembered that benzodiazepines are now often available to buy illegally via the Internet, where the dose and constituents are unknown and unregulated, thus providing a possible clinical challenge in care management.

In many countries, including the UK, prescriptions for benzodiazepines as anxiolytics have fallen over the past two decades, whereas prescriptions for their use as hypnotics are little changed. In contrast, benzodiazepine prescribing has soared in the United States in recent years. Despite warnings about their prescription, particularly for long-term use, benzodiazepines continue to be widely prescribed, with highest prevalence in the elderly (Crome et al., 2011; Olfson, King, & Schoenbaum, 2015). This is despite the well-documented risk of reduced mobility and driving skills and increased falls and confusion in older adults. Shorter-acting benzodiazepines at high doses are associated with amnesia. And, as mentioned, benzodiazepines and alcohol are often important factors in fatal overdose.

Table 7.2. Some common benzodiazepines

Nonproprietary name	Proprietary name (common)	Active metabolites	Approximate half-life	Approximate equivalent dose (mg)
Diazepam	Valium	Several	2–4 days	5
Chlordiazepoxide	Librium	Several	2–4 days	12.5
Nitrazepam	Mogadon	None	12–24 hours	5
Clonazepam	Rivotril, Klonopin	Several	1–2 days	0.25
Lorazepam	Ativan	None	8–12 hours	0.5
Temazepam	Normison, Restoril	None	8 hours	10
Oxazepam	Oxanid	None	8–12 hours	10
Alprazolam	Xanax	Several	12 15 hours	0.25

Source: Joint Formulary Committee, British National Formulary (2015)

Prescribing benzodiazepines other than for alcohol detoxification is controversial in alcohol dependence; in general, they should not be used. Better and safer pharmacological (e.g., selective serotonin reuptake inhibitors [SSRIs]) and psychosocial (e.g., CBT) alternative treatments are recommended over benzodiazepines for conditions such as anxiety or insomnia. Some individuals with alcohol problems may be taking benzodiazepines for their anxiety or insomnia, but this is risky unless they take them exactly as prescribed. This distinction must be sought at assessment in order to inform an appropriate management plan. Benzodiazepine misuse may not be as widespread in those with alcohol dependence as many people fear (Chick & Nutt, 2012; Ciraulo & Nace, 2000; Ciraulo, Sands, & Shader, 1988). Their use does not appear to increase the risk of alcohol misuse or relapse. Although not advocating widespread prescribing of benzodiazepines, in specialist services, there may be some patients (e.g., terminally ill, end-stage liver failure) whose alcohol consumption may benefit from careful use of a benzodiazepine.

Treatment of comorbid alcohol and benzodiazepine misuse or dependency requires consultation with the patient about the best approach. For comorbid dependence, alcohol and benzodiazepine detoxification may be undertaken simultaneously or in series, with the alcohol detoxification first. When benzodiazepines are used in a "binge" pattern (large quantities not on a daily basis), individuals may not be dependent. A benzodiazepine detoxification may not be required in this situation, and prescribing a benzodiazepine substitute should only be initiated after careful consideration. Misuse of other drugs, such as opioids, is generally also present. An in-patient admission may therefore be required to fully assess an individual's polydrug use and to develop an appropriate treatment plan.

Alcohol and Z-drugs

The "Z-drugs" are commonly used sleeping tablets and include zolpidem (Ambien, Stilnoct; time to peak levels ~2½ hrs), zopiclone (Zimovane; ~2 hrs), and zaleplon (Sonata; ~ 1hr). They are putatively nonbenzodiazepine medications, but they target the benzodiazepine receptor in the brain. Like benzodiazepines, only short-term use of Z-drugs is recommended. They can be purchased on the Internet and have abuse potential.

There is limited evidence on the prevalence of Z-drug misuse, although dependence has been reported (Lingford-Hughes et al., 2012). They are recommended for short-term treatment of insomnia (NICE, 2004). There is limited evidence about how Z-drugs may be used alongside alcohol, but it is appropriate to apply the same principles as set out earlier for benzodiazepines.

Alcohol and "club drugs": Novel psychoactive substances

The term "club drugs" describes psychoactive drugs used in clubs and at raves, music festivals, and other venues. They include a wide range of substances with differing pharmacology and effects. They include illicit drugs such as MDMA, cocaine, gamma-hydroxybutyrate (GHB), ketamine, and mephedrone, as well as so-called "legal highs" such as "benzofury."

There are six main groups of novel psychoactive substances (NPS): synthetic cannabinoids, synthetic cathinones, ketamine, phenethylamines, piperazines, and plant-based substances, as well as seventh group of miscellaneous substances. New drugs emerge regularly, with the number of NPS on the global market more than doubling during 2009–13 (United Nations Office on Drugs and Crime, 2014).

Given the range of drugs, their potential interactions with alcohol, and the fact that new ones appear regularly, clinicians should ask specifically about these drugs at assessment: their names, how they are used, and why. For most NPS, there is no test available to check for their presence, and thus management of any suspected clinical presentation such as intoxication or withdrawal relies on symptomatic treatment (e.g., for agitation, sedation, etc.). Helping patients to reduce or quit this group of drugs is mainly through using psychosocial approaches, although for some of these substances (e.g., GBH), medication is required to safely manage withdrawal.

Some combinations, such as GHB and alcohol, are associated with high risk of overdose and respiratory depression. On the other hand, the sodium salt of GHB, sodium oxybate, is licensed in some countries for the treatment of alcohol dependence and has been used to treat alcohol withdrawal and for relapse prevention. Ketamine is another club drug sometimes used in combination with alcohol that has therapeutic potential in other contexts (as an anaesthetic and perhaps as a treatment for depression as well).

Alcohol and nonmedical use of prescription drugs

Research in the United States has shown that nonmedical use of prescription opioids, stimulants, tranquillizers, and sedatives is more prevalent among individuals with AUDs (McCabe et al., 2006). Most of this polydrug use is simultaneous use. Young adults (18–24 years), particularly those with a history of binge drinking or alcohol dependence, showed higher past-year prevalence rates for such medication than did adults older than

Table 7.3. Tips for clinicians

- Have a good working knowledge of alcohol and other drugs.
- Always take a complete alcohol and other drug history.
- Update history regularly.
- Organize spot urinary or oral fluid drug screens where indicated.

25 years of age. Clinicians should ensure that when young people with alcohol problems present for treatment a thorough drug history is taken. Further work is needed to understand the associated individual and situational risk factors.

Two new medications, gabapentin and pregabalin, have recently been introduced to treat peripheral and central neuropathic pain, fibromyalgia, partial epilepsy, and generalized anxiety disorder. As an alternative to opioids or benzodiazepines, they appear attractive to prescribers when considering how to manage these conditions in addicted patients. However, there are increasing anecdotal reports of their abuse and misuse alone and with alcohol; therefore, prescribing should be considered and monitored carefully (Schifano, 2014). In addition, they are being studied as a treatment for alcohol dependence, withdrawal, and relapse prevention, as well as other dependencies (see Chapters 11 and 13).

Alcohol and other drugs as one domain: The practical implications

As has already been described, polydrug use raises fundamental questions about the nature of addiction (West, 2001). Should dependence be viewed as a condition that spans more than one substance instead of multiple substance-specific conditions residing in the same person (Gossop, 2001; West, 2001)? This has profound implications for treatment. For instance, should we routinely try to help alcohol dependent individuals in recovery to quit smoking, too?

Several of the most immediate implications of this perspective have already been discussed in earlier sections of this chapter. At this point, it may, however, be useful to bring together the core implications; in Table 7.3 we draw attention to some matters of special clinical relevance.

Implications for training and service organization

Anyone taking professional responsibility for the treatment of alcohol problems should recognize that polydrug use is pervasive, and the alcohol treatment clinician should possess a good working knowledge of other drug problems (and vice versa). There may be a continuing place for specialized drug or specialized alcohol treatment services, but the intensity of specialization must not be of such a degree as to be out of tune with clinical realities. For many problem drinkers who enter treatment, their medical and psychosocial comorbidity cannot be understood on the basis of their alcohol consumption/dependence alone. Clinical assessment must take into account the complexities of any polydrug use, and the treatment intervention must be tailored accordingly. Many of these individuals also have anxiety, depression, post-traumatic stress disorder (PTSD), and other psychiatric disorders, and may present, in the first instance, to general psychiatric services. Psychiatric services should also be able to assess individuals with polydrug use and factor this into their treatment programmes.

Working with polydrug users requires cross-discipline liaison and collaboration. Complex patients with complex problems do not always respect specialist demarcations. Inadequate training may mean that individuals with combined alcohol and other drug problems, particularly those who also have psychiatric comorbidity, find it difficult to obtain treatment, are incompletely evaluated and treated, and are effectively abandoned because they don't meet rigid criteria for treatment services. However, this is a cop-out for services. Treatment services wishing to face the challenge of polydrug use successfully must develop the capacity to integrate alcohol, drug, and psychiatric treatment to meet the needs of these complex individuals.

A prime responsibility for prevention

Clinicians who treat patients with drinking problems have a special responsibility not to do their patients damage through the careless prescription of sedatives and minor tranquillizers. It is likewise important that anyone treating opioid-dependent patients should advise them on use of alcohol and the dangers of binge or harmful use with heroin, as well as alcohol-dependence itself. At the very least, it is important to provide alcohol and drug users with information on the effects of specific drugs and combinations of drugs and, in particular, how to manage emergencies (European Monitoring Centre for Drugs and Drug Addiction, 2009).

Diagnosis and screening

With a patient whose presenting problem is with one type of substance, an open eye should be kept on the possible existence of problems with other drugs. It is, for instance, less than useful to concentrate exclusively on a patient's drinking while failing to detect the fact that massive quantities of benzodiazepines or cannabis are being consumed.

A complete alcohol and other drug use history should be obtained, remembering that relevant drugs can also be bought via the Internet or head shops as well as prescribed. The evolution of use and dependence for every drug taken should be charted, including alcohol. In this way, the sequence and pattern of alcohol and other drug use can be mapped out: for example, solvents as a child, alcohol and later amphetamines in the teenage years, cocaine and heroin as an adult. A history of the combinations of drugs used should be taken (alcohol and cannabis, alcohol and cigarettes, alcohol and cocaine, and so on). It will be helpful to work out whether the scale of drug(s) used amounts to dependence or not. Polydrug users who are dependent on one or two drugs may use other drugs in a problematic but nondependent way. When presenting for treatment, these patients can be clear in their minds as to which drugs are currently posing the greatest problems and, when asked, are able to rank them in a hierarchical fashion. This may be different to your view as their clinician. Therefore, sensitive clinical engagement will be required to use and possibly modify their perspective to map out a workable treatment plan.

Many clients presenting to alcohol services may have a history of intravenous drug use and will need assessment of risk behaviour and counselling with respect to testing for hepatitis B and C and HIV status. Routine urine or oral fluid testing should be more widely employed. The history should be updated at regular intervals.

Treatment goals

As discussed, polydrug use is generally more difficult to treat than an uncomplicated AUD, with the possible exception of comorbid tobacco smoking. Staff should be trained to deal with polydrug users and their problems, and services should focus on behaviour rather than on substances. Although there is little research on what treatments are effective, therapists working within treatment programmes that take the concept of chemical dependence as a central tenet would probably advise a patient who has encountered difficulties, with either alcohol or other drugs, to avoid all nonprescribed mood-altering chemicals for ever after. For many patients, this is the best advice, although it is unlikely to be acceptable for all (some former heroin addicts may, for instance, later use alcohol moderately and safely). The insistence that patients should be made aware of the dangers of crossing over from one substance to another is very appropriate. It should also be recognized that some patients may not want to tackle the totality of their polydrug use. For those individuals, it is important to set out the risks and to continue to work with them so that they are in the best position to take responsibility for their drug use, to the point where they may agree ultimately to come off everything.

A constant two-way vigilance

When seeing a patient or client for the first time, when planning and carrying through a treatment programme and when assessing success, the patient and clinician should be thinking in terms of alcohol and other drugs and not just alcohol or just other drugs.

References

Apantaku-Olajide, T., Darker, C. D., & Smyth, B. P. (2013). Onset of cocaine use: Associated alcohol intoxication and psychosocial characteristics among adolescents in substance abuse treatment. *Journal of Addiction Medicine*, **7**, 183–188.

Babor, T. F. (2004). Brief treatments for cannabis dependence: Findings from a randomized multisite trial. *Journal of Consulting and Clinical Psychology*, **72**(3), 455.

Barrett, S. P., Darredeau, C., & Pihl, R. O. (2006). Patterns of simultaneous polysubstance use in drug using university students. *Human Psychopharmacology: Clinical and Experimental*, **21**, 255–263.

Brady, K. T., Sonne, E., Randall, C. L., Adinoff, B., & Malcolm, R. (1995). Features of cocaine dependence with concurrent alcohol use. *Drug and Alcohol Dependence*, **39**, 69–71.

Carroll, K. M., Nich, C., Ball, S. A., McCance, E., & Rounsavile, B. J. (1998). Treatment of cocaine and alcohol dependence with psychotherapy and disulfiram. *Addiction*, **93**, 713–728.

Carroll, K. M., Nich, C., Ball, S. A., McCance, E., Frankforter, T. L., & Rounsaville, B. J. (2000). One-year follow-up of disulfiram and psychotherapy for cocaine-alcohol users: Sustained effects of treatment. *Addiction*, **95**, 1335–1349.

Carroll, K. M., Power, M. -E. D., Bryant, K., & Rounsaville B. (1993). One-year follow-up status of treatment-seeking cocaine abusers. *Journal of Nervous and Mental Disease*, **181**, 71–79.

Carroll, K. M., Rounsaville, B. J., & Bryant, K. J. (1993). Alcoholism in treatment seeking cocaine abusers: Clinical and prognostic significance. *Journal of Studies on Alcohol*, **54**, 199–208.

Carter, J. L., Strang, J., Frissa, S., Hayes, R. D., SELCoH Study Team, Hatch, S. L., & Hotopf, M. (2013). Comparisons of polydrug use at national and inner city levels in England: Associations with demographic and socioeconomic factors. *Annals of Epidemiology*, **23**, 636–45.

Chick, J., & Nutt, D. J. (2012). Substitution therapy for alcoholism: Time for a reappraisal? *Journal of Psychopharmacology*, **26**(2), 205–212.

Ciraulo, D. A., & Nace, E. P. (2000). Benzodiazepine treatment of anxiety or insomnia in substance abuse patients. *American Journal on Addictions*, **9**(4), 276–284.

Ciraulo, D. A., Sands, B. F., & Shader, R. I. (1988). Critical review of liability for benzodiazepine abuse among alcoholics. *American Journal of Psychiatry*, **145**, 1501–1506.

Connor, J. P., Gullo, M. J., White, A., & Kelly, A. B. (2014). Polysubstance use: Diagnostic challenges, patterns of use and health. *Current Opinion in Psychiatry*, **27**, 269–75

Crome, I., Brown, A., Dar, K., Janikiewicz, S., Rao, T., & Tarbuck, A. (2011). *Our invisible addicts: First report of the Older Persons' Substance Misuse Working Group of the Royal College of Psychiatrists.* London: Royal College of Psychiatrists.

Daeppen, J. -B., Smith, T. L., Danko, G. P., Gordon, L., Landi, N. A., Nurnberger J. I. Jr, ... Schuckit, M. A. (2000). Clinical correlates of cigarette smoking and nicotine dependence in alcohol dependent men and women. *Alcohol and Alcoholism*, **35**, 171–175.

Darke, S., Degenhardt, L., & Mattick, R. (2007). *Mortality amongst illicit drug users: Epidemiology, causes and intervention.* Cambridge: Cambridge University Press.

Daskalopoulou, M., Rodger, A., Phillips, A. N., Sherr, L., Speakman, A., Collins, S., ... Lampe, F. C. (2014). Recreational drug use, polydrug use, and sexual behaviour in HIV-diagnosed men who have sex with men in the UK: Results from the cross-sectional ASTRA study. *Lancet HIV*, **1**, e22–e31.

Dreifuss, J. A., Griffin, M. L., Frost, K., Fitzmaurice, G. M., Potter, J. S., Fiellin, D. A., ... Weiss, R. D. (2013). Patient characteristics associated with buprenorphine/naloxone treatment outcome for prescription opioid dependence: Results from a multisite study. *Drug and Alcohol Dependence*, **131**(1), 112–118.

European Monitoring Centre for Drugs and Drug Addiction. (2009). *Polydrug use: Patterns and responses.* Luxembourg: Office for Official Publications of the European Communities.

Fiore, M. C., Jaén, C. R., Baker, T. B., Bailey, W. C., Bennett, G., Benowitz, N. L., ... Williams, C. (2009). *Treating tobacco use and dependence: 2008 Update. Quick reference guide for clinicians.* Rockville, MD: U.S. Department of Health and Human Services.

Gossop, M. (2001). A web of dependence. *Addiction*, **96**, 677–678.

Gossop, M., Manning, V., & Ridge, G. (2006). Concurrent use of alcohol and cocaine: Differences in patterns of use and problems among users of crack cocaine and cocaine powder. *Alcohol and Alcoholism*, **41**, 121–125.

Grant, B., & Dawson, D. (1997). Age at onset of alcohol use and its association with DSM-IV alcohol abuse and dependence: Results from the National Longitudinal Alcohol Epidemiologic Survey. *Journal of Substance Abuse*, **9**, 103–110.

Han, C., McGue, M. K., & Iacono, W. G. (1999). Lifetime tobacco, alcohol and other substance use in adolescent Minnesota twins: Univariate and multivariate behavioural genetic analyses. *Addiction*, **94**, 981–993.

Harris, J., Best, D., Man, L. H., Welch, S., Gossop, M., & Strang, J. (2000). Change in cigarette smoking among alcohol and drug misusers during in-patient detoxification. *Addiction Biology*, **5**, 443–450.

Hartman, R., Brown, T., Milavetz, G., Spurgin, A., Pierce, R. S., Gorelick D. A., Gaffney, G., & Huestis, M. A. (2015). Cannabis effects on driving lateral control with and without alcohol. *Drug and Alcohol Dependence*, **154**, 25–37

Hayford, K. E., Patten, C. A., Rummans, T. A., Schroeder, D. R., Offord, K. P., Croghan, I. T., ... Hurt, R. D. (1999). Efficacy of bupropion for smoking cessation in smokers with a former history of major depression or alcoholism. *British Journal of Psychiatry*, **174**, 173–178.

Heil, S. H., Badger, G. J., & Higgins, S. T. (2001). Alcohol dependence among cocaine-dependent outpatients: Demographics, drug use, treatment outcome and other characteristics. *Journal of Studies on Alcohol*, **62**, 14–22.

Herbst, E. D., Harris, D. S., Everhart, E. T., Mendelson, J., Jacob, P., & Jones, R. T. (2011). Cocaethylene formation following ethanol and cocaine administration by different routes. *Experimental and Clinical Psychopharmacology*, **19**, 95–104.

Humphreys, K., Blodgett, J. C., & Roberts, L. W. (2015). The exclusion of people with psychiatric disorders from medical research. *Journal of Psychiatric Research*, **70**, 28–32.

Humphreys, K., & Gifford, E. (2006). Religion, spirituality and the troublesome use of substances. In W. R. Miller & K. Carroll (Eds.), *Rethinking substance abuse: What the science shows and what we should do about it* (pp. 257–274). New York: Guilford.

Joint Formulary Committee. (2015). *British National Formulary (BNF) 69*. London: BMJ Publishing Group Ltd and Royal Pharmaceutical Society.

Kalman, D., Herz, L., Monti, P., Kahler, C. W., Mooney, M., Rodrigues, S., & O'Connor, K. (2011). Incremental efficacy of adding bupropion to the nicotine patch for smoking cessation in smokers with a recent history of alcohol dependence: Results from a randomized, double-blind, placebo-controlled study. *Drug and Alcohol Dependence*, **118**, 111–118.

Karam-Hage, M., Strobbe, S., Robinson, J. D., & Brower, K. J. (2011). Bupropion-SR for smoking cessation in early recovery from alcohol dependence: A placebo-controlled, double-blind pilot study. *American Journal of Drug and Alcohol Abuse*, **37**, 487–490.

Kedia, S., Sell, M. A., & Relyea, G. (2007). Mono-versus polydrug abuse patterns among publicly funded clients. *Substance Abuse Treatment, Prevention and Policy*, **2**, 33.

Kelly, A. B., Chan, G. C., White, A., Saunders, J. B., Baker, P. J., & Connor, J. P. (2014). Is there any evidence of changes in patterns of concurrent drug use among young Australians 18–29 years between 2007 and 2010?. *Addictive Behaviors*, **39**(8), 1249–1252.

Lembke, A., & Humphreys, K. (2015). A call to include people with mental illness and substance use disorders alongside "regular" smokers in smoking cessation research. *Tobacco Control*. Advance online publication. doi:10.1136/tobaccocontrol-2014-052215

Leri, F., Bruneau, J., & Stewart, J. (2003). Understanding polydrug use: Review of heroin and cocaine co-use. *Addiction*, **98**, 7–22.

Le Strat, Y., Ramoz, N., & Gorwood, P. (2010). In alcohol-dependent drinkers, what does the presence of nicotine dependence tell us about psychiatric and addictive disorders comorbidity? *Alcohol and Alcoholism*, **45**(2), 167–172.

Lingford-Hughes, A. R., Welch, S., Peters, L., Nutt, D. J., & British Association for Psychopharmacology, Expert Reviewers Group. (2012). BAP updated guidelines: Evidence-based guidelines for the pharmacological management of substance abuse, harmful use, addiction and comorbidity: Recommendations from BAP. *Journal of Psychopharmacology*, **26**, 899–952.

Madden, P. A., & Heath, A. C. (2002). Shared genetic vulnerability in alcohol and cigarette use dependence. *Alcoholism: Clinical and Experimental Research*, **26**, 1919–1921.

Martin, C. S., Clifford, P. R., Maisto, S. A., Earleywine, M., Kirisci, L., & Longabaugh, R. (1996). Polydrug use in an inpatient treatment sample of problem drinkers. *Alcoholism: Clinical and Experimental Research*, **20**, 413–417.

Martin, G., Macdonald, S., Pakula, B., & Roth, E. A. (2014). A comparison of motivations for use among users of crack cocaine and cocaine powder in a sample of simultaneous cocaine and alcohol users. *Addictive Behaviors*, **39**, 699–702.

McCabe, S. E., Cranford, J. A., & Boyd, C. J. (2006). The relationship between past-year drinking behaviours and non-medical use of prescription drugs: Prevalence of co-occurrence in a national sample. *Drug and Alcohol Dependence*, **84**, 281–288.

McKee, S. A., & Weinberger, A. H. (2013). How can we use our knowledge of alcohol-tobacco interactions to reduce alcohol use? *Annual Review of Clinical Psychology*, **9**, 649–674.

McKetin, R., Chalmers, J., Sunderland, M., & Bright, D. A. (2014). Recreational drug use and binge drinking: Stimulant but not cannabis intoxication is associated with excessive alcohol consumption. *Drug and Alcohol Review*, **33**, 436–445.

Midanik, L. T., Tam, T. W., & Weisner, C. (2007). Concurrent and simultaneous drug and alcohol use: Results of the 2000 National Alcohol Survey. *Drug and Alcohol Dependence*, **90**, 72–80.

Moss, H. B., Chen, C. M., & Yi, H. Y. (2014). Early adolescent patterns of alcohol, cigarettes, and marijuana polysubstance use and young adult substance use outcomes in a nationally representative sample. *Drug and Alcohol Dependence*, **136**, 51–62.

Myers, M. G., & Kelly, J. F. (2006). Cigarette smoking among adolescents with alcohol and other drug use problems. *Alcohol Research and Health*, **29**, 221–227.

National Highway Traffic Safety Administration. (1999). *Marijuana & alcohol combined increase impairment* (Traffic Safety Facts Banner No. 201). Washington, DC: U.S. Department of Transportation.

NICE, National Institute for Health and Clinical Excellence. (2004). *Zaleplon, zolpidem and zopiclone for the management of insomnia* (NICE technology appraisal guidance 77). London: Author.

NICE, National Institute for Health and Clinical Excellence. (2013). *Smoking cessation in secondary care: Acute, maternity and mental health services* (NICE Public Health Guidance 48). London: Author.

Nocente, R., Vitali, M., Balducci, G., Enea, D., Kranzler, H. R., & Ceccanti, M. (2013). Varenicline and neuronal nicotinic acetylcholine receptors: A new approach to the treatment of co-occurring alcohol and nicotine addiction? *American Journal on Addictions*, **22**, 453–459.

Olfson, M., King, M., & Schoenbaum, M. (2015). Benzodiazepine use in the United States. *JAMA Psychiatry*, **72**, 136–142.

Otomanelli, G. (1999). Methadone patients and alcohol abuse [review]. *Journal of Substance Abuse Treatment*, **16**, 113–121.

Pelucchi, C., Gallus, S., Garavello, W., Bosetti, C., & La Vecchia, C. (2006). Cancer risk associated with alcohol and tobacco use: Focus on upper aero-digestive tract and liver. *Alcohol Research & Health*, **29**, 193–198.

Pettinati, H. M., Kampman, K. M., Lynch, K. G., Xie, H., Dackis, C., Rabinowitz, A. R., & O'Brien, C. P. (2008). A double blind, placebo-controlled trial that combines disulfiram and naltrexone for treating co-occurring cocaine and alcohol dependence. *Addictive Behaviors*, **33**, 651–667.

Prochaska, J. J., Delucchi, K., & Hall, S. M. (2004). A meta-analysis of smoking cessation interventions with individuals in substance abuse treatment or recovery. *Journal of Consulting and Clinical Psychology*, **72**(6), 1144.

Roux, P., Lions, C., Michel, L., Cohen, J., Mora, M., Marcellin, F., … ANRS Methaville Study Group. (2014). Predictors of non-adherence to methadone maintenance treatment in opioid-dependent individuals: Implications for clinicians. *Current Pharmaceutical Design*, **20**, 4097–4105.

Rubio, G., Manzanares, J., Jiménez, M., Rodríguez-Jiménez, R., Martínez, I., Iribarren, M.M., … Palomo, T. (2008). Use of cocaine by heavy drinkers increases vulnerability to developing alcohol dependence: A 4-year follow-up study. *Journal of Clinical Psychiatry*, **69**, 563–570.

Schifano, F. (2014). Misuse and abuse of pregabalin and gabapentin: Cause for concern? *CNS Drugs*, **28**, 491–496.

Smith, G. W., Farrell, M., Bunting, B. P., Houston, J. E., & Shevlin, M. (2011). Patterns of polydrug use in Great Britain: Findings from a national household population survey. *Drug and Alcohol Dependence*, **113**, 222–228.

Srivastava, A., Kahan, M., & Ross, S. (2008). The effect of methadone maintenance treatment on alcohol consumption: A systematic review. *Journal of Substance Abuse Treatment*, **34**, 215–223.

Staines, G. L., Magura, S., Foote, J., Deluca, A., & Kosanke, N. (2001). Polysubstance use among alcoholics. *Journal of Addictive Disorders*, **20**, 53–69.

Substance Abuse and Mental Health Services Administration (SAMHSA). (2002). *The DASIS (Drug and Alcohol Services Information System) report: Polydrug admissions – 2002*. Rockville, MD: Office of Applied Studies.

United Nations Office on Drugs and Crime (UNODC). (2014). *World drug report 2014* (United Nations publication, Sales No. E.14. XI.7). Vienna: United Nations.

West, R. (2001). Multiple substance dependence: Implications for treatment of nicotine dependence. *Addiction*, **96**, 775–776.

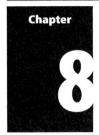

Introduction, settings, and roles

The preceding chapters of this book provide the background information for the following chapters that will describe the actual treatment of drinking problems. Historically, there has been a tendency to focus on the specialist field of treatment – alcoholism hospitals, recovery homes, addiction treatment clinics, and the like – but only a small minority of people with drinking problems is actually in contact with these sorts of services (Substance Abuse and Mental Health Services Administration, 2014). We take a far broader view in this book of where problem drinkers may find help (Figure 8.1).

The outermost layer of Figure 8.1 comprises informal influences on problem drinkers: the work colleague who advises that a career may be damaged if drinking is not stopped, the husband who supports his wife as she tries to get away from the bottle,

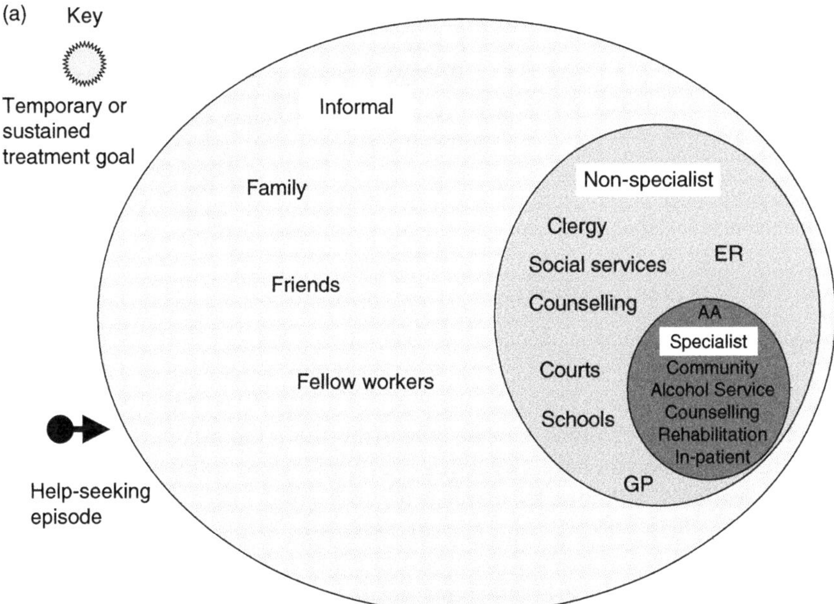

Figure 8.1: Treatment influences and trajectories. The light-tinted area represents the informal influences on problem drinkers, the medium-tinted area is the nonspecialist sectors and the dark-tinted innermost circle is the specialist sector. Different treatment trajectories are depicted (a–c) on and between these treatment settings. AA, Alcoholics Anonymous; ER, Emergency Room; GP, general practitioner.

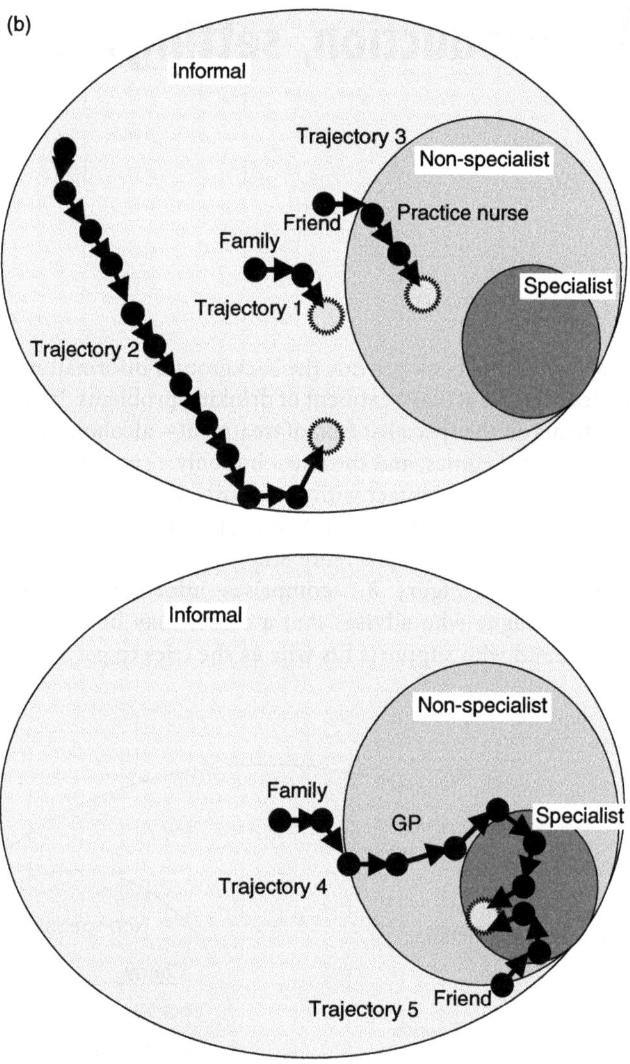

Figure 8.1: (cont.)

the friends who praise or mock a newly abstinent chum's lifestyle, the Internet questionnaire that asks "Do you have a drinking problem?" These influences were addressed primarily in Section 1, although their role is felt in Section 2 because informal influence can spur or deter help-seeking from formal sources of help, as shown in Figure 8.1's inner two circles.

The middle area of Figure 8.1 is the nonspecialist sector, those agencies that may offer support or apply pressure (or both) to problem drinkers even though their raison d'être is not related to alcohol. The hidden majority of problem drinkers daily rub shoulders with fellow members of their community in these settings; for example, when they consult their primary care doctors or have the misfortune to attend the Emergency Room. Therefore,

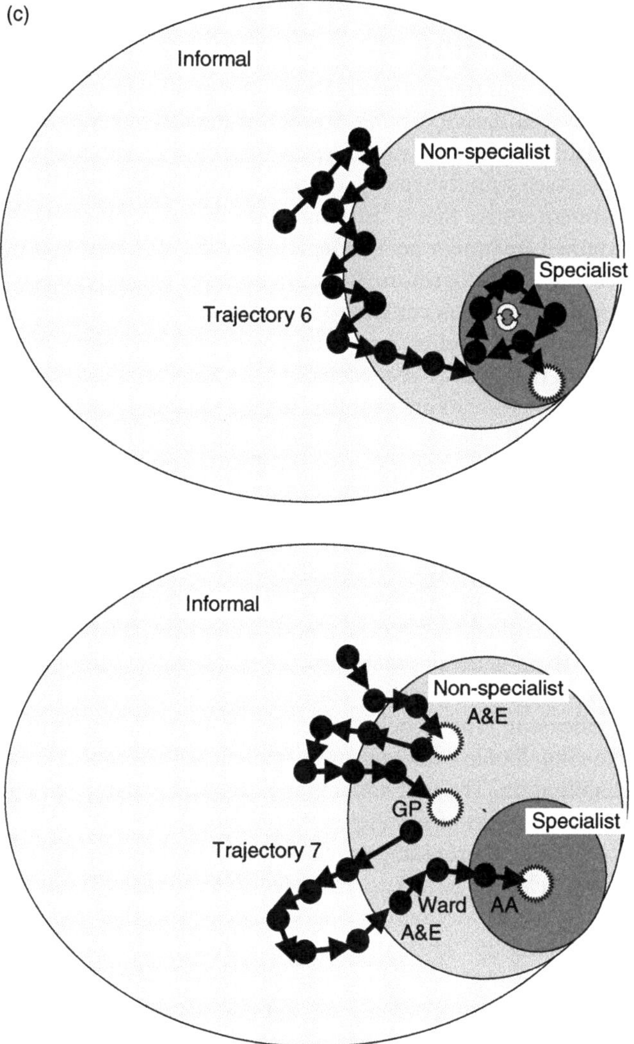

Figure 8.1: (cont.)

any approach to the treatment of drinking problems must consider the many different settings in which these develop and present. These settings are described in detail in Chapter 9.

Finally, the innermost circle of Figure 8.1 is the specialist sector, namely professional services (see Chapter 13) and mutual-help programmes (see Chapter 14) with the explicit purpose of helping problem drinkers. Their location at the centre of the diagram is not specialist narcissism. Rather, it reflects specialist treatment being where a small minority of all drinking problems is handled and, indeed, that the other influences in the larger circles of the chart are often sufficient to bring a drinking problem to heel.

Trajectories of help-seeking and progress or regress in the drinking problem

The help-seeking pathway of most individuals will not be straightforward but in fact rather "messy" because they will derive varying degrees of parallel support from informal, nonspecialist, and specialist sources that vary over the time course. Although multiple sources of treatment can be accessed simultaneously, the position of the treatment arrow on Figure 8.1 highlights the treatment source that is "making the running" at any one particular time. The temporary or sustained treatment goal is depicted by the star, and many treatment paths may not terminate in one. Furthermore, there are multiple permutations of these treatment trajectories that occur in various combinations, with associated gaps, pauses, and delays. Whilst the treatment arrows build into a trajectory that is unique for that individual, characteristic patterns may also be recognized.

Many will manage their drinking problem without accessing specialist or nonspecialist services, using the informal support of family and friends to achieve their goal, either rapidly as shown by trajectory 1 in Figure 8.1b or over a longer period as depicted in trajectory 2. Others will approach nonspecialist services, such as their practice nurse, who may assist by using a brief intervention (trajectory 3). An example of the stepped-care model is presented in trajectory 4, in which specialist alcohol treatment is reserved for those who do not respond to simpler approaches (Bower & Gilbody, 2005). In this example, concerned relatives advise the individual to cut down, and, when this fails for the second time, the individual consults their general practitioner who provides community detoxification. Several weeks later, the patient relapses, continuing drinking during a second attempted community detoxification. The general practitioner then refers them to the specialist services, and, following detailed assessment, in-patient detoxification is arranged followed by residential rehabilitation. The individual then successfully maintains a prolonged period of abstinence with the support of Alcoholics Anonymous.

Some see stepped care as providing specialist input to those who have "failed" at other approaches, thereby delaying access to the needed treatment. Therefore, an important aspect of stepped care is a mechanism for self-correction that monitors progress and provides for the "stepping up" of treatment as required. In addition, accurate assessment in the early stages of presentation is vital because this can identify an individual who needs direct access to specialist care and thereby prevent the delay and negative impact associated with multiple failures at lower intensity interventions. Indeed, in trajectory 5 in Figure 8.1b, a friend at work who has experienced a drinking problem advised the individual to attend the open-access assessment clinic with the local community alcohol team; the team recommends a course of individual counselling. An early accurate assessment enabled this individual to be identified and referred to a supportive resource.

The "messy" treatment of drinking problems

The majority of treatment trajectories will not be joined up, direct, or efficient, and many will represent "messy" treatment. For example, in trajectory 6 in Figure 8.1c, the individual experienced multiple inputs from informal sources, including family, friends, the local church, and work colleagues, before presenting to their general practitioner and undergoing several community detoxifications. They were eventually referred to the local specialist alcohol team, where they underwent multiple rounds of in-patient, group, and individual treatment before they finally achieved abstinence. This trajectory includes zigzag patterns, during which the individual goes backward and forward between services: this is sometimes termed "ping-pong" treatment. There are also loops in which the patient repeatedly circulates between services: these people are sometimes labelled "revolving-door" patients. In this case, the individual finally broke out of the revolving-door loop and achieved their treatment goal of stable abstinence. But this is not always the case, and some may access different levels of treatment throughout their lives. As such, therapists may maintain their enthusiasm for this work by hoping that this occasion might be the one in which the individual finally succeeds.

A further common complication is the changing of goals as treatment progresses. In trajectory 7 in Figure 8.1c, the person initially wishes to pursue moderate drinking and, after presenting to the local Emergency Room, they achieve this following a brief intervention by the alcohol liaison worker. Subsequently, they lose their job; the drinking escalates and can no longer be reined in. Further attempts at maintaining moderate drinking with support from their general practitioner fail and they disengage. They do not attend the practice for several months, finally presenting again with features of physical dependence on alcohol. This time, they reluctantly recognize that they cannot control their alcohol consumption and opt for community detoxification – which they complete, only to relapse after several weeks. A year later, they present again in the Emergency Room with a head injury. Fortunately, the drinking history is noted, and they undergo medically assisted detoxification, following which they achieve stable abstinence for several months with the support of a SMART Recovery mutual help group.

It is worth taking a moment just to imagine the different patterns that can exist and to identify the individual treatment trajectories of those people who have shared their treatment histories with you. For many problem drinkers, the treatment journey will be desultory and complex; at times simultaneously accessing support across the informal, nonspecialist, and specialist domains, whilst at other times, a single source may be the most helpful. Different helpers may give differing advice – indeed, sometimes directly contradictory advice. The course of treatment may be punctuated with pauses by the individual or imposed waits by the care system. Specific patterns can be discerned as the drinking problem unfolds and suitable treatment is sought and delivered. Retrospectively, the presentation of the drinking problem and the consolidation of the previous treatment experience can be plotted on the individual's life map. The chapters that follow explore the various components of these different treatment trajectories that together make up the breadth of the treatment of drinking problems.

References

Bower, P., & Gilbody, S. (2005). Stepped care in psychological therapies: Access, effectiveness and efficiency. Narrative literature review. *British Journal of Psychiatry*, **186**, 11–17.

Substance Abuse and Mental Health Services Administration. (2014). *Results from the 2013 National Survey on Drug Use and Health: Summary of national findings* (NSDUH Series H-48, HHS Publication No. (SMA) 14-4863). Rockville, MD: Substance Abuse and Mental Health Services Administration.

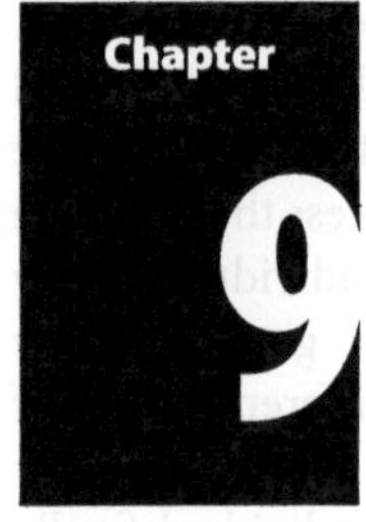

Case-finding and intervention outside of specialty settings

Specialty alcohol clinical settings are an important focus of this book and are obviously an appropriate location in which to pursue the treatment of drinking problems. But individuals with drinking problems – sometimes identified, sometimes not – are scattered across a range of health and social service settings, typically in far larger numbers than are present in a nation's specialty alcohol care sector. This chapter describes screening procedures that can identify such cases, presents interventions that can be applied in even short-term clinical contacts outside the specialty sector, and provides guidelines for determining when care collaboration with specialty services is called for.

Why nonspecialists should screen for and intervene with drinking problems

To the probation officer, school counselor, or primary care nurse, worrying about drinking problems may seem a distraction from their "day job." What good does it do for nonspecialists to get involved in the treatment of drinking problems, and, in any event, isn't that someone else's responsibility? Such attitudes are short-sighted for at least three reasons.

First, many interventions directed at problems other than drinking in nonspecialty settings fail precisely because of an unrecognized drinking problem. Alcohol misuse is a causal or exacerbating factor in countless problems that come to the attention of health and social service professionals: unhappy marriages, family violence, unemployment, anxiety disorders, injuries, school failure, and cardiovascular illness, to name but a few (see Section 1). When the drinking problem is not addressed, the attempts to tackle the presenting problem may be ineffective or even cause harm. The "depression" will not respond to the prescribed antidepressant, a peptic ulcer will fail to heal, a distressed marriage will rapidly deteriorate, leaving the helping professional puzzled and frustrated. Thus, rather than being a distraction from the main clinical goals of nonspecialist clinicians, tackling drinking problems can facilitate the achievement of those goals.

Second, nonspecialist settings provide the chance to influence low-level drinking problems before they become serious. Specialist alcohol services in most countries tend to serve individuals with quite severe drinking problems (Humphreys & Tucker, 2002). In many cases, this end state could have been forestalled by intervention earlier in the life course. A serious discussion with a guidance counsellor when college drinking has just started to harm academic performance, advice to cut down from a physician at the first report of occasional tiredness after an evening's drinking, support from an employee assistance programme after a few late arrivals to work on Monday mornings may only nudge the life

Table 9.1. Nonspecialist settings in which drinking problems are prevalent

- Criminal justice system
- Workplace
- School, colleges, universities
- Primary care
- Emergency rooms
- Hepatology clinics
- Sexual health clinics
- Geriatric care settings
- General psychiatry/mental health clinics

course slightly. But even a small intervention made early enough can have a pronounced long-term impact, akin to how a small turn of an ocean liner's wheel as it leaves Boston Harbour can make it arrive in Liverpool rather than Brest.

Third, nonspecialist settings can be the bridge to specialty care for individuals with severe but as yet undetected drinking problems. Not all drinking problems can be managed by nonspecialists, making specialty treatment desirable. Yet because of stigma, lack of information, or ambivalence about change, even the most severely impaired drinkers may hesitate to directly access a designated alcohol treatment programme. With proper screening and referral, however, the office of a trusted GP or employee assistance programme staff member can be the entry route to potentially life-saving care for a greatly troubled individual.

Nonspecialist settings in which drinking problems are prevalent

Table 9.1 lists settings in which drinking problems are prevalent, if not necessarily recognized. We include on the list the special case of general psychiatry services in which drinking problems are overlooked despite the capacity to treat them. Each setting is described in more detail in the next sections.

Criminal justice

Although many people believe that illegal drugs drive most crime and incarceration, no drug competes with alcohol in these respects. Domestic violence, reckless driving, and child abuse are just three of many crimes strongly associated with excessive alcohol consumption (see Chapter 4). The criminal justice system is thus de facto among the largest handlers of people with drinking problems. Assessment of the use of alcohol and other drugs is therefore an essential part of any psychiatric consultation in the criminal justice system, including competency assessments, child custody hearings, and evaluations of dangerousness.

The workplace

The emergence of in-house employee assistance programmes was both a reaction to and an illuminator of the high prevalence of alcohol problems in many companies. Alcohol is the hidden factor behind many cases of absenteeism, job conflicts, and worksite accidents. Workforces with a particularly high prevalence of alcohol problems – and therefore a particular opportunity for intervention – include the military, law enforcement, and the alcohol industry itself.

Schools, colleges, universities

Educational institutions at all levels are profoundly affected by drinking problems. In primary school, a drinking problem in the family may be the force driving the child who is chronically late, anxious, socially rejected, or physically aggressive. In adolescence and young adulthood, problem drinking by students themselves is frequently commingled with problems of academic achievement and social behaviour. The widespread anxiety about adolescent use of illicit drugs should not overshadow the fact that, in many communities, alcohol is a more pervasive adolescent problem.

Primary care

Within the healthcare system, the primary care setting is probably the greatest missed opportunity to address drinking problems, which are in some way implicated in perhaps 25 percent of all visits. Yet recognition of drinking problems is often not given priority, and it is even less frequently the subject of intervention.

Accident and emergency departments

Another critical opportunity for intervention in the healthcare system is the emergency room (Crawford et al., 2004; Havard, Shakeshaft, & Sanson-Fisher, 2008). A growing body of work has documented that drinking problems are prevalent among individuals injured in a range of accidents including, but not limited to, road traffic accidents. The shock of the injury can provide a "teachable moment" during which long-ignored pleas for attention to drinking are finally heard.

Hepatology clinics

Although every hepatologist is aware that chronic heavy drinking is a leading cause of cirrhosis of the liver, hepatology clinics do not always sufficiently screen nor intervene with drinking problems. This is not merely a matter of detecting cases of severe drinking, but also of advising abstinence for lower level drinkers to whom such consumption can be unusually dangerous (e.g., those with hepatitis C).

Sexual health clinics

A night's heavy drinking is often behind an unintentional pregnancy, as well as the contraction of a sexually transmitted disease. These risks arise in consensual sexual relationships when condoms or other forms of contraception are forgotten or simply disregarded. They are also prevalent in sexual assaults, for which intoxicated individuals may be targeted by perpetrators. As the prevalence of heavy alcohol consumption among young women has risen, intervention for women in sexual health and obstetric clinics has become more important, not only for the women themselves, but also, in cases of pregnancy, for the developing foetus (see Chapter 5).

Geriatric care settings

One less appreciated effect of the ageing of the Baby Boom generation is a rise in elderly people who have a substance use disorder (Crome et al., 2011). Such problems can be the source of presenting complaints of confusion and poor memory in a geriatrician's practice or of depression or agitation in a nursing home. Addressing alcohol problems in this population assumes particular importance in those cases where the individual is taking a prescribed medication that interacts with alcohol.

The special case of general psychiatry/mental health services

> I was in psychoanalysis for depression 3 days a week for 20 years. I killed a pint of bourbon almost every night throughout it, but my analyst never even asked me about my drinking.

> There is no point addressing symptoms without getting at their root cause. That's why I don't get distracted by how much patients drink. Once their emotional conflict is resolved in therapy, they won't need to self-medicate their pain any more, and the drinking will stop on its own.

These comments, the first by an elderly psychiatric patient, the second by a young psychiatry resident, illustrate a sad reality in many mental health settings not specifically dedicated to alcohol treatment: despite the presence of trained psychiatrists, psychologists, social workers, and counsellors, drinking problems are often completely ignored. The reasons for the oversight are partly ideological and partly practical.

Freudian theory, which remains influential with many mental health professionals, holds that heavy drinking is not a problem, per se, but a side effect of a psychodynamic conflict. Freud himself conveyed great scepticism about whether alcoholic patients could ever form a therapeutic alliance that would promote change. This combination of dismissing the importance of drinking on the one hand and being nihilistic about the prospects of intervention on the other has been absorbed into much of the mental health field and remains a considerable ideological barrier to intervention in some settings.

At a practical level, training in psychiatry, psychology, and allied fields often devotes little attention to drinking problems, despite their prevalence in psychiatric settings. Many mental health professionals thus feel incompetent to address problem drinking and hence never broach the subject with patients.

More positively, once drinking is recognized and taken seriously, virtually everything that can be done in a specialist alcohol clinic can be accomplished in a general mental health programme. This would include, for example, all the therapeutic processes and tactics described in Chapter 12.

Screening and case-finding

Drinking problems often go undetected in nonspecialist care settings (Cheeta et al., 2008). If the element of drinking is allowed to remain hidden, it will defeat efforts to help the patient, client, student, or employee. This section starts with a review of clinical strategies for enhancing the detection of problem drinking, followed by a review of biological assays and standardized screening questionnaires.

The use of disarming questions

It is useful to have a few disarming questions about drinking problems that can be fed into any assessment in an almost throwaway fashion. The scene is often best set by a casual introductory remark such as, "I always ask everyone about drinking – it can be important to feel that one can talk about one's drinking without being got at." This implies that questions in this area are routine rather than the patient being singled out as a special case, and this is coupled with an immediate indication that anything the patient reveals will be sympathetically heard.

One useful disarming question is "When did you have your last drink?" because it cannot be fobbed off with a yes/no answer. "How would you describe your drinking?" has the same virtue. An open-ended invitation to reveal current concerns can also be effective: "Please tell me about any worries you have related to your drinking – you know, any rows, troubles at home, health problems, things of that sort."

Questions that feel out the possibility of worry or trouble are more likely to provide a way into fruitful dialogue than are mechanistic questions along such lines as, "Do you drink?" The latter type of interrogation does not immediately reach across barriers toward what the patient is feeling and experiencing. It is too readily deflected by a bland answer, such as "Just socially."

Remembering who may be especially at risk

To bear in mind a list of who may be especially at risk is useful, provided the clinician does not become blinkered to the wider truth that drinking problems can affect both sexes and, either directly or indirectly, people of any age and every occupation. With that proviso, an awareness of a particular occupational hazard is then important (see Chapter 3). The separated, or divorced person; those considered to be at risk of suicide; the recently bereaved; and certain ethnic groups also go on this "at-risk" list. The person who is homeless and drifting is also likely to have a drinking problem.

Common social presentations

One should always be on the look out for a hidden drinking problem with the client or patient who is frequently changing house, jobs, or relationships. Family presentations are common – marital disharmony or family violence, the spouse presenting with depression or the children with truanting, school failure, antisocial behaviour or neurotic symptoms. Criminal offences also suggest the need to ask about drinking.

Common psychiatric clues

Here, the essential background list derives from Chapters 6 and 7. In particular, one should be alert to the possibility of a drinking problem when the patient or client complains rather nonspecifically of "bad nerves," insomnia, or depression. Phobic symptoms, paranoid symptoms, and dementia or delirium may all be alcohol-related. A drug problem may also be associated with a drinking problem. A suicidal gesture or act of deliberate self-harm always demands enquiry into drinking.

Common medical clues

An account of the medical complications of heavy drinking is given in Chapter 5. In practical terms, one should be particularly alert if a patient repeatedly asks for a 'certificate', is a frequent visitor to the doctor's office on a Monday morning, is suffering from malnutrition, is complaining of any gastrointestinal disorder or liver problem, has otherwise unexplained heart trouble, or is presenting with "epilepsy" of late onset. Bruising also may be a clue, as may burns that resulted from a cigarette being dropped on the skin while the drinker was intoxicated. Accidents of any sort may be alcohol-related, and 20 percent of those involved in road traffic accidents may be classified as problem drinkers (Mayou & Bryant, 1995).

Not overlooking the obvious

The patient may declare the diagnosis by the smell of alcohol on their breath, by the bottle sticking out of their pocket, by their flushed face and bloodshot eyes, or by their tremor, but even the fact that they are obviously intoxicated can be overlooked if the possibility of drinking is not held in mind. The patient who makes jokes about their drinking should have those jokes taken seriously. Similarly obvious presentations may be seen on a visit to the home: bottles and glasses lying around, decoration neglected, and furniture reduced to a few sticks; the home may be a sad parody of a stage-set portraying decay. It would, however, be a mistake to think only in terms of such flagrant presentations and therefore overlook subtler clues.

Taking advantage of technology

Sophisticated, evidence-based screeners for drinking problems are available as Internet web pages and smartphone apps (see, e.g., www.checkyourdrinking.net), and patients are increasingly comfortable screening themselves and even receiving an ensuing brief intervention online where indicated (Cucciare et al., 2013; Cunningham et al., 2009). A fixed terminal in the waiting room of a clinic can easily mount such software and help open the conversation about the role of problem drinking in a service recipient's life.

Laboratory tests

A number of laboratory tests are useful in the screening of populations for possible drinking problems – within, for instance, a routine medical examination when staff are recruited or undergo annual health checks. Laboratory tests are not by themselves diagnostic but are useful to help confirm a diagnosis in the individual case where excessive drinking is suspected but has not been admitted. A battery of tests will generally perform better than any single test. Indeed, a properly chosen array of currently available tests should detect more than 90 percent of people with an at least moderately severe drinking problem (Hashimoto et al., 2013; Niemela, 2007). A negative result does not rule out the possibility that excessive drinking has begun to adversely affect the individual's life, and false positives also occur. Laboratory tests need to be interpreted shrewdly and in the context of all those considerations listed earlier.

Sensitivity and specificity

Two characteristics of individual tests define their usefulness in detecting and diagnosing cases. The *specificity* of a test refers to the extent to which a positive result is indicative of the condition of interest. In this case, the condition of interest may be heavy drinking, drinking problems, or alcohol dependence, depending on the circumstances and reasons for screening. A nonspecific test for heavy drinking, for example, would show a positive result not just in heavy drinking but in a range of other unrelated disorders as well. The ideal test would be 100 percent specific, indicating that it only became positive as a result of heavy drinking. The *sensitivity* of a test indicates the extent to which it reliably detects every case of the condition of interest. For our present purpose, we would like a 100 percent sensitive test, which would always be positive in every case of heavy drinking, drinking problems, or alcohol dependence (as appropriate).

To date, no one has devised a 100 percent specific and 100 percent sensitive test for heavy drinking, drinking problems, or alcohol dependence. Different tests are more or less specific and sensitive, and these parameters vary with the group under study (e.g., dependent or hazardous drinkers). The extent to which these tests will serve practical diagnostic needs depends on the prevalence of heavy drinking, drinking problems, or alcohol dependence in the population in which they are being used. To understand this better, let us consider a fictitious illustration:

> A new test for heavy drinking, "alcoholin," has 95 percent specificity and 60 percent sensitivity. It is used to screen 1,000 apparently healthy employees at their annual medical review. Let us assume that 10 percent of these employees are actually drinking sufficient amounts of alcohol to be a cause for concern. How useful will the new test be?
>
> Out of 1,000 employees, 10 percent (n = 100) are drinking too much, and 60 percent of these (n = 60) will be correctly identified by the test as being "heavy drinkers." However, out of the whole group of 1,000, 5 percent (n = 50) will be identified as positive due to nonspecific (i.e., not alcohol-related) results of the test. Therefore, a total of 110 people will be identified by the test, and only 60 of these (55 percent) will actually be drinking too much. The "alcoholin" test is therefore of limited usefulness and must be followed by other tests and by more detailed inquiries in order to confirm whether or not each of the individuals testing positive actually is drinking too much. Furthermore, 40 people who are drinking excessively will not be identified by the test.

The problems illustrated by this example become more severe as the ratio of those with versus without the disorder departs further from 1 (i.e., as the base rate of disorder departs in either direction from 50 percent). Thus, if the prevalence of heavy drinking were only 1 percent, only 1 in 9 of those who tested positive with the same test would actually be heavy drinkers. Conversely, if used in a population where almost everyone had a drinking problem, then more than 9 out of 10 would test positive, including most of the few non-problem drinkers in the sample.

Screening tests for heavy drinking

Let us now consider the actual tests used to screen for heavy drinking in populations, as well as to monitor clinical progress in ongoing cases. The most useful tests are described in the following sections.

Mean corpuscular volume

Mean corpuscular volume (MCV) is a measure of the size of red blood cells, which may increase in response to heavy drinking due to a poorly understood mechanism affecting the developing cells. Sensitivity is 20–30 percent in hazardous drinkers and 40–50 percent in dependence, with a specificity of 64–100 percent (Conigrave, Saunders, & Whitfield, 1995). The sensitivity in women is higher.

If MCV has been elevated as a result of heavy drinking, it may remain raised for several months after a reduction or cessation of alcohol consumption. This is because of the relatively long life of red blood cells (about 120 days); the average cell size reduces as those of normal size replace the large red blood cells. Other causes of a raised MCV that affect the specificity include vitamin B_{12} deficiency, folic acid deficiency, liver disease, blood disorders, hypothyroidism, and smoking (Niemela, 2007).

Liver function tests

Serum gamma-glutamyl transferase (GGT) is an enzyme that the body produces in response to alcohol ingestion. Serum aspartate aminotransferase (AST) and serum alanine aminotransferase (ALT) are also indicators of alcoholic hepatotoxicity, which may be elevated as a result of heavy drinking. Of these, GGT is generally considered the most useful as a screening test for heavy drinking. However, the sensitivity of 20–50 percent in hazardous consumption and 60–90 percent in dependence, along with a specificity of 55–100 percent (Conigrave et al., 1995), has led to its value being questioned. In many laboratories, GGT measurement requires a specific request because it is not included in routine liver function tests. If GGT has been elevated due to drinking, as in a relapse, it will fall again after abstinence is established. This occurs more rapidly than the restoration of MCV, with the level falling to approximately half after approximately 2–4 weeks of abstinence (Hashimoto et al., 2013). It may still take several weeks to return to normal depending on the level to which it had been raised.

Non–alcohol-related causes of a raised GGT include liver disease (alcohol-induced or otherwise), with the greatest increases being associated with biliary obstruction (blockage of bile flow from any cause), obesity, diabetes, pancreatitis, hyperlipidaemia, cardiac failure, severe trauma, nephrotic syndrome, renal rejection, and other drugs (e.g., barbiturates, anticonvulsants, statins, and anticoagulants; Niemela, 2007). With more serious liver damage, other biochemical parameters, such as the albumin level, clotting factors, and bilirubin, will also be altered; in such cases, there may be enduring abnormalities of some levels, even after prolonged abstinence.

Carbohydrate-deficient (desialylated) transferrin

Carbohydrate-deficient (desialylated) transferrin (CDT) is a variant of a serum protein that transports iron around the body. The usual transferrin molecule contains three or more sialic acid residues, a carbohydrate. Excessive alcohol consumption is associated, by reasons not clearly understood, with the stripping off of some of these residues. Levels are increased in response to heavy drinking. Its sensitivity as a test of hazardous consumption is 26–62 percent and for dependence 65–95 percent with a specificity greater than 90 percent (Conigrave et al., 1995). This is arguably better than most other tests, and therefore CDT is considered by some to be the best available screening test for heavy drinking (Fagan et al., 2014; Hashimoto et al., 2013; Piano et al., 2014). Similar to GGT, an elevated CDT takes approximately 2 weeks to fall to half its level on stopping drinking (Niemela, 2007).

Blood alcohol concentration

Blood alcohol concentration (BAC) returns to zero quickly with abstinence: in humans, the average rate of clearance of alcohol from the blood is 15 mg/100 mL per hour or, very approximately, 1 UK unit per hour. This results in a fairly low sensitivity when used as a screening test for habitual heavy drinking. Depending on the time and context of testing, as well as the threshold alcohol concentration used to define a positive result, moderate social drinkers will also be detected, thus making BAC fairly nonspecific as well. Blood alcohol (or breath alcohol as an indirect measure) is therefore not often used as a screening test in the same fashion as GGT or CDT. However, BAC is related to impairment of psychomotor performance and therefore provides a particularly valuable measure in the workplace and in other safety-sensitive contexts (e.g., driving). The BAC may also have an underestimated utility as a screening test in the clinical setting. Even if not used as a screening test, BAC may be a useful confirmatory investigation. For instance, a high BAC at 9 a.m. could contradict a patient's report that she "only had a few drinks" the previous evening. Likewise, for patients who receive a day pass from a residential treatment facility, a BAC test upon return can detect violations of abstinence rules. Finally, the finding of a high BAC in the absence of evident intoxication suggests a high level of tolerance and is therefore important presumptive evidence for habitual heavy drinking.

Other potential biomarkers of alcohol consumption

Other biomarkers of alcohol misuse are currently being evaluated and may be introduced into future clinical practice. These include acetaldehyde adducts, phosphatidylethanol, and sialic acid in blood along with 5-hydroxytryptophol and ethyl glucuronide in urine (see Niemela, 2007; Hashimoto et al., 2013). Ethyl glucuronide can also be detected in other tissues such as hair, and this raises the possibility of a new sampling method to detect alcohol misuse that has thus far been limited to the detection of other drugs. Currently, the role of hair analysis in accurately reflecting drinking remains to be established and is more commonly used in forensic than in routine clinical settings (Boscolo-Berto et al., 2013).

Laboratory tests: An overall judgment

It will be apparent that none of the tests just mentioned offers improvement over the fictitious "alcoholin" test. In fact, "alcoholin" could easily be GGT or CDT. All these tests are limited in their usefulness as screening instruments, and, in some circumstances, standardized questionnaires (discussed later) may fare better at lower cost (Drummond, Ghodse, & Chengappa, 2007). Laboratory tests will be of greatest assistance to both clinician and patient if used in full awareness of the strengths and weaknesses of each; in this field of practice, there are skills to be learnt in using this technology to best advantage.

Screening questionnaires

A number of screening questionnaires have been devised in recent decades with the intention of detecting hazardous and harmful drinking as well as dependence in nonmedical settings. The development of the Alcohol Use Disorders Identification Test (AUDIT) was supported by the World Health Organization (Babor, Higgins-Biddle, Saunders, & Montiero, 2001). It was designed for use by healthcare workers in both developed and developing countries and is available in multiple languages. It shows good sensitivity and specificity and is useful in screening for hazardous and harmful drinking in non–treatment-seeking populations.

The AUDIT is administered as a brief (10-item) structured interview or self-report instrument and comprises questions about recent alcohol consumption (3 items), alcohol-related problems (4 items), and alcohol dependence (3 items). A score of eight or higher denotes hazardous drinking (or worse) worthy of further intervention and assessment. Based on the score generated by the AUDIT, the associated manual provides guidance for the management of any identified alcohol problem (Babor et al., 2001). The AUDIT is also available as an even briefer 5-item questionnaire, which has almost 80 percent sensitivity and 95 percent specificity in screening for hazardous alcohol intake and formal alcohol disorders (Piccinelli et al., 1997). The AUDIT-C is another shorter version comprising the first three AUDIT consumption items only (Bush et al., 1998).

Other validated questionnaires include the Fast Alcohol Screening Test (FAST) and the Paddington Alcohol Test (PAT). Both were developed for use in the busy emergency room (Hodgson et al., 2002; Smith, Touquet, Wright, & Das Gupta, 1996).

Older screening tools, including CAGE and the Michigan Alcoholism Screening Test (MAST), are better at picking up more extreme or dependent drinkers rather than hazardous or harmful drinkers (Mayfield, MacLeod, & Hall, 1974; Selzer, 1971). CAGE is an acronym derived from taking the first letter from the keywords of each of the four items that compose the CAGE questionnaire, and it also acts as a handy mnemonic: Felt you needed to *C*ut down, *A*nnoyed by other people criticizing one's drinking, *G*uilty about drinking, and needing an *E*ye-opener first thing in the morning. The MAST is a 24-item questionnaire also published in a 10-item brief form (BMAST; Pokorny, Miller, & Kaplan, 1972). Both the CAGE and the MAST focus on lifetime experiences of alcohol use. The MAST, for instance, has among its items delirium tremens and hospital admission for drinking. However, they show remarkably good sensitivity and specificity for "excessive drinking" as well as for "alcoholism" and may be superior to laboratory tests when used as screening instruments (Bernadt et al., 1982).

Two screening instruments have been developed for use with pregnant women, the T-ACE (Sokol, Martier, & Ager, 1989) and the TWEAK (Russell, 1994). They each perform rather better than the CAGE and MAST, with the 5-item TWEAK being more sensitive and less specific than the 4-item T-ACE.

All screening questionnaires can be administered by a trained clinician, but, in many settings, costs and convenience will make it more sensible for them to be self-completed (with clinical follow-up, if needed). Internet and smartphone technology makes it fairly easy to have some questionnaires completed electronically, with the results transmitted to the patient's record if appropriate. However, the older method of paper-and-pencil will always suffice, and, with some populations (e.g., elderly individuals), this may also be preferred by the individuals completing the questionnaire.

Practical conclusions on screening and case-finding

Table 9.2 summarizes the relative utility of various methods for detection and diagnosis of drinking problems. To a large extent, each method's utility for detection and screening is determined by its sensitivity, and its utility for diagnosis depends on its specificity. However, both parameters are important in both contexts. Cost, convenience, flexibility, and the ability to interface with electronic health records are also important.

In both specialty and nonspecialty settings, no screening tool eliminates the need for careful clinical enquiry as a means for detecting problem drinking. Information gained in this way may valuably be supported by the discerning use of appropriate laboratory investigations, breath alcohol testing, and questionnaires.

Where a large, healthy population must be screened, as, for example, in the occupational setting, even a brief clinical interview may not be possible, and questionnaires are therefore advantageous. But where the potential consequences of detection include disciplinary procedures or other adverse consequences, self-report questionnaires may not be valid. In such circumstances, laboratory tests such as GGT, MCV, or CDT can give useful information. Where the maintenance of a safe environment is of concern, such as for transportation workers or healthcare professionals suspected of having a drinking problem, blood or breath alcohol testing may also be effective.

Table 9.2. Advantages and disadvantages of different screening procedures

Procedure	Advantages	Disadvantages
Clinical interview	Flexibility	Subjectivity
	Potentially high specificity	Dependent on clinical skill and time/trouble taken
	Potential to detect cases that laboratory tests or questionnaires will miss	Poor sensitivity if the subject is embarrassed or covering up
		Can be time-consuming
Laboratory tests	Objective	Limited sensitivity and specificity (CDT arguably best, but GGT not much worse)
	Quick and convenient for screening large numbers of subjects	CDT is expensive (GGT much cheaper)
	If positive, useful to monitor subsequent progress	Do not detect social/ psychological problems
	Detect heavy use/some tissue toxicity (e.g., liver/blood)	
Breath alcohol estimation	Objective	Rapid clearance of alcohol from the blood/breath limits sensitivity
	Cheap and convenient	Detects alcohol use, not problems per se (i.e., poor specificity)
	Good for detecting drinking in safety-sensitive context (e.g., drinking and driving)	
	Useful to confirm history and monitor progress	
Questionnaires	More standardized than clinical interview	Subject to honesty of the respondent
	Cheap, convenient, and adaptable to electronic reporting	Limited sensitivity and specificity (but better than laboratory tests)

Triage decisions and intervention once a drinking problem is identified in a nonspeciality setting

When a drinking problem has come to light, the helping professional must make a judgement as to whether the appropriate decision is to attempt to manage the problem on site or to refer the problem drinker to specialist alcohol services. This section discusses this triage process and how to proceed in each of these situations.

How to determine whether the case will be handled in a nonspecialist setting

Sometimes practical realities dictate that a case will be treated in a nonspecialist setting, not because it is optimal but because needs must. In the hustle and bustle of the emergency room, a one-time, brief chat may be all that can be done even with a severely dependent drinker. In rural areas, constraints of travel time may reduce access to specialty care, which is disproportionately sited in urban and suburban areas. There is little to be lost from trying an intervention in such cases, as long as the clinician does not communicate false hope or implicitly minimize the severity of the problem.

When a specialty referral is practical, the most compelling reason for nonetheless handling someone with a drinking problem in a nonspecialist setting is that therapeutic gains can be made with the more limited level of intervention that can typically be accomplished there. There is no firm rule for making such judgements, but two general guidelines are supported both by research and by common sense. The lower the severity of the drinking problem and the greater the patient's social capital (e.g., a job, a marriage, a network of friends), the greater the likelihood that a modest intervention can nudge the course of drinking down a safer road (Moyer, Finney, Swearingen, & Vergun, 2002).

In cases where an advance judgement of whether specialist care is required is not easily made, the clinician should make the matter empirical: that is, provide the nonspecialist interventions (described in the next section) and then assess the impact. If the drinking problem responds to the intervention, so much the better. If not, the poor outcome provides information for both the clinician and patient that the problem is too severe to respond to this level of care, and elevation to the next step in the care system is the logical response. Indeed, from a public health viewpoint, it is probably a good strategy for all but the most obviously impaired problem drinkers to receive lower intensity interventions as a first step, such that specialist services are conserved for those who most need them.

The concept of stepped care being invoked here is a perfectly reasonable one that has long guided medical care and public health planning in many countries. In the alcohol field, however, it has faced some practical problems that have impeded its impact. Many nonspecialist providers do not want to treat even minor alcohol problems, whether because they feel incompetent to do so, look down on patients with drinking problems, or feel scarred by prior experiences (in their clinical or personal life) with problem drinkers. This leads some of them to over-refer patients reflexively to specialist alcohol services the moment even a relatively minor alcohol problem comes to light. In addition to the problems this can create in overloading specialist services, it sends a potent meta-message to the patient: "Your drinking problem is so severe or so shameful (or both), that while I, your doctor, can handle whatever other problems you have, at this I throw up my hands."

Resistance to specialist referral can also come from the other end of the patient–doctor interaction. For most health conditions, referral to a specialist is experienced as a chance to get expert help and superior care. Few patients with a heart condition, for example, would react with anger if their general practitioner said, "Just to be sure you get the care you need, I'm going to refer you to a cardiologist who has much more experience with your condition than I have." Yet many people with drinking problems have no interest in specialist care. They may fear consequences to their reputation if they are seen entering the door of a "rehab," turn up their nose at being in group therapy with "chronic drunks," or simply may be unable to accept that their alcohol problem is indeed too severe to be handled by a nonspecialist. In such cases, the clinician can still make efforts to manage the problem in the nonspecialist setting but should still communicate that a referral would be better in order not to collude with the patient in denying the severity of the problem.

When a patient is transferred to a specialist setting, either based on the initial triage decision or in light of a poor outcome from nonspecialist intervention, the referring clinician should be aware that this is a point at which many patients go missing. Sometimes this reflects an unwillingness to change, but, in many cases, it also reflects practicalities. In making the referral, it is therefore quite important for the clinician to explore mundane questions with the patient: "Are there alcohol services close to where you live?", "Do you have a means to get there?"; "If it's a residential programme, is it possible for you to be away from work and family responsibilities?" As a general rule, the closer the programme is, the more rapidly it can accept the patient and the simpler the bureaucratic procedures (e.g., is there a mountain of new forms the patient must complete, or can the patient's medical record simply be moved over to the new setting?), the more likely the patient is to follow-through on the referral.

Finally, as with all referrals to specialists, the clinician should stay in touch with the specialist rather than say, "Out of sight out of mind." For their part, specialists in the alcohol treatment programme have to keep the lines of communication as open as possible with the referring generalists and not become (as one referring physician put it) "a black hole from which none of my patients ever returns." With other serious disorders, such as cancer and heart disease, the general practitioner is informed of progress in specialty care and asked to follow-up later with monitoring. To the extent that practicality and confidentiality rules allow, the same should be true in the treatment of drinking problems.

Intervention within the nonspecialist setting

The three mainstays of nonspecialist intervention are the provision of information about safe drinking guidelines, brief motivational interviewing, and medical management. Each can also be part of more comprehensive specialist treatment, but they are discussed here because they are well suited to the constraints of most nonspecialist settings (e.g., primary care).

Provision of information on safe drinking, with special attention to particularly vulnerable patients

Safe drinking guidelines were reviewed in Chapter 1 and need not be repeated here. As such, guidelines are simple and easy to convey and can motivate change; there is little excuse for a patient with a drinking problem leaving any of the settings discussed in this chapter without having been exposed to the guidelines, even if only in a handout or through a website link.

When sharing general guidelines, their focus on the typical individual should be emphasized. Certain vulnerable patients, for example those who are pregnant, have hepatitis C, or have a history of disabling depression, incur risk from alcohol consumption even within the constraints of healthy drinking guidelines developed for the general population.

Brief motivational intervention

The term brief motivational intervention (BMI) is being used here as a grab bag of techniques alternatively called *brief intervention*, *motivational interviewing*, and BMI.

These techniques were initially developed and tested in the UK and are now employed in a wide range of developed and developing nations. All variants of these interventions assume that contacts between the provider and the patient will be one to three in number, including instances in which later contacts are telephone or videophone calls from the clinician or someone else in the practice (e.g., a nurse in a general practitioner's office).

In some respects, BMI is an attitude as much as a technique, being developed explicitly in contrast with the (albeit somewhat stereotyped) image of the alcoholism counsellor who labels every patient "alcoholic," demands lifetime abstinence, and accuses anyone who disagrees as being in denial. In BMI, rather than a making a moral judgement or being confrontational or hectoring, the clinician is concerned, warm, and matter of fact. The patient's perceptions of the benefits of drinking are acknowledged rather than debated. The exchange is respectful and to the point, with the responsibility for making the ultimate decision about drinking placed explicitly on the patient. The patient is also responsible for setting change goals, with the clinician reinforcing small steps (e.g., avoiding drinking and driving, not drinking 2 days in a row, alternating soft drinks with alcoholic drinks during drinking sessions) rather than insisting on an all-or-nothing approach.

One helpful mnemonic for the components of BMI is FRAMES (Miller & Sanchez, 1993). Table 9.3 describes each technique in some detail. The nature and rationale for each is as follows.

Feedback can be powerful because heavy drinkers often underestimate the risks of their drinking, as well as how their drinking compares to that of the general population. Normative feedback – for example, noting that a patient's alcohol consumption is in the 90th percentile of the population – can be motivating insofar as many individuals dislike being outside sociobehavioural norms. Risk-related information can also enhance motivation by inducing appropriate anxiety about possible harms. As mentioned, such norm-related feedback is available free online (http://www.checkyourdrinking.net).

Placing *responsibility* on the patient is partly an acknowledgment of reality (the patient is ultimately in the driver's seat) and partly a considered clinical tactic. When they feel pressed to change, many individuals will defend their drinking or otherwise engage in a power struggle with the clinician. Saying flat out, "Of course whether you change is entirely up to you. I can provide advice but I can't decide for you" defuses any potential battles of this sort. Furthermore, the perception of having control enhances both motivation to change and the sense of being able to accomplish it (Kanfer & Schefft, 1988).

Advice to change and the *menu* of alternative strategies must be offered completely in the spirit just described, with respect for the patient's autonomy. Thus, not, "You must stop drinking right now!" but, "I recognize that change is difficult, but I'd be failing in my job as your physician if I didn't advise you to take a hard look at how your drinking is compromising your health." A menu of alternatives in some sense bridges advice provision with respect for autonomy in that, although the patient is given a range of choices, all of them are aligned with the clinician's fundamental advice to recognize the current drinking as problematic and make some change in it.

The *empathic* style and enhancement of the patient's *self-efficacy* work together to reduce resistance to change and increase confidence that it can be accomplished. They also create a positive relationship between the clinician and patient that can facilitate future contacts.

Do such clinical tactics really work? BMI can be used in many contexts; for the present purposes, the question is how effective it is in nonspecialist settings. A meta-analysis of

Table 9.3. The FRAMES mnemonic for brief motivational intervention

Feedback: The clinician conveys in a factual, nonjudgmental fashion the level of risk associated with the patient's drinking. Feedback may include the results of laboratory tests, including for medical problems upon which heavy drinking has an exacerbating effect (e.g., hypertension). In addition to oral feedback, written materials are commonly provided.

Responsibility of the patient: The clinician explicitly acknowledges that the patient has the power to change and that no one else can make him or her do so. Responsibility for goal-setting is also specifically allotted to the patient.

Advice to change: The clinician communicates concern about the current level of drinking and provides advice to reduce risk; for example, to avoid drinking in particular situations or to reduce or eliminate alcohol consumption.

Menu of change strategies: A range of options should be presented to the patient, including formal alcohol treatment, attendance at mutual-help groups, and use of self-help manuals and websites. For many patients, a range of interim goals that the patient can attempt on his or her own can be useful; for example, keeping a diary of drinking, strictly limiting drinking to particular times of day (e.g., never before 6 p.m.) or days of the week (e.g., never the evening before a work or school day), and switching from regular to low-strength beer.

Empathetic counselling style: Confrontation and condemnation are completely avoided. The patient's emotions, including those that might mitigate against change (e.g., fear of failure, enjoyment of drinking), are respectfully acknowledged. The clinician reflects the patient's emotions in order to communicate understanding; for example, "You would like not to deal with hangovers and vomiting in the mornings, but you also enjoy the way heavy drinking makes you feel while you are doing it."

Self-efficacy enhancement: The clinician communicates confidence in the patient's abilities. To enhance motivation, the clinician specifically reinforces any verbal commitment to change; for example, "You said you had been thinking of making a change, and maybe this is the right time."

Adapted from Miller & Sanchez (1993).

34 outcome studies conducted in such settings (typically primary care) found strong evidence of benefit, with significant reductions both in drinking-related problems and in alcohol consumption at follow-ups of less than 3 months, 3–6 months, and 6–12 months (Moyer et al., 2002). A subsequent analysis confined to nonphysician clinicians found less strong but still significant effects (Sullivan et al., 2011). And, of course, whether a BMI succeeds or fails, the result will be informative as to what next steps, if any, are required.

Medical management

Medical management (sometimes termed "chronic disease management") is a well-established model of care for many chronic illnesses. It does not compete with BMI as a strategy and, indeed, can follow after it. Care is ongoing in this model but, unlike with traditional alcohol treatment, the primary provider is a nonspecialist (e.g., a general practitioner, nurse practitioner, physician's assistant), and the sessions are shorter. A manual describing this intervention in detail is available free of charge from the U.S. National Institute on Alcohol Abuse and Alcoholism (Pettinati et al., 2004).

The initial session of medical management can last as long as 45 minutes and comprises a diagnostic interview, a review with the patient of the health and social effects of the drinking, and a consideration of the medication options available (see Chapter 13). Follow-up appointments occur every week or two and are shorter in duration, perhaps 15–20 minutes. These are not psychotherapy sessions but instead a focused review of drinking since the last visit, medication compliance, and side effects and overall functioning. Concurrent involvement in mutual help groups is encouraged but is not essential for medical management. If the drinking problem becomes more severe, the decision may be made to transfer the patient to the more extensive services available in a specialty alcohol programme.

Summary

A care system that only provides help for drinking problems within alcohol treatment programmes will have a suboptimal impact on public health. Helping professionals who don't work in alcohol programmes can enhance public health and their own success by making alcohol intervention part of their work. A range of instruments is available to detect drinking problems in nonspecialist settings, as are some evidence-based approaches for intervention. Particularly when drinking problems are at the lower end of severity, nonspecialists can make a positive impact on the course of drinking problems.

References

Babor, T. F., Higgins-Biddle, J., Saunders, J. B., & Montiero, M. G. (2001). *AUDIT: The Alcohol Use Disorders Identification Test: Guidelines for use in primary health care* (2nd ed.). Geneva: World Health Organization.

Bernadt, M. W., Mumford, J., Taylor, C., Smith, B., & Murray, R. M. (1982). Comparison of questionnaire and laboratory tests in the detection of excessive drinking and alcoholism. *Lancet*, **8267**, 325–328.

Boscolo-Berto, R., Viel, G., Montisci, M., Terranova, C., Favretto, D., & Ferrara, S. D. (2013). Ethyl glucuronide concentration in hair for detecting heavy drinking and/or abstinence: A meta-analysis. *International Journal of Legal Medicine*, **127**, 611–619.

Bush, K., Kivlahan, D. R., McDonnell, M. B., Fihn, S., & Bradley, K. A. (1998). The AUDIT alcohol consumption questions (AUDIT-C): An effective brief screening test for problem drinking. *Archives of Internal Medicine*, **158**, 1789–1795.

Cheeta, S., Drummond, C., Oyefeso, A., Phillips, T., Deluca, P., Perryman, K., & Coulton, S. (2008). Low identification of alcohol use disorders in general practice in England. *Addiction*, **103**, 766–773.

Conigrave, K. M., Saunders, J. B., & Whitfield, J. B. (1995). Diagnostic tests for alcohol consumption. *Alcohol and Alcoholism*, **30**, 13–26.

Crawford, M., Patton, R., Touquet, R., Drummond, C., Byford, S., Barrett, B., ... Henry, J. A. (2004), Screening and referral for brief intervention of alcohol-misusing patients in an emergency department: A pragmatic randomised controlled trial. *Lancet*, **364**, 1134–1139.

Crome, I., Brown, A., Dar, K., et al. (2011). *Our invisible addicts: First report of the Older Persons' Substance Misuse Working Group of the Royal College of Psychiatrists*. London: Royal College of Psychiatrists.

Cucciare, M. A., Weingardt, K. R., Ghaus, S., Boden, M. T., & Frayne, S. M. (2013). A randomized controlled trial of a web-delivered brief alcohol intervention in Veterans Affairs primary care. *Journal of Studies on Alcohol and Drugs*, **74**, 428–436.

Cunningham, J., Wild, T. C., Cordingley, J., van Mierlo, T., & Humphreys, K. (2009). A randomized controlled trial of Internet-based intervention for alcohol abuse. *Addiction*, **104**, 2023–2032.

Drummond, C., Ghodse, H., & Chengappa, S. (2007). Investigations in alcohol use disorders. In E. Day (Ed.), *Clinical topics in addictions* (pp. 113–129). London: Royal College of Psychiatrists.

Fagan, K. J., Irvine, K. M., McWhinney, B. C., Fletcher, L. M., Horsfall, L. U., Johnson, L., … Powell, E. E. (2014). Diagnostic sensitivity of carbohydrate deficient transferrin in heavy drinkers. *BMC Gastroenterology*, **22**(14), 97.

Hashimoto, E., Riederer, P. F., Hesselbrock, V. M., Hesselbrock, M. N., Ukai, W., Thibaut, F., … Saito, T. (2013). Consensus paper of the WFSBP task force on biological markers: Biological markers for alcoholism. *World Journal of Biological Psychiatry*, **14**, 549–564.

Havard, A., Shakeshaft, A., & Sanson-Fisher, R. (2008). Systematic review and meta-analysis of strategies targeting alcohol problems in emergency departments: Interventions reduce alcohol-related injuries. *Addiction*, **103**, 368–376.

Hodgson, R. J., Alwyn, T., John, B., Thom, B., & Smith, A. (2002). The FAST Alcohol Screening Test. *Alcohol and Alcoholism*, **37**, 61–66.

Humphreys, K., & Tucker, J. (2002). Towards more responsive and effective intervention systems for alcohol-related problems. *Addiction*, **97**, 126–132.

Kanfer, F. H., & Schefft, B. K. (1988). *Guiding the process of therapeutic change*. Champaign, IL: Research Press.

Mayfield, D., MacLeod, G., & Hall, P. (1974). The CAGE questionnaire: Validation of a new alcoholism screening instrument. *American Journal of Psychiatry*, **131**, 1121–1123.

Mayou, R., & Bryant, B. (1995). Alcohol and road traffic accidents. *Alcohol and Alcoholism*, **30**, 709–711.

Miller, W. R., & Sanchez, V. C. (1993). Motivating young adults for treatment and lifestyle change. In G. Howard (Ed.), *Issues in alcohol use and misuse by young adults*. South Bend, IN: University of Notre Dame Press.

Moyer, A., Finney, J. W., Swearingen, C. E., & Vergun, P. (2002). Brief interventions for alcohol problems: A meta-analytic review of controlled investigations in treatment-seeking and non-treatment-seeking populations. *Addiction*, **97**, 279–292.

Niemela, O. (2007). Biomarkers in alcoholism. *Clinica Chimica Acta*, **377**, 39–49.

Pettinati, H. M., Weiss, R. D., Miller, W. R., Donovan, D., Ernst, D.B., & Rounsaville, B.J. (2004). *Medical Management (MM) treatment manual*. Bethesda, MD: National Institute on Alcohol Abuse and Alcoholism.

Piano, S., Marchioro, L., Gola, E., Rosi, S., Morando, F., Cavallin, M., … Angeli, P. (2014). Assessment of alcohol consumption in liver transplant candidates and recipients: The best combination of the tools available. *Liver Transplantation*, **20**, 815–822.

Piccinelli, M., Tessari, E., Bortolomasi, M., Piasere, P., Semenzin, M., Garzotto, N., & Tansella, M. (1997). Efficacy of the alcohol use disorders identification test as a screening tool for hazardous alcohol intake and related disorders in primary care: A validity study. *British Medical Journal*, **314**, 420–424.

Pokorny, A. D., Miller, B. A., & Kaplan, H. B. (1972). The brief MAST: A shortened version of the Michigan Alcoholism Screening Test. *American Journal of Psychiatry*, **129**, 342–345.

Russell, M. (1994). New assessment tools for risk taking during pregnancy: T-ACE, TWEAK and others. *Alcohol Health and Research World*, **18**, 55–61.

Selzer, M. L. (1971). The Michigan Alcoholism Screening Test: The quest for a new diagnostic instrument. *American Journal of Psychiatry*, **127**(12), 1653–1658.

Smith, S. G. T., Touquet, R., Wright, S., & Das Gupta, N. (1996). Detection of alcohol misusing patients in accident and emergency departments: The Paddington Alcohol Test (PAT). *Journal of Accident and Emergency Medicine*, **13**, 308–312.

Sokol, R. J., Martier, S. S., & Ager, J. W. (1989). The T-ACE questions: Practical prenatal detection of risk-taking. *American Journal of Obstetrics and Gynaecology*, **160**, 863–870.

Sullivan, L. E., Tetrault, J. M., Braithwaite, R. S., Turner, B. J., & Fiellin, D. A. (2011). A meta-analysis of the efficacy of nonphysician brief interventions for unhealthy alcohol use: Implications for the patient-centered medical home. *American Journal of Addictions*, **20**, 343–356.

Chapter 10

Assessment of patients with drinking problems

The previous chapter dealt with case-finding through the use of screening tools, which are in themselves a form of brief assessment. This chapter describes how to conduct more thorough patient evaluations, for example prior to the commencement of psychotherapy in a psychiatric or addiction care setting. A properly conducted assessment is critical both for the selection of treatment and its goals, but also because it is the first opportunity to create a therapeutic alliance with the patient and to communicate important information to him or her. For this reason, clinicians should remember that even the assessment before the intervention is in fact an intervention in its own right.

Practically, the assessment process should explore what the individual wants or expects, gather the information based on which the drinking problem can be identified, and explore any factors that may complicate the presentation and management, including the physical, psychiatric, or social. On the basis of this assessment, a mutually agreed treatment plan should be negotiated.

This chapter seeks to cover practical issues related to the art and technique of such history-taking. However, more research-oriented and structured approaches are provided by diagnostic instruments such as the Diagnostic Interview Schedule (DIS), the Structured Clinical Interview for DSM-V, and the Comprehensive International Diagnostic Interview (CIDI) (World Health Organization, 1993). This chapter is cast in the form of a series of working guidelines. As such, the framework builds on the general format for psychiatric history-taking (University of London, Institute of Psychiatry & Bethlem Royal Hospital and the Maudsley Hospital, 1987). History-taking is a rewarding aspect of clinical work, and the reader should not be daunted by the details of this presentation. In particular, anyone coming to this type of work for the first time should not attempt to absorb everything that is being said here at one sitting. Consequently, for those very much constrained by time, there follows a description of what might reasonably be achieved in a 15-minute assessment. Then, having outlined the patient interview, the chapter will describe a parallel approach to history-taking from the partner. Tables will provide a summary of the key points in history-taking, both for the person presenting with the problem and for the partner. Finally, a scheme for the construction of a case formulation is provided.

Case history as initiation of treatment

Taking a history from an individual should not only be a matter of obtaining facts to be written down in the case notes. It is an interaction between two people, and it ought to be as meaningful for the person who answers the questions as for the questioner. The patient should be invited to use the occasion as a personal opportunity to review the past and present and to make sense of what may previously have been a chaotic array of happenings. When skillfully administered, an assessment alone can help change the drinker's attitudes, enhance commitment, and clarify goals (Thom et al., 1992).

Assessment is therefore the beginning of treatment (Novey, 1968). The relationship between patient and clinician begins at this moment, and, if the occasion is mishandled, the patient may not attend for a second appointment. A positive relationship has been shown between the perceived quality of the initial assessment and patient receptiveness with subsequent willingness to engage in treatment (Fiorentine, Nakashima, & Anglin, 1999; Hyams, Cartwright, & Spratley, 1996).

Setting the tone

Handling the initial contact with someone who has a drinking problem does not stand entirely apart from work with any other type of patient. However, it may have been especially difficult for this person to get themselves so far as to recognize that they have a need for help and then to keep the first appointment. To reveal that one is not fully in control of drinking can feel like an admission of failure, and patients may be highly ambivalent about walking into the interview room (indeed, more often than not, pressure from someone else was required to get them there).

Clinicians should therefore not assume that their own goodwill and value is self-evident to a new patient. Some patients may even be looking for a reason to quickly judge that this is all a waste of time and that the first contact should justifiably also be the last. Special care must be put into showing ordinary courtesies: to introduce oneself, to walk up the corridor to the interview room with the patient rather than five paces in front, to take a coat and hang it up, to show that person toward a comfortable chair, and turn off the mobile phone are small but telling gestures. It may be useful to say, "I'm glad you've decided to come, and I hope that this meeting will be helpful for you."

Case notes have to be recorded and a semi-structured approach is useful. The procedure should be as informal and unthreatening as possible rather than a cross-examination. The first question should always be something like, "What can we do for you?" There should then be a willingness to listen to the answer while looking at the person who is talking. The answer may be discursive or brief, may bear on the drinking or deal with other issues, but the patient is setting the scene in the way that he or she finds helpful. It can be useful to explore the circumstances that have led to this appointment being made.

Finally, the clinician can defuse tension up front by saying something like "After today's session, we will each have a better understanding of the situation and can then decide together whether we should continue forward with treatment." Such clarifying of expectations generally helps patients relax as they realize that, so to speak, they are being asked only to go on a first date rather than having to commit to marriage within a moment of meeting the clinician.

The clinician can then proceed to taking a formal history. A statement such as the following can be made:

> "I've listened to what you are saying carefully. If you don't mind, it would help if I asked you some questions and made notes. I'm going to assume that all your answers are as honest and as open as you can possibly make them. If there's anything too difficult to talk about, let me know, and I'll respect your feelings."

This might seem to be emphasizing the ordinary assumption of the therapeutic position in a way that is overdrawn. But if history-taking is clumsily handled and the initial relationship not sympathetically established, the interview will be interpreted as an attack, and defences will rapidly be brought into play. The likely result will be the gathering of poor-quality information and the confirmation of the stereotype that problem drinkers "never tell the truth."

Background history

Although the discussion here divides the assessment into background history and drinking history, the two are often related. In the *background* section, many matters are touched on that will inevitably elicit information on drinking and drinking problems, and such information should be jotted down rather than discarded or ignored because it does not come tidily at the right moment. The *drinking* section, as well as eliciting further new information, then gives the opportunity to bring together and explore the relevance of the material that the patient gave earlier. This chapter focuses primarily on assessment of drinking but the reader should bear in mind the material in prior chapters regarding medical complications (Chapter 5), comorbid psychiatric disorders (Chapter 6), and use of drugs other than alcohol (Chapter 7). The clinician must keep an eye open for any or all of those problems arising in the assessment and investigate them (or seek consultation from other professionals) when they do.

Because time is often at a premium, data on strictly factual aspects of the patient's life should be gathered in advance of the clinical assessment either via paper-and-pencil forms or through an electronic assessment package on a computer. Such facts include the patient's age, marital status, race/ethnicity, level of education, number and age of children, number and age of siblings and of parents, occupation, and religious affiliation if any. The clinician should then refer to this material during the assessment, both to communicate that the information provided is being attended to and also to know where clinical attention should be directed for further information gathering (e.g., "I see that you were divorced last year and that you have a 14-year-old daughter. Is your daughter living with you and how would you describe your relationship with her?").

Family history

1. *For both parents.* Present relationship with parents, if living; date and cause of death if deceased; quality of relationships offered to patient in childhood; parents' drinking and attitudes toward alcohol; parents' use of other drugs and experience of any psychiatric illness. Enquiry may also be needed into drinking and other drug problems and psychiatric illness in the wider family.
2. *Siblings.* Present contact with patient and quality of relationship. Current or past psychiatric problems or drug/alcohol problems.
3. *Childhood environment.* Reconstruction of the home atmosphere during childhood and the social and cultural milieu in which this home was embedded. Sources of stress (e.g., marital conflict) should be explored but so too should any perceived strengths of the family of origin. Where relevant, childhood relations with other important adult figures should be explored (e.g., step-parents, grandparents, aunts, uncles).

The purpose of this section is to obtain a preliminary understanding of the crucial early relationships and experiences that may have contributed to the shaping of the individual's strengths or vulnerabilities and their relationship with alcohol. Attention should be paid to any positive features of the patient's family history rather than subtly guiding the patient to weave a narrative of woe that culminates in the current difficulties.

Personal history

1. *Adjustment in childhood.* This assessment should include the psychological and social strengths of the individual as child, as well as any challenges. For example, the good times of childhood, what gave them hope, their ability to make friends, signs of mastery, the proud moments, and their sources of love. Difficulties in childhood should also be explored, including problems relating to other children, conduct disorder, dyslexia, trauma, and childhood illness.
2. *Education.* Academic performance and social adjustment at school – how the patient got on with other children and with teachers, school refusal or truancy, whether they were bullied, literacy, and exam certificates obtained. To ask, "What were you best at?" will help confer a sense of self.
3. *Occupational history and nature of present occupation.* Has employment history been stable or unstable? Is current work satisfying, and does it involve any alcohol exposure? Have co-workers and supervisors shown any awareness of the patient's drinking?
4. *Significant romantic relationships and marriage.* Status of current relationship and drinking of the partner and perceived cause of the ending of any prior marriages and/or significant marriage-like relationships. When asking questions in this domain, clinicians should be careful not to make assumptions that makes it difficult for patients to be forthcoming. For example, current and past relationships should not be presumed heterosexual, nor should the clinician consider questions about current romantic relationships at an end simply because the patient mentions being married.
5. *Children.* Closeness of the patient to children and parenting abilities; perceived impact of drinking on the children and their reaction to the drinking. Drinking by children should also be explored where appropriate.
6. *Finances and housing.* The economic impact of drinking; the estimated amount of money spent on drink per week.
7. *Leisure.* The way in which the person usually spends their leisure time; proportion of such time that does and does not involve drinking. Ask if any enjoyable leisure activities have been curtailed.
8. *Forensic history.* Public drunkenness offences, drink driving, and all other convictions or pending court appearances. The relationship between the drinking and the offending may need to be explored, as should any connection between drinking and violent behaviour, whether it has resulted in arrest or not.
9. *Friendships and social network.* Nonfamily members who can be relied on for practical and/or emotional support; drinking by such network members; frequency of feeling lonely and wanting more social contact.
10. *Motivations and values.* The patient's moral code; what and who they consider most important in their life. In exploring these issues, the clinician should treat religiously derived and secular values and motivations with comparable respect and attention.

Previous illnesses

1. *Physical illness, operations, and accidents.*
2. *Psychiatric illnesses.*

Information is needed under both subheadings, with emphasis on identification of alcohol-related health problems. Under the heading of *psychiatric illness*, specific inquiry should always be made for any history suggesting experience of depressive illness or pronounced mood swings, generalized or situational anxiety, obsessional disorder, post-traumatic stress disorder (PTSD), suicide attempts, and drug-taking.

Drinking history

A detailed account of everything that has happened over a lifetime's drinking is unattainable and unnecessary. Rather, the goal is to understand the individual's drinking in longitudinal perspective, including milestones, major transitions, phases of the drinking career, and the broadly related influences on it. This picture needs to be built up through exploring three different but closely related dimensions of the person's life.

The evolution of drinking

The task here is to chart the major phases in drinking quantities and patterns, from first experiences of alcohol to the present. Useful lines of questioning (any of which might honestly be answered "never" in some cases) may relate to such issues as:

First drinking other than the occasional sip in childhood?
First buying own drink?
First drinking most weekends?
First drinking spirits?
Any periods completely off drinking?
First drinking every day?
First drinking in the morning?
First time not able to remember what happened while drinking?
First time needing a drink to stop withdrawal symptoms?
First drinking in present pattern?

Evolution of drink-related problems

Apart from noting objective impacts on health and social functioning, there are two special questions which are often useful:

When did you yourself first realize drinking was a problem?
Looking back now with greater understanding, when in fact do you think drinking really became a problem?

With hindsight, patients will nearly always distinguish between the first self-awareness of there being a problem (precipitated perhaps by some catastrophic event) and an earlier date now recognizable as the period when drinking was undramatically beginning to, say, erode the happiness of a marriage or interfere with work.

Evolution of pressures and circumstances

The dimension that has to be charted under this heading is concerned with an understanding of the pressures and circumstances that have caused, contributed to, or shaped the evolving drinking patterns, dependence, and problem experience. Questioning has to sense out influences that were already operating when the patient began to drink (parental example, peer group pressures, cultural influence, etc.) and then go forward to understand the subsequent impact of environment, life events, personal relations, mental state, and other relevant factors. This exploration should comprise both factors co-occurring with increased drinking as well as those associated with reductions in consumption/periods of abstinence. Examples of appropriate questions about how drinking changed at different points are numerous:

When you first left home?
At college?
When you were married?
After the children were born?
When the children left home?
When you were promoted to manager?
When you were fired from your job?
When you worked abroad?
After your partner left you?
After you developed depression?
When you retired?

The typical recent heavy drinking day

Review of the evolution in drinking history seeks to build an understanding that is *longitudinal* – the present is understood in its historical perspective. Reconstruction of the typical drinking day, on the other hand, focuses exclusively on the present and the cross-sectional rather than the longitudinal view. The styles of enquiry are correspondingly different. When reconstructing the evolution of the problem, it is the broad sweep that is important and the reconstruction of how drinking has interacted with a life path. Analysis of the typical day requires, in contrast, a minute and focused enquiry directed at present behaviour. This understanding should be so exact that, in the mind's eye, it is possible to project a film of the patient's day.

Establishing the notion of "typical"

First, the concept involved has to be conveyed to the patient. He or she is asked to identify (1) *a recent period* when drinking was, in terms of their own definition, (2) *heavy*, with the drinking then of a kind that they would generally consider to be (3) *typical* of their recent drinking. The patient has to identify the exact period they have in mind – "the way I was drinking until 2 weeks ago when I lost my job and had to cut down." What has to be emphasized is the actuality, rather than any generalized abstractions that have no real time base. Most patients find it possible to identify such a period, but for others there is so much variability in their drinking pattern that what is typical is difficult to define, and this in itself is a reality that has to be described.

Waking and events around waking

Having explained the ground rules, it is necessary to establish at what time the patient usually wakes. Enquiry is then made into the events immediately around the time of waking because it is here that evidence will be obtained of withdrawal symptoms, withdrawal relief drinking, and other signs and symptoms that help to elucidate the patient's degree of dependence.

Subsequent hour-by-hour time-table

The patient is then taken through a reconstruction of the day as follows:

1. *The background structure of daily activities.* For instance, what time they leave the house in the morning, what train they catch, what time they get to work, when they take their lunch break, and so on.
2. *The time-table of drinking.* With the framework now provided by the structure of the day, the next task is to fit in a full description of the day's drinking. What time does the patient take their first drink, how much do they drink, and over what duration? This enquiry is then taken forward, step by step, through the day. In each instance, to a description of actual alcohol intake is added a note of where the drinking takes place and with whom (if anyone) the patient is drinking. Note also has to be made of the patient's ideas about the determinants of each drinking occasion – whether to relieve or avoid withdrawal symptoms, to lessen anxiety or other unpleasant inner feelings, whether in the setting of business or for the companionship of the pub, or for any other reason. A final aspect of drinking that has to be time-tabled is the experience of intoxication and whether, at any point of the day, the patient would consider that drink is interfering with ordinary functioning.

Perceived influence of drinking on mood and behaviour

Some patients are not aware that drinking alters how they feel and act, whereas others will describe a transformation. The issue has to be examined, both in terms of positive and negative effects. Positively, someone may, for instance, see themselves as more outgoing, sexier, confident, and fun when drinking. On the negative side, the "Jekyll and Hyde" effects may include irritability and loss of control over temper (including violence), suspiciousness, moroseness, self-pity, or lack of feeling for others. Because, by definition, observation of one's intoxicated behaviour is made in an impaired state, the clinician should be aware that the patient's perception of changed behaviour may differ from that of observers (e.g., the drinker finds himself delightfully brash and witty; everyone else considers him cruel and boorish).

Probing and checking

Careful probing is essential when assessing current drinking:

CLINICIAN: All right, you say you have 3 pints of lager at lunch-time. How long do you spend in the pub at lunch time?

PATIENT: Noon till 2 p.m., sometimes 3 p.m.

CLINICIAN: So, you are there until 2 p.m. or 3 p.m.?

PATIENT: Say, 2:30 p.m.

CLINICIAN: Three pints in two and a half hours seems quite slow drinking.

PATIENT: If I'm there 12 to 2:30, I suppose it would be 4 or 5 pints. I was thinking of when I have a short lunch break. It's more often a long liquid lunch these days.

CLINICIAN: You say 4 or 5 pints – could it be more?

PATIENT: No, I'd get too bloated. I don't think I'd ever go above 5 pints.

CLINICIAN: Anything else besides lager at lunch time?

PATIENT: I might have a couple of whiskies.

CLINICIAN: Why "a couple" – could it be more?

PATIENT: No, I'll have just a couple of whiskies to round things off when I've finished with the lager. Not more than a couple.

CLINICIAN: Double or single measures?

PATIENT: Doubles.

CLINICIAN: Ever leave out the whisky?

PATIENT: No, it's pretty regular.

Putting quantity consumed against time spent drinking, sometimes checking stated consumption against money usually spent, comparing reported alcohol consumption prior to attending with breathalyser readings, testing the stated upper limit by offering a higher or lower one, going through other alcoholic beverages than the one first named, and relating the stated drinking to the company and other circumstances, all provide useful methods for checking that can help to establish a valid picture.

Totalling the daily intake

Information on quantity drunk throughout the day can be summed to total daily intake. Because of uncertainties in size of drink poured, broad variations in alcohol content for drinks within any beverage type (beer, wine, or spirits), and international differences on the size of a standard drink, the summated figure is at best an approximation rather than an exact index. For research purposes, the most satisfactory approach is to express the total in terms of grams absolute alcohol, but in the clinical setting the idea of *units or standard drinks* provides a useful basis (see Chapter 1).

Bringing together any evidence of dependence

Much information relevant to establishing whether and to what degree the patient is alcohol-dependent will have been obtained from questioning in the areas of *evolution* and *drinking day*. It is, however, necessary to have in the history a place where evidence on possible dependence is reviewed and brought together.

The picture of the alcohol dependence syndrome and its degrees of variation has been fully discussed in Chapter 1, and the headings used in that chapter to describe the core elements of the syndrome provide the framework for this section of the history-taking. Brief notes are added here on the practical approach to questioning in each instance.

Narrowing of the drinking repertoire

Useful questions relate to the sameness or otherwise of drinking during weekdays as opposed to weekends or during the working week as opposed to holidays.

Salience of drinking

Reconstructing the evolution of the patient's drinking will have implicitly provided an account of the progressive importance of alcohol in their life and their progressive ability to discount other considerations. An attempt should also be made to sense out with the patient how salient drinking has become in the here and now. Useful questions are, for instance:

Just how important has drinking become for you?

Is drinking more or less important for you than eating?

Is drinking more important than people?

A particular phrase in the patient's answers may suddenly and empathetically convey the reality of their drink-centredness: "When my husband said he would leave me if I went on drinking, I had the sly thought, well, if he leaves me, there will be more time and money for drinking."

Here, it is often useful to ask a question like, "What are the good things that drinking does for you?" In this way, one gains a sense of the functional significance of alcohol for that patient; for example, whether they see themselves as drinking for company and the pleasures of the bar-room environment, for the "high" state and directly pleasurable effects of intoxication, for relief of unpleasant feelings, or for a combination of these reasons. The dependent drinker may insist that they have ceased to get any pleasure out of drinking or even say that they hate every drink – they are caught on a treadmill.

Increased tolerance (or evidence of decreased tolerance)

Many patients will say that they can "drink a lot without getting drunk," and the quantity that is habitually taken is itself evidence of tolerance. If, at a later stage in the drinking career, a severe decline in tolerance is experienced, this is often reported as a worrying happening.

Withdrawal symptoms

Questioning here has to deal with the frequency and intensity of common withdrawal symptoms: tremor, nausea, sweating, mood disturbance. These symptoms may be experienced not only on waking but also with partial alcohol withdrawal during the waking day. Any history of subacute hallucinatory experiences, delirium tremens, or withdrawal fits should also be noted.

Relief or avoidance of withdrawal symptoms by further drinking

Questioning here must cover the frequency with which the patient drinks to relieve or avoid withdrawal and the perceived urgency for such a drink.

Subjective awareness of compulsion to drink

Matters that may bear on the assessment of subjective experience were discussed in Chapter 1. Craving may be most intense during withdrawal, but there may be rumination on drink and the need to protect the drink supply pretty well throughout the day.

Reinstatement after abstinence

Questioning here should focus on the actualities of what happened on recent occasions when the patient was abstinent and then went back to drinking again – when they came out of prison perhaps; when they came out of the hospital; or when, after a period of involvement with Alcoholics Anonymous, they "had a slip." How quickly were they again experiencing withdrawal symptoms or needing to take a morning drink?

Standard diagnostic systems

The *Diagnostic and Statistical Manual of Mental Disorders* (DSM-5) criteria for alcohol use disorder (American Psychiatric Association, 2013) and the International Classification of Disease (ICD-10) criteria for alcohol dependence (World Health Organization, 1992, 1997) are reproduced in Chapter 1. Both sets of criteria are useful in standardizing diagnostic practice, nationally and internationally, and they carry authority. However, the ICD criteria have a drawback from the clinician's point of view in that they picture dependence as an all-or-none rather than as a dimensional state. Categorical formulae are proposed at the cost of clinical subtlety. The DSM-V is superior in this respect and will be particularly appreciated by clinicians working in settings where many patients have significant but not highly severe drinking problems.

Questionnaires for measuring dependence

As mentioned in the prior chapter, the Alcohol Use Disorder Identification Test (AUDIT) is valuable for measuring drinking problems at the lower end of severity. Standardized instruments have also been designed to rate the degree of alcohol dependence, including the Alcohol Dependence Scale (Skinner & Horn, 1984), the Short Alcohol Dependence Data questionnaire (Raistrick, Dunbar, & Davidson, 1983), and the Severity of Alcohol Dependence Questionnaire (Stockwell et al., 1979; Stockwell, Murphy, & Hodgson, 1983). The practitioner will do well to gain a working familiarity with just one such approach so that scores can be readily related to their clinical meaning.

Bringing together evidence on the consequences of drinking

The introduction of the patient to this section of history-taking could be as follows: "Let's try to bring together the ways in which alcohol may have been having any sort of positive and negative effect on your life – on your physical health, or your job, or your relationships, or your life satisfaction or anything else. You've already told me a lot about separate problems, but now let's try to make out the whole list."

If, for example, the impact of drinking on the patient's marriage were to arise in a particular case, the discussion might be as follows:

CLINICIAN: You told me that your wife walked out on you because of your drinking.

PATIENT: If it hadn't been for the drinking, we might have made a go of it. I'm not saying we *would* have made a go of it. We *might* have made a go of the marriage.

There is a question here that could be explored with this patient later at greater length, but, for purposes of this initial history, it is sufficient to establish that the patient accepts as a fair assessment that, without the drinking he "might have made a go of the marriage." A clumsy interrogation that faced him with no more than a sort of yes/no alternative would not have given him an opportunity to convey and define in a personally meaningful way the impact of drinking on his marriage.

Standardized questionnaires completed by the patient or by the patient and clinician together can be quite useful in this part of the assessment, including the Drinker Inventory of Consequences (DrInC; Miller, Tonigan, & Longabaugh, 1995). The Alcohol Problems Questionnaire (APQ) is another validated, standardized inventory that exists in a fuller version that includes sections on marriage, children, and employment and in a shorter form that excludes these areas (Drummond, 1990; Williams & Drummond, 1994). Both scales can make a useful contribution to the overall assessment, with the meaning of any scored items discussed with the patient.

Questioning in this section should be aimed at involving the patient in a candid review of the available data. Each relevant fact is adduced with the patient's exploration of its significance and the degree to which alcohol was involved. The list ends up as his own assessment, rather than it being the therapist's private clinical note.

BOX 10.1 From the pages of history: The invention of the t-test

> I was mixed up with a lot of large scale experiments partly agricultural but chiefly in an Experimental Brewery. The agricultural (and indeed almost any) Experiments naturally required a solution of the mean/S.D. problem and the Experimental Brewery which concerns such things as the connection between analysis of malt or hops, and the behaviour of the beer, and which takes a day to each unit of the experiment, thus limiting the numbers, demanded an answer to such questions as 'If with a small number of cases I get a value r, what is the probability that there is really a positive correlation of greater than (say) −25 T.'
>
> Extract of 15 September 1915 letter of W. S. Gosset to R. A. Fisher

> I am enclosing a letter which gives a proof of my formulae for the frequency distribution of z (= x/a), where x is the distance of the mean of n observations from the general mean and s is the S.D. of the n observations. Would you mind looking at it for me; I don't feel at home in more than three dimensions even if I could understand it otherwise.
>
> Extract of 12 September 1912 letter of W. S. Gosset to Karl Pearson

Throughout this book are many scientific findings regarding, for example, how people with drinking problems differ from people without such problems and how one treatment differs in effectiveness from another. Typically, such conclusions rest on comparisons of samples drawn from a larger population. Such inferences depend on comparing observed differences to a standardized distribution, which helps the researcher determine the validity of assumptions about a population from which the sample was drawn. One of the most widely used methods of making such comparisons is the *Student's t-test*, which funnily enough emerged from the alcohol industry.

Guinness Brewery, producer of some of the world's best-loved beers, hired an Oxford University chemistry graduate named William Sealy Gosset in 1899. Among Gosset's responsibilities was to judge the quality of brewing methods based on small quantities of stout. He developed for this purpose a formal statistical test, which he published in the prestigious journal *Biometrika*. Because Guinness did not allow its staff to publish their work, Gosset adopted the humble pseudonym "Student" (1908). However, as the extracts of the preceding

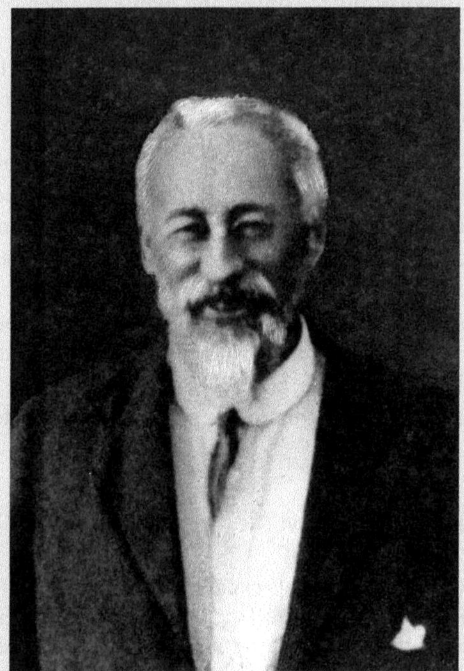

Figure 10.1: William Sealy Gosset. Courtesy of Guinness/Diageo.

letters show, Gosset's true identity was well-known to the greatest statisticians of his day, including Sir Ronald Fisher and Karl Pearson (the letters were discovered and published by Karl's son Egon many years after they were written; Pearson 1968). Gosset continued to make significant contributions to statistics for the rest of his career. By the time of his death in 1937, his place in the pantheon of statistical giants was well-established, and today most researchers in the world – of alcohol or otherwise – will at some point be exposed to Student's t-test, even if they don't know its origins in Irish brewing history.

History of and current reasons for help-seeking

Enquiry should be made both about help sought by the patient in the past and help being given at present. It is then essential to understand the patient's reasons for coming to this present consultation – the pressures they see themselves as experiencing (a court order or threats from a partner, for instance), what crisis may suddenly have precipitated the immediate help-seeking, or what inner sense of need is driving the motivation. Once more, the process of history-taking is an experience for the patient as well as it giving information to the clinician. The patient is exploring the question of why he or she is in this room and is trying to understand the ambiguous, confused, or contradictory motivations that have brought them here. Such knowledge is an important basis for later work. The history has to be taken with an awareness that motivation is often ambivalent: the patient both wants to go on drinking and wants to stop drinking. These conflicting forces should be identified and labeled rather than the reality of conflict being evaded.

Physical examination and investigations

Physical examination and laboratory investigations will be part of the assessment routine in a medical setting. In a social work or probation office, this aspect of assessment is not within expected practice, but there would be an advantage to such agencies in ensuring that the patient receives a physical examination from a medical professional with the results fed back. This insistence on the importance of making a medical connection may go against the usual working methods of some nonmedical agencies and be seen as burdensome. However, the likelihood of physical disorder in the patient with a drinking problem puts that person in a different category from many other social work clients.

What might go into a 15-minute assessment?

The way that constricted time is best used must be, to an extent, patient- and setting-specific. The following notes offer some general suggestions:

1. *Despite pressures of time, do not lose sight of the fact that assessment should be an indication of treatment.* Give the patient initial free time to talk, try to understand why this person has come to see you, respond to them positively and give encouragement, round off the interview, and identify productive next steps.
2. *Concentrate on the present.* Try to get a sense of present drinking level, current and recent problems with drinking, present life situation, and recent help-seeking.
3. *Estimate degree of dependence on alcohol.* Information on presence and intensity of any withdrawal symptoms can provide a useful short-cut.
4. *Set proximate goals* in relation to moderation of drinking, abstinence, and/or seeking of additional support.
5. *Always seek to identify any possibility of comorbid diagnosis.* Concomitant depression, anxiety, traumatic injuries, and drug-taking should always be on the checklist.
6. *In a medical setting, carry out blood tests* (see Chapter 9). A quick physical examination may be needed.
7. *Make another appointment,* keep in touch, monitor progress, offer to see the partner, and network with other agencies that could help the patient.

Assessment with the partner or other significant individual in the patient's life

For a range of reasons, patients do not always provide full or accurate information during an assessment. If the patient consents, it is therefore extremely useful for the clinician to talk to an important person in the patient's life who has knowledge of the patient's drinking. Most commonly, this individual will be a partner, but the many other possibilities include a grandfather who is raising an adolescent whose parents are absent, a sibling with a particularly close relationship to the patient, and a member of the clergy who has known and counselled the patient since childhood. Whether this assessment is conducted with the patient present or independently depends on the specifics of the case and the clinician's judgement of whether the other informant has any fear of contradicting the patient or will be seen by the patient as an ally in the development of an accurate assessment.

Structuring the interaction requires sensitivity and flexibility. In some cases, it will quickly become apparent that the informant has serious difficulties of his or her own, for example, in a couple where both members of a romantic relationship drink to excess as a shared activity. The clinician may be tempted to plunge into a full assessment of the informant's life, but this is inappropriate if the informant is in contact to help the patient but has no interest in pursuing treatment of his or her own. However, it is entirely appropriate for a clinician to express concern about problems in the informant's life and to offer separate or conjoint treatment, as appropriate.

Case formulation and treatment planning

After a thorough assessment, the clinician's task is to pull together a large and diverse range of information into a coherent case formulation. A well-constructed formulation is a creative act of empathy rather than just an ordering of information under headings.

The additional investment of time to develop a case formulation pays handsome returns. The clinician is directionless until the formulation is made. Furthermore, when the notes and questionnaires are put aside for a few weeks and the patient reattends treatment, the freshness of understanding has often faded unless the formulation has been written. The original formulation will also be of great use if a case is reopened after a gap of a year or two or if the patient's case is eventually taken over by a different care provider.

A formulation should not be of inordinate length or it defeats its purpose. Ideally, the formulation should be a summary of key information consumable in less than 10 minutes that explains the evolution and current state of the patient's predicament; his or her strengths, weaknesses, and aspirations; and the environmental supports and impediments to change. It is entirely appropriate, particularly early in treatment, for the formulation to include a note that certain areas of the patient's life remain to be explored in further detail and what this will require (e.g., a referral to a neuropsychologist for a cognitive assessment).

Reference has already been made to the necessity of the formulation serving the needs of the patient as well as the therapist. Before making final notes on the formulation, there should have been an interchange in which the therapist says, "What we have talked through is valuable ... I see it this way ... What we ought to do is perhaps this ... How do you see it? ... Can we agree then? ..." Such discussion ensures that not only is the clinician standing back from the data and gaining a whole view, but that the patient is doing the same, and they are doing so together.

Once completed and reviewed with the patient, the formulation becomes the basis for selecting the appropriate goals and modality of treatment. On the basis of what has already been laid out in the preceding sections of the formulation, it should be possible to set up a series of specific treatment goals. At least one goal should concern drinking behaviour, but other goals may be about other important life domains such as family and work.

With as much specificity as possible, the clinician and patient should then agree to a course of treatment that follows from the case formulation and the goals of the intervention. "Treat the alcohol problem" is not a sufficiently specific treatment plan; something like

"Meet once or twice a week for cognitive-behavioural therapy directed at returning to moderate drinking" is better. Plans to evaluate progress or lack of progress at a designated point are typically valuable, and the treatment goals and modality may be revisited in light of what is evident at that time.

Assessment: The essential business

Assessment is a process that, if skillfully and humanely conducted, should be both rewarding and challenging for the person who has come into the consulting room. It should allow patients to see the evolution of their drinking within their life course. It may illuminate problems that are serious, painful, and/or embarrassing, but it should at the same time give hope. Assessment is at best a small but important new step in a longer journey, but it should help the patient leave the room with the crucial sense that he is beginning to understand what needs to be done for him to make changes and that change is possible.

References

American Psychiatric Association. (2013). *Diagnostic and statistical manual of mental disorders* (5th ed.). Washington, DC: Author.

Drummond, D. C. (1990). The relationship between alcohol dependence and alcohol-related problems in a clinical population. *British Journal of Addiction*, **85**, 357–366.

Fiorentine, R., Nakashima, J., & Anglin, M. D. (1999). Client engagement in drug treatment. *Journal of Substance Abuse and Treatment*, **17**, 199–206.

Hyams, G., Cartwright, A., & Spratley, T. (1996). Engagement in alcohol treatment: The client's experience of, and satisfaction with, the assessment interview. *Addiction Research*, **4**, 105–123.

Miller, W. R., Tonigan, J. S., & Longabaugh, R. (1995). *The Drinker Inventory of Consequences (DRInC)*. Retrieved from the National Institute of Alcohol Abuse and Alcoholism website: http://pubs.niaaa.nih.gov/publications/ProjectMatch/match04.pdf

Novey, S. (1968). *The second look: The reconstruction of personal history in psychiatry and psychoanalysis*. Baltimore, MD: Johns Hopkins Press.

Pearson, E. S. (1968). Some early correspondence between W. S. Gosset, R. A. Fisher and Karl Pearson, with notes and comments. *Biometrika*, **55**, 445–457.

Raistrick, D. S., Dunbar, G., & Davidson, R. J. (1983). Development of a questionnaire to measure alcohol dependence. *British Journal of Addiction*, **78**, 89–95.

Skinner, H. A., & Horn, J. L. (1984). *Alcohol dependence scale: User's guide*. Toronto, Canada: Addiction Research Foundation.

Stockwell, T., Hodgson, R., Edwards, G., Taylor, C., & Rankin, H. (1979). The development of a questionnaire to measure severity of alcohol dependence. *British Journal of Addiction to Alcohol and Other Drugs*, **74**, 79–87.

Stockwell, T., Murphy, D., & Hodgson, R. (1983). The Severity of Alcohol Dependence Questionnaire: Its use, reliability and validity. *British Journal of Addiction*, **78**, 145–155.

Student. (1908). The probable error of a mean. *Biometrika*, **6**, 1–25.

Thom, B., Brown, C., Drummond, C., Edwards, G., Mullan, M., & Taylor, C. (1992). Engaging patients with alcohol problems in treatment: The first consultation. *British Journal of Addiction*, **87**, 601–611.

University of London, Institute of Psychiatry & Bethlem Royal Hospital and the Maudsley Hospital. (1987). *Psychiatric examination: Notes on eliciting and recording clinical information in psychiatric patients* (2nd ed.). Oxford: Oxford University Press.

Williams, B. T., & Drummond, D. C. (1994). The Alcohol Problems Questionnaire: Reliability and validity. *Drug and Alcohol Dependence*, **35**, 239–243.

World Health Organization. (1992). *The ICD-10 classification of mental and behavioural disorders: Clinical descriptions and diagnostic guidelines*. Geneva: Author.

World Health Organization. (1993). *Composite International Diagnostic Interview (CIDI): Interviewer's manual.* Geneva: Author.

World Health Organization. (1997). *The ICD-10 classification of mental and behavioural disorders: Diagnostic criteria for research.* Geneva: Author.

Chapter 11 Withdrawal states and their clinical management

Many individuals who have sustained serious problems as a result of their drinking have not developed dependence and will not experience significant physiological disturbance upon withdrawal. A further important group will show dependence to a slight or moderate degree but will still not suffer from withdrawal symptoms that are to any major extent debilitating. On the other hand, there are individuals who will feel wretched during withdrawal, and a small group for whom withdrawal will precipitate life-threatening disturbances. Many individuals who are problem drinkers may not know about alcohol withdrawal symptoms, and therefore exploration of symptoms is required.

Given the diversity in possible withdrawal experiences, it makes no sense to approach the clinical management of withdrawal in terms of a fixed regime for all comers. A spectrum of likely withdrawal experiences suggests a corresponding need for a spectrum of clinical approaches. Many patients will need no medication at all to help them come off alcohol, whereas, for many others, withdrawal can be safely managed on an out-patient basis with appropriate medication. In only a minority will safe withdrawal from alcohol require admission to either a hospital or residential rehabilitation setting to receive more intensive monitoring of a withdrawal and medication regimen. The clinical significance of withdrawal is, first, therefore, the demand it makes on the clinician to see the different needs of different patients and to manage minor withdrawal states without unnecessary fuss while at the same time learning to recognize the necessity for very great care in managing the potentially dangerous situation. This chapter discusses clinical management of withdrawal in terms of different regimes for different intensities of need.

Significance of withdrawal as a barrier to "coming off"

Some patients will present themselves as unable to come off alcohol because of their incapacity to cope with the withdrawal symptoms. This plea may be entirely genuine, but their degree of withdrawal and any associated complications should be confirmed by appropriate assessment. A patient who has previously experienced an attack of delirium tremens (DTs; "the horrors") may know full well that when they are in a state of severe relapse there is a grave risk of precipitating a further attack of delirium if they attempt to stop drinking abruptly. For such individuals – and similarly for those who have experienced a seizure during alcohol withdrawal – their request for in-patient admission should be carefully considered. On the other hand, there are patients with less severe degrees of dependence whose belief that they cannot stop drinking without being hospitalized should be kindly resisted. It is important for such patients to learn that they can cope with withdrawal at home, with appropriate medication and support. This will result in minimal upheaval and will also not reinforce the idea that they are incapable of dealing with withdrawal and relapse themselves without repeated admissions. Unnecessary admissions, which engender sickness behaviour, are best avoided. In any case, with fewer dedicated units for alcohol detoxification available in the United Kingdom and United States, safe and appropriate out-patient management is increasingly required.

Withdrawal and clinical teamwork

Given that medication may be prescribed for out-patient withdrawal, and given also the potential seriousness of the major withdrawal experience that demands in-patient admission, the medical practitioner clearly has an important role to play in treatment. If the patient is being handled primarily by nonmedical staff, this implies the need for good medical liaison. The counsellor in an agency with no medically trained staff must, for instance, know when to make the rapid out-patient/community alcohol team referral or call on the advice of the general practitioner with whom there is a working relationship.

Withdrawal in context

Mere stopping drinking or drying out is not by itself an effective way of helping a patient, and whatever is done about withdrawal only has its meaning within the context of other strategies for aiding the patient. Clinical management of withdrawal, although essential, does not in itself constitute treatment of the drinking problem. When plans for withdrawal are being made during their initial assessment and goal-setting, the withdrawal phase is easily placed within the wider frame about what relapse prevention support they require. When, however, withdrawal is being dealt with in response to relapse and in an atmosphere of crisis, it is easy to react precipitously and forget the context within which decisions about withdrawal management ought to be made. Questions that should be asked in such circumstances centre on what relapse prevention plans the patient had and what happened, as well as what needs to be done differently and what use the patient is to make of this help. There should be as much discussion as possible about the patient's expectations and their responsibility in this particular aspect of the contract to help. What plans has the patient got for the far side of withdrawal?

A checklist for managing alcohol withdrawal

Does the patient want to stop drinking?

To put this item first in the checklist may seem an overemphasis of the obvious, but it is not uncommon for an individual to not realize that "detox" means they have agreed to stop drinking. It may be that the doctor has given the patient medication to treat withdrawal because the doctor believes that the patient ought to come off alcohol, rather than because the patient seriously intends to come off alcohol. The patient leaves the interview with a prescription for a bottle of benzodiazepines, which they will use to supplement continued alcohol consumption at even greater risk than before.

Is it safe to conduct withdrawal in an out-patient setting?

This decision is made without difficulty when, as commonly happens, the patient is not severely dependent. They are, for instance, suffering from morning shakes of only moderate

Table 11.1. Indicators that suggest in-patient detoxification may be appropriate

- Severe dependence
- History of complicated withdrawal, delirium tremens, or withdrawal seizures, particularly in presence of previous medically assisted withdrawals
- Previous failed community detoxification
- Lives alone or in unsupportive home environment
- Serious medical (e.g., epilepsy) or psychiatric (e.g., psychosis, severe cognitive impairment) comorbidity
- Other substance dependence, particularly opioid
- Pregnancy
- Malnourished

intensity that have been present for not much longer than 6 months, and they came off alcohol for 2 weeks on their own initiative and without any untoward happenings a month ago. A brief review with the patient of such points as these will usually settle the question of whether out-patient withdrawal is appropriate and whether medication should be prescribed. A similarly quick answer can be reached in the other direction if there is a previous history of major withdrawal experience and the patient has now reinstated dependence of serious degree. It is decisions lying in the middle ground that can be challenging to the novice clinician, who should discuss the situation with those experienced in managing alcohol withdrawal. Handling this problem will, as ever, depend on a relationship with the patient that allows open discussion of the issues involved. Nevertheless, it should be possible to manage safely and effectively the majority of patients in the community (Collins, Burns, Van den Berk, & Tubman, 1990; Stockwell et al., 1991).

In addition to severity of dependence, a number of other specific pointers may offer further guidance regarding the safety of a community detox. Has out-patient management failed previously, and, if so, why? Is there any specific medical reason why community detoxification may be hazardous; for example, a history of DTs or withdrawal seizures? Is the home environment sufficiently supportive, both in terms of family or friends who may summon help if needed and in terms of support for treatment of the drinking problem? This is discussed further later.

A summary of the indicators that suggest detoxification might be more safely and effectively conducted in an in-patient setting is given in Table 11.1. These are only an indication though, and, particularly during assessment, it is important to ascertain if complications of alcohol withdrawal occurred with medication for detoxification or not. Many patients may experience complications that, in the presence of such medication, are much reduced or absent and therefore in-patient admission may not be required. In addition, in-patient facilities range from general medical hospitals to psychiatric nonspecialist wards to residential rehabilitation facilities. Therefore, the clinician needs to carefully consider what treatment and support the available in-patient facilities offer in relation to what their patient requires.

Are there likely to be withdrawal symptoms that require clinical management?

Just as a clinician would not admit a patient for in-patient detoxification without first ensuring that it is needed (i.e., severe withdrawal symptoms are likely), a medically managed out-patient detoxification should not be undertaken without first determining that withdrawal symptoms are likely to be more than minimal. Some patients will be able to stop drinking with only minimal discomfort, and the clinician's job is to reassure, support, and reassess if symptoms worsen. This might seem a too obvious point if it were not common to find patients routinely being offered benzodiazepines without any enquiry being made into their true needs.

What is the best time?

Completing successful alcohol withdrawal without adequate time or support is likely to be challenging. For instance, those who want to detox in the midst of a busy job or childcare commitments and in the full setting of usual drinking pressures are not giving themselves the best chance of success. Discussion may suggest that they set aside time or take time off work or use holiday leave especially for this purpose. To suggest this degree of planning may usefully help to focus commitment.

Is the environment and support adequate?

The environment should be properly supportive whether the patient is detoxifying at home or as an in-patient. Support includes not just emotional and practical help but also an environment free from problem drinkers and from people who encourage problem drinking by the patient. General and psychiatric nursing skills have to be employed to help the patient through what may be a few unpleasant days, and the ability of the patient to tolerate this experience will depend in part on the sort of friendliness and support which they are being offered. To mobilize support from other patients and from visiting relatives can also be valuable.

Although there are plenty of people who at some time in their lives have been so determined to deal with their drinking that they have come off alcohol in such adverse surroundings as a "wet" or drinking hostel for the homeless, it is always useful to think through with the patient how environmental supports may be deployed to maximize the chances of success. If there is a partner available to give support, that person should be brought into the discussion, and his or her active engagement may have benefit for both partners. This may also be the moment when a patient will be particularly able to accept the usefulness of Alcoholics Anonymous (AA) or similar organization: getting out perhaps to a meeting and hearing how others dealt with this problem or receiving a phone call from another member to give a feeling of contact and fellowship, with a follow-through to more continuing involvement. The patient should have had a physical examination and recent blood tests. It is important that his or her general practitioner is kept in the picture. For those undertaking their detoxification in the community, what support can the community alcohol team offer (e.g., daily appointments over the period of a few days or daily visits from a nurse as well as low-intensity support groups)?

Which medication?

Some practical aspects for the use of medication for medically assisted withdrawal will be discussed in this section, both to provide background information for the person other than the doctor who wants to understand this aspect of the patient's treatment and to emphasize points of immediate medical concern.

Benzodiazepines

A drug of the benzodiazepine group is commonly the first choice for clinical management of alcohol withdrawal, although alternatives are available (e.g., anticonvulsants; see Kosten & O'Connor, 2003; Lingford-Hughes, Welch, Peters, & Nutt, 2012; Management of Substance Use Disorders Workgroup, 2009; National Institute for Health and Clinical Excellence, 2011). Longer acting benzodiazepines such as chlordiazepoxide or diazepam are helpful in preventing alcohol withdrawal seizures and delirium. It is best for the prescribing clinician to become familiar with one medication from this group to develop a sense of the likely needed dosages in particular circumstances, rather than switching medications. The skilled use of medication to ameliorate severe withdrawal distress or limit risk of seizures or delirium is a matter of titrating the dose against the symptoms. The withdrawal symptoms occur because the level of alcohol in the brain is falling, and these symptoms will be ameliorated when the level of prescribed medication is high enough to compensate. What one is in fact doing is substituting the alcohol with the medication, and it is often necessary and rational in the severe case to increase the medication dose boldly. Particularly with larger doses of medication, appropriate and competent monitoring should be conducted.

The dose and frequency of medication should be discussed with the patient and, if they are an out-patient, with anyone else supporting them. Instructions should written down as well as communicated verbally.

Prescribing regimes

Benzodiazepines can be prescribed in a number of ways. The most common mode of treatment is a tapering dose regime. For instance, chlordiazepoxide (Librium) may be prescribed in an initial dose of say 10–30 mg 3 or 4 times per day in an out-patient setting, reducing by 10 mg/d. Lower doses may be indicated for less severely dependent individuals, whereas higher starting doses may be required by in-patients due to their severe dependence and high risk of complications (e.g., 40–60 mg 3 or 4 times per day). Diazepam (Valium) is also commonly used. If there is an immediate need to bring severe symptoms under control, lorazepam may be given by intramuscular injection, with an initial dose of 25–30 μg/kg. Alternatively, diazepam may be given by slow intravenous injection or as a rectal suppository or enema.

A prescription should not be given for more than 3–7 days, and prescribing should not be allowed to trail on unnecessarily once the patient has withdrawn. A community or in-patient detoxification regime generally lasts about a week and rarely longer than 10 days (Lingford-Hughes et al., 2012).

Alternatively, in patients without a history of complications, a symptom-triggered regime can be instituted whereby medication is only given when symptoms emerge (Saitz et al., 1994). This approach requires skilled monitoring and should not be undertaken in its absence (Lingford-Hughes, et al., 2012; National Institute for Health and Clinical Excellence, 2010, 2011). A third method is "front-loading," which involves giving a loading dose of diazepam and following this with doses every 90 minutes or so until the patient is lightly sedated (Sellers et al., 1983).

It should again be stressed that what is "enough" is determined by clinical observation of response rather than by any rulebook. If the patient becomes excessively drowsy or if there is a large fall in blood pressure, drugs should be cut back or temporarily withheld. Such an approach is far more in the patient's interests than a blind reliance on heavy mixed medication schedules that will be unnecessarily extreme in many instances and yet insufficient in other cases.

If it has been necessary in the acute phase to load the patient with medication, one is then in effect subsequently carrying out medication withdrawal rather than an alcohol withdrawal procedure. This implies gradually tailing off the drug dose at a rate that will not produce significant additional withdrawal symptoms. The rate of reduction must once more be patient-specific and in accord with monitored symptoms.

Special populations

Healthy older patients going through managed withdrawal should be able to tolerate longer-acting benzodiazepines. However, they are more likely to experience concurrent physical illness, are at higher risk of developing medical complications (e.g., delirium), and are vulnerable to oversedation. Close monitoring is therefore advisable, although using short-acting benzodiazepines such as oxazepam or lorazepam in this age group can also be considered (Lingford-Hughes et al., 2012).

Short-acting benzodiazepines should also be considered in patients with alcohol-related liver disease. The extent of the elevation in biochemical markers (γ-glutamyl transferase [GGT], aspartate aminotransferase [AST]) will help guide decisions about dose level.

Medically supervised withdrawal of alcohol dependent pregnant women is ideally carried out in an in-patient setting, with input from medical and obstetric services to maximizes the health and safety of both the mother and the fetus. Pregnant women with alcohol dependence are likely to present later in the pregnancy (e.g., mid to late second trimester) and may be using other drugs as well. A risk–benefit assessment of alcohol withdrawal symptoms versus the prescription of benzodiazepines should be carried out. This involves taking a comprehensive history of alcohol and drug use and of withdrawal symptoms, carrying out a physical examination and obtaining laboratory investigations. The trimester of pregnancy should be noted. The use of benzodiazepines should be avoided where possible. However, they are less teratogenic than anticonvulsants and are only needed for a short period of time. If they are required, it is probably wise to use a short-acting variety (Flannery, Wolff, & Marshall, 2006; Substance Abuse and Mental Health Services Administration, 1993).

Monitoring is very important

Competent routine monitoring provides the basis for clinical management that is alert, flexible, and able to be rapidly escalated in case of need. There is much to be said for the use of standardized scales to facilitate this process, and a number of suitable instruments are available. The revised Clinical Institute Withdrawal Assessment for Alcohol Scale (CIWA-Ar; Sullivan et al., 1989) is a 10-item scale that can be completed in about 5 minutes. It scores the severity of nausea, tremor, sweating, anxiety, agitation, headache, orientation, and sensory disturbances. A brief online course providing training in the CIWA-Ar is available at no charge (http://www.ci2i.research.va.gov/paws/default.htm). The 8-item Mainz Alcohol Withdrawal Scale is also available (Banger et al., 1992). Careful monitoring, combined with supportive care, can reduce the need for medication (Shaw et al., 1981).

In an in-patient setting, a sensible procedure may be for the nurses to make at least 8-hourly observations on all withdrawing patients for the first 3 days, but this may need to be more frequent during the first 24 hours. If seen daily in an out-patient setting, it is similarly sensible to check blood pressure, pulse, and temperature. Observations may be discontinued with the agreement of the medical and nursing team once readings are stable and within normal range. Every now and then, a patient who has given an incomplete history and who is expected to show only mild withdrawal will unexpectedly develop more severe symptoms. Routine observations over the first few days are therefore essential. If, however, a patient is not being seen daily, they and whoever is supporting them should be advised to seek urgent medical review if symptoms do not respond to medication.

In addition to rating withdrawal symptoms, at the start of alcohol detoxification, breath alcohol should be measured. Taking two measurements at least 20 minutes apart allows an estimation of the actual blood alcohol concentration and also confirms the rate of fall of blood alcohol. This is important for several reasons. First, if estimated blood or breath alcohol is high, there may be a danger of interaction with prescribed medication during the first few hours of detoxification and particular care must be taken with prescribing during this period. Second, if the patient has consumed a significant amount of alcohol immediately before arriving, their blood alcohol levels may still be rising. This should generate even greater caution in the immediate prescribing and administration of medication. However, there is no "safe" breath alcohol level because an alcohol dependent patient may have high levels (e.g., three times the legal driving limit) and yet experience significant withdrawal symptoms. Therefore, when deciding whether to give medication, the breathalyzer level *and* whether it is changing, *and* the severity of withdrawal symptoms should be taken into account.

Alternative medications

A number of other drugs have been used in the management of alcohol withdrawal, including anticonvulsants (Lingford-Hughes et al., 2012; National Institute for Health and Clinical Excellence, 2010, 2011). Because studies of anticonvulsants have typically involved small numbers and heterogeneous populations, no definite conclusions about their effectiveness can be made (Polycarpou, Papanikolau, Ioannidis, & Contopoulos Ioannidis, 2009). Some anticonvulsants, including carbamazepine, topiramate, and lamotrigine, have shown promise in reducing alcohol withdrawal symptoms. There is still insufficient evidence for the utility of other drugs in this class, such as gabapentin and vigabatrin (McKeon, Frye, & Delanty, 2008).

Phenothiazines and other major tranquilizers or antipsychotics have no part to play in the routine treatment of alcohol withdrawal and only add to the risks.

Vitamins

Patients who have been drinking heavily and neglecting their diet are at increased risk of acute Wernicke's encephalopathy developing with disastrous suddenness due to the extra metabolic load during alcohol withdrawal (see Chapter 5). All patients should be assessed whether they are at risk of thiamine (vitamin B_1) deficiency (e.g., missed meals, signs of peripheral neuropathy such as "pins and needles"). If there are no concerns, the prescription of oral vitamins is not an absolute requirement of withdrawal treatment, but oral supplements (e.g., thiamine, 100 mg/d) are generally given during detoxification and thereafter until a good diet is achieved.

If, however, there are concerns that a patient is at risk of thiamine deficiency, it is a wise prophylactic measure to give parenteral thiamine supplements either as an intramuscular injection or a slow intravenous infusion because there is evidence that absorption is particularly poor in this group of patients (Thomson, Baker, & Leevy, 1970). Such parenteral administration is therefore essential where there is any specific cause for concern (Cook & Thomson, 1997; Thomson & Marshall, 2006). For example, in cases of malnutrition, peripheral neuropathy, or signs and symptoms of Wernicke-Korsakoff syndrome, it is particularly important to employ this approach. Because the diagnosis of Wernicke's encephalopathy is easily missed, a presumptive diagnosis should be made and treatment instituted, with a low threshold of suspicion (Cook, Hallwood, & Thomson, 1998; Thomson et al., 2008). A presumptive diagnosis should be made in any patient undergoing alcohol withdrawal who shows signs of acute confusion, ataxia, ophthalmoplegia, memory disturbance, hypothermia, or hypotension.

The correct dose of prophylactic thiamine is a subject of debate, and local guidelines may differ. Because alcohol dependence is associated with other vitamin deficiencies, preparations generally contain these in addition to at least 250 mg of thiamine. For instance, if using Pabrinex one pair of its 2 mL and 5 mL ampoules of high-potency parenteral B vitamins is administered intramuscularly once or twice daily for 3–5 days, is likely to be effective in those at risk in order to prevent the onset of Wernicke-Korsakoff syndrome (Day et al., 2008).

As a medical emergency, Wernicke's encephalopathy is best treated in a medical setting. At least 500 mg of thiamine should be given and is two pairs of ampoules of Pabrinex's high-potency parenteral B vitamins 3 times daily for at least 2 days or until there is no improvement (Cook et al., 1998; Thomson et al., 2008). Intravenous administration should be by infusion over 30 minutes. Parenteral thiamine should always be administered before an oral or intravenous glucose load. Thiamine is a cofactor for enzymes involved in glucose metabolism, thus there is a risk of precipitating Wernicke's encephalopathy if glucose is given before thiamine in at-risk individuals.

Administration of parenteral vitamins has become much less popular following reports of very rare but sometimes severe adverse allergic reactions, even though these were with older preparations that have fallen out of use. It must not be forgotten that Wernicke's encephalopathy is potentially fatal and that the sequelae can be severely disabling (Day et al., 2008; Kopelman, Thomson, Guerrini, & Marshall, 2009). In a properly supervised setting, where some patients may be at particular risk of Wernicke-Korsakoff syndrome, the balance of risks and benefits will usually be in favour of parenteral vitamin supplementation. However, parenteral administration of B-complex vitamins should only be given in settings where treatment for anaphylaxis is available if necessary.

In addition to thiamine deficiency, patients may be also have low levels of other vitamins or dysregulated electrolytes or salts in their blood (e.g., sodium or potassium). A thorough medical assessment and review is therefore necessary.

Alcohol withdrawal seizures

Averting withdrawal seizures

The effective use of benzodiazepines, particularly long-acting preparations such as diazepam or chlordiazepoxide, should be sufficient to minimize the development of withdrawal seizures, and it is usually neither necessary nor useful to give additional medication for this purpose (Hillbom, Pieninkeroinen, & Leone, 2003; Lingford-Hughes et al., 2012; Ntais et al., 2005). The use of an anticonvulsant in combination with a benzodiazepine does not appear to confer added benefit, and such polypharmacy may result in unnecessary side effects and uncertainties. Phenytoin does not prevent alcohol withdrawal seizures and is therefore not indicated (Hillbom et al., 2003). Anticonvulsants are not recommended as long-term treatment for alcohol withdrawal seizures.

Treating withdrawal seizures

Seizures usually occur within the first 24–48 hours of admission, but they may also ensue during the course of delirium (see Chapter 5) or even while the patient is still drinking if there is a rapid fall in blood alcohol concentration. They are less likely to develop if the patient has been adequately treated with long-acting benzodiazepines, particularly diazepam (Brathan et al., 2005; Ntais et al., 2005). There is evidence that lorazepam but not phenytoin reduces the risk of a subsequent seizure (Brathan et al., 2005).

Predisposing factors for alcohol withdrawal seizures include a history of such seizures, multiple detoxification episodes, concurrent epilepsy, hypokalaemia, and hypomagnesaemia. Other contributing factors include head injury, hypoglycaemia, and stroke. If a sequence of seizures occurs or status epilepticus develops (a run of seizures in continuous succession), intravenous medication will have to be given to bring the situation rapidly under control and the usual measures deployed as for any patient suffering from epilepsy.

The treatment of DTs

DTs usually occurs after about 72 hours of stopping drinking. This section deals with technical issues that are mainly the concern of medical and nursing staff, but it may again be of interest to other professionals to acquaint themselves with at least the outlines of how such problems are handled. See Chapter 5 for a full discussion of the causes and clinical features of DTs.

Ideally, the onset of delirium should have been prevented by adequately treating severe alcohol withdrawal symptoms with benzodiazepines. If severe withdrawal is adequately managed with appropriate drug doses, the risk of DTs will in many instances be aborted. However, despite the best efforts, hospital admission and alcohol withdrawal will sometimes precipitate DTs, and cases of already established delirium will also sometimes present directly for admission. Once a fully developed attack of DTs is under way, it is uncertain whether any treatment will actually shorten the course of the disorder, but there is persuasive evidence that the difference between competent and less competent treatment may be the survival as opposed to the death of the patient. The dangers of death from DTs should not be exaggerated, but they do exist.

The following sections list matters to be kept in mind when treating this condition (and see also Table 11.2).

What setting for treatment?

Given the risks to life, patients suffering from this condition should have the benefit of being treated in a setting where the medical and nursing staff are as experienced as possible. When

Table 11.2. Important requirements in the treatment of DTs

- In-patient environment, preferably with experienced staff
- Careful assessment and monitoring for comorbid physical and psychiatric disorders – especially head injury, intercurrent infection, liver disease and hepatic coma, gastrointestinal bleeding, and acute Wernicke–Korsakoff syndrome
- Chlordiazepoxide is the preferred drug treatment
- Careful monitoring of body temperature, fluids, electrolytes, and blood sugar
- Parenteral vitamin supplementation
- Availability of emergency medical facilities

DTs occurs on a psychiatric ward or in-patient alcohol unit, there may be uncertainty as to whether the patient should remain on that ward or be transferred to a general medical unit. The decision can only be made in the light of an appraisal of the skills and resources available in either setting.

Whatever the setting in which the patient is to be treated, the basic elements that must be provided are much the same. First-rate nursing is required, both for observation and for care. The situation must be one where a potentially disturbed patient can be cared for without staff becoming flustered, and there must be precaution against a patient sustaining accidental injury while in a state of confusion. A safe nursing environment must be established with no possibility of the patient falling out of the window, tumbling down a flight of stairs, or wandering off the ward. A patient who is only uncertainly in contact with reality is going to be helped by friendliness, reassurance, and by good room lighting rather than a side room with shadowy corners.

Depending on the mental health legislation of the country concerned, it may be necessary to consider compulsory admission if the patient refuses to stay in the hospital. The risks to such a patient, should they be allowed to take their own discharge, would be considerable, and there should be no hesitation to arrange an assessment for compulsory detention. In the UK, this would be considered under the Mental Capacity Act and, on occasions, a section of the Mental Health Act. In the United States, individual states establish guidelines for involuntary admission. Note that it is the DTs, not alcohol dependence, which would justify detention against the patient's will.

What underlying or complicating conditions may be missed?

Although the need for an alcohol detoxification itself can be missed, so, too, can the need for treatment of other medical conditions that become evident during or after the process. Patients who die in DTs perhaps most often do so as a result of a medical complication that has been overlooked. Such oversight, unless actively guarded against, can easily come about when all energies are being concentrated on dealing with the immediate and acutely worrying presentation. The patient is probably in no condition to give an accurate history or an account of other symptoms.

The conditions that must be recognized are many, and no checklist can substitute for full initial examination and subsequent continued watchfulness. But conditions particularly to be borne in mind include the possibility of head injury, intercurrent infection (particularly chest infection), liver disease and hepatic coma, gastrointestinal bleeding, and the acute onset of the Wernicke's encephalopathy. The picture may also be complicated if the patient has been taking another depressant.

Choice of medication

Much the same considerations apply here as with choice of drugs for treatment of less severe withdrawal symptoms. A great deal of research has been aimed at determining which medication is likely to be most useful in treating DTs. On the whole, it seems best to employ a long-acting benzodiazepine. Chlordiazepoxide may be given in a dose up to 400 mg daily by mouth in divided doses. Where a rapid response is required, it may be necessary to supplement this with intramuscular, intravenous, or rectal medication, as described earlier. Phenothiazines and other major tranquilizers should not be used routinely because they have the potential to lower seizure threshold and are associated with higher mortality and longer duration of delirium when compared with other sedative-hypnotic agents (Mayo-Smith et al., 2004). They may, exceptionally, be used to reduce agitation, but only when a review of benzodiazepine dosage has been carried out.

Fluids and electrolytes

Patients who are overactive, sweating, and feverish (and perhaps also suffering from gastrointestinal disturbance) are candidates for serious disturbances in fluid and electrolyte balance, which must therefore be monitored. A dangerous fall in potassium level must be averted, and there have been suggestions that decreased magnesium levels are a particular likelihood in DTs (Turner et al., 1989). Blood sugar levels should also be watched. Although an intravenous line may have to be set up, so far as possible fluid and electrolyte correction should be managed by oral administration: keeping an intravenous line in position with a delirious patient can present problems.

Vitamin deficiency

Given the dangers of Wernicke–Korsakoff syndrome, there can be no doubt that the patient with DTs should receive appropriate doses of intravenous or intramuscular thiamine for several days (as described earlier). With the virtual impossibility at an early stage of distinguishing the signs and symptoms of DTs from those of Wernicke's encephalopathy, a presumptive diagnosis of the latter condition should be made, and treatment instituted accordingly.

Life support

Emergency facilities must be available in the event of acute circulatory failure. A rare complication is hyperthermia, with the temperature suddenly rising to 40.5°C or higher. Hepatic coma is sometimes precipitated when the previously malnourished patient begins to take protein.

A case history

A 33-year-old man, living alone, asked his social worker for help with "coming off" alcohol. A previous episode of withdrawal, a year earlier, had failed because he recommenced drinking while still taking medication prescribed for his withdrawal symptoms. He therefore reluctantly agreed that, on this occasion, he would go into a hospital for detoxification. On arrival on the, ward he was intoxicated, with a BAC of 350 mg/100 mL. An hour later, a repeat measurement indicated a decrease to 335 mg/100 mL, at which point the patient was starting to sweat and suffering from a coarse tremor. Regular observations of withdrawal symptoms were commenced using the CIWA-Ar. Chlordiazepoxide was prescribed, commencing with a cautious dose of 25 mg in view of the high breath alcohol. In view of the evidence of poor nutritional status, a high-dose B-complex vitamin preparation was also prescribed for intramuscular administration once daily for 5 days.

Over the first 24 hours, a total of 250 mg chlordiazepoxide was administered to the patient orally, and this was effective in keeping him reasonably comfortable, albeit he was rather sleepless for the first night on the ward. Tapering doses of chlordiazepoxide were prescribed over succeeding days, and the drug was discontinued completely after 5 days on the ward.

The patient was discharged after 7 days. By this time, after encouragement and advice from the ward staff, he had made his own arrangements to be admitted to a residential rehabilitation facility in another part of the country. Arrangements had also been made by the medical staff for him to receive investigation and treatment for a suspected peptic ulcer. The ward psychologist had taught him some basic anxiety management techniques because he had indicated that he often drank in response to symptoms of anxiety due to various life stresses.

Withdrawal from drugs other than alcohol

Some patients may be dependent on other drugs in addition to their dependence on or misuse of alcohol (see Chapter 7). In these circumstances, appropriate medical management of substitution or withdrawal from drugs other than alcohol must be provided. It is not possible to describe here in detail the clinical management required for all other types of drugs. However, a few comments may be in order in relation to dependence on benzodiazepines and opioids, and the interested reader is referred to more detailed sources for further information in relation to these and other drugs (Lingford-Hughes et al., 2012; Management of Substance Use Disorders Workgroup, 2009; National Institute for Health and Clinical Excellence, 2010, 2011). For both drugs, either a simultaneous detoxification is done along with alcohol detox, or their substitution dose is optimized.

Benzodiazepine dependence is usually best managed in the community, with gradual dose reduction being undertaken over a period of weeks or months (Higgitt, Lader, & Fonagy, 1985; Lingford-Hughes et al., 2012; Schweizer & Rickels, 1998). However, where concomitant alcohol withdrawal is involved, admission may be required in order to ensure appropriate monitoring and prescribing during the acute phase of alcohol and early benzodiazepine withdrawal. It is usually best to convert other benzodiazepines into the equivalent dosage of a long-acting preparation, such as diazepam or chlordiazepoxide, and then to adjust the dose of this single drug in accordance with alcohol withdrawal symptoms. Managing the doses of several benzodiazepines prescribed concomitantly can be confusing at best and dangerous at worst. Whereas benzodiazepines are usually discontinued after 7–10 days in cases of acute alcohol withdrawal alone, concomitant benzodiazepine dependence will usually require that the patient be discharged to the community on a lower dose, which is then gradually tailed off over a period of weeks or months. Carbamazepine may be helpful in managing withdrawal from high doses of benzodiazepines (Lingford-Hughes et al., 2012). Alternatively, if the patient is stable on their benzodiazepine dose and detoxification is not currently planned, but they require an alcohol detoxification (e.g., due to admission for surgery or an accident), then a typical benzodiazepine reducing regimen could be added.

Similarly, if a patient is opioid dependent and detoxification is not appropriate, their substitution dose and medication can be optimized (Lingford-Hughes et al., 2012). Alternatively, a gradual dose reduction of the drug in question (e.g., methadone, buprenorphine, or codeine) is used over a period of weeks or months (Lingford-Hughes et al., 2012). Alternatively, other drugs may be prescribed to ameliorate symptoms of acute opioid withdrawal. Among the drugs used in this way are lofexidine (Bearn, Gossop, & Strang, 1996; National Institute for Health and Clinical Excellence, 2007*a*, 2007*b*).

Withdrawal symptoms in summary

From what has been said in this chapter, it must be evident that the clinical skills required to respond effectively to the range of alcohol withdrawal pictures that will be encountered involve the ability to deploy a range of techniques apposite to varied presentations. The proper use of medication can sometimes be very important, but this should not lead to any neglect of the importance of support and encouragement. The trust and the relationships established during the management of the crisis can be valuably carried through to the next phase of treatment.

References

Banger, M, Philipp, M., Herth, T., Hebenstreit, M., & Aldenhoff, J. (1992). Development of a rating scale for quantitative measurement of the alcohol withdrawal syndrome. *European Archives of Psychiatry and Clinical Neuroscience*, **241**, 241–246.

Bearn, J., Gossop, M., & Strang, J. (1996). Randomised double-blind comparison of lofexidine and methadone in the in-patient treatment of opiate withdrawal. *Drug and Alcohol Dependence*, **43**, 87–91.

Brathan, B., Ben-Menachem, E., Brodtkorb, E., Galvin, R., Garcia-Monco, J. C., Halasz, P., … EFNS Task Force on Diagnosis and Treatment of Alcohol-Related Seizures. (2005). *EFNS guideline on the diagnosis and management of alcohol-related seizures: Report of an EFNS task force*. Vienna, Austria: European Foundation of Neurological Societies.

Collins, M. N., Burns, T., Van den Berk, P. A. H., & Tubman, G. F. (1990). A structured programme for out-patient alcohol detoxification. *British Journal of Psychiatry*, **156**, 871–874.

Cook, C. C. H., Hallwood, P. M., & Thomson, A. D. (1998). B vitamin deficiency and neuropsychiatric syndromes in alcohol misuse. *Alcohol and Alcoholism*, **33**, 317–336.

Cook, C. C. H., & Thomson, A. D. (1997). B-complex vitamins in the prevention and treatment of Wernicke–Korsakoff syndrome. *British Journal of Hospital Medicine*, **57**, 461–465.

Day, E., Bentham, P., Callaghan, R., Kuruvilla, T., & George, S. (2008). *Thiamine for Wernicke–Korsakoff syndrome in people at risk from alcohol abuse. The Cochrane Collaboration*. Chichester, UK: John Wiley & Sons.

Flannery, W., Wolff, K., & Marshall, E. J. (2006). Substance use disorders in pregnancy. In V. O'Keane, T. Seneviratne, & M. Marsh (Eds.), *Psychiatric disorders and pregnancy: Obstetric and psychiatric care* (pp. 197–222). London: Taylor and Francis.

Higgitt, A. C., Lader, M. H., & Fonagy, P. (1985). Clinical management of benzodiazepine dependence. *British Medical Journal*, **291**, 688–690.

Hillbom, M., Pieninkeroinen, I., & Leone, M. (2003). Seizures in alcohol-dependent patients: Epidemiology, pathophysiology and management. *CNS Drugs*, **17**, 1013–1030.

Kopelman, M. D., Thomson, A. D., Guerrini, I., & Marshall, E. J. (2009). The Korsakoff syndrome: Clinical aspects, psychology and treatment. *Alcohol and Alcoholism*, **44**, 148–154.

Kosten, T. R., & O'Connor, P. G. (2003). Management of drug and alcohol withdrawal. *New England Journal of Medicine*, **348**(18), 1786–1795.

Lingford-Hughes, A. R., Welch, S., Peters, L., & Nutt, D. J. (2012). BAP updated guidelines: Evidence-based guidelines for the pharmacological management of substance abuse, harmful use, addiction and comorbidity: Recommendations from BAP. *Journal of Psychopharmacology*, **26**(7), 899–952.

Management of Substance Use Disorders Workgroup. (2009). *VA/DOD clinical practice guideline for the management of substance abuse disorders (Schedule S: Stabilization and withdrawal management)*. Washington, DC: Departments of Defense and Veterans Affairs.

Mayo-Smith, M. F., Beecher, L. H., Fischer, T. L., Gorelick, D.A., Guillaume, J.L., Hill, A., … Working Group on the Management of Alcohol Withdrawal Delirium, Practice Guidelines Committee, American Society of Addiction Medicine. (2004). Management of alcohol withdrawal delirium: An evidence-based practice guideline. *Archives of Internal Medicine*, **164**, 1405–1412.

McKeon, A., Frye, M. A., & Delanty, N. (2008). The alcohol withdrawal syndrome. *Journal of Neurology, Neurosurgery, and Psychiatry*, **79**, 854–862.

National Institute for Health and Clinical Excellence. (2007*a*). *Drug misuse: Opiate detoxification management of drug misusers in the community and prison settings* (NICE Clinical Guideline 57). London: Author.

National Institute for Health and Clinical Excellence. (2007*b*). *Methadone and buprenorphine for the management of opioid dependence* (NICE technology appraisal guidance 114). London: Author.

National Institute for Health and Clinical Excellence. (2010). *Alcohol-use disorder: Physical complications* (NICE Clinical Guideline 110). London: Author.

National Institute for Health and Clinical Excellence. (2011). *Alcohol dependence and harmful alcohol use* (NICE Clinical Guideline 115). London: Author.

Ntais, C., Pakos, E., Kyzas, P., & Ioannidis, J. P. (2005). Benzodiazepines for alcohol withdrawal. *Cochrane Database of Systematic Reviews*, CD005063.

Polycarpou, A., Papanikolau, P., Ioannidis, J. P., & Contopoulos Ioannidis D. (2009). Anticonvulsants for alcohol withdrawal. *Cochrane Database of Systematic Reviews*, CD005064.

Saitz, R., Mayo-Smith, M. F., Roberts, M. S., Redmond, H. A., Bernard, D. R., & Calkins, D. R. (1994). Individualized treatment for alcohol withdrawal. A randomized double-blind controlled trial. *Journal of the American Medical Association*, **272**, 519–523.

Schweizer, E., & Rickels, K. (1998). Benzodiazepine dependence and withdrawal: A review of the syndrome and its clinical management. *Acta Psychiatrica Scandinavica*, **98**(Suppl 393), 95–101.

Sellers, E. M., Naranjo, C. A., Harrison, M., Devenyi, P., Roach, C., & Sykora, K. (1983). Diazepam loading: Simplified treatment of alcohol withdrawal. *Clinical Pharmacology and Therapeutics*, **34**, 822–826.

Shaw, J. M., Kolesar, G. S., Sellers, E. M., Kaplan, H. L., & Sandor, P. (1981). Development of optimal treatment tactics for alcohol withdrawal. I. Assessment and effectiveness of supportive care. *Journal of Clinical Psychopharmacology*, **1**, 382–388.

Stockwell, T., Bolt, L., Milner, I., Pugh, P., & Young, I. (1991). Home detoxification from alcohol: Its safety and efficacy in comparison with inpatient care. *Alcohol and Alcoholism*, **26**, 645–650.

Substance Abuse and Mental Health Services Administration (SAMHSA). (1993). *Pregnant, substance-using women: Treatment Improvement Protocol (TIP) series 2* (DHHS Publication No. (SMA) 95–3056). Rockville, MD: US Department of Health and Human Services.

Sullivan, J. T., Sykora, K., Schneiderman, J., Naranjo, C. A., & Sellers, E. M. (1989). Assessment of alcohol withdrawal: The revised Clinical Institute Withdrawal Assessment for Alcohol Scale (CIWA-Ar). *British Journal of Addiction*, **84**, 1353–1357.

Thomson, A. D., Baker, H., & Leevy, C. H. (1970). Patterns of 35 S-thiamine hydrochloride absorption in the malnourished alcoholic patient. *Journal of Laboratory and Clinical Medicine*, **76**, 34–45.

Thomson, A. D., Cook, C. C. H., Guerrini, I., Sheedy, D., Harper, C., & Marshall, E. J. (2008). Wernicke's encephalopathy: "Plus ca change, plus c'est la meme chose." *Alcohol and Alcoholism*, **43**, 180–186.

Thomson, A. D., & Marshall, E. J. (2006). The treatment of patients at risk of developing Wernicke's encephalopathy in the community. *Alcohol and Alcoholism*, **41**, 158–167.

Turner, R. C., Lichstein, P. R., Peden, J. G., Busher, J. T., & Waivers, L. E. (1989). Alcohol withdrawal syndromes: A review of pathophysiology, clinical presentation, and treatment. *Journal of General Internal Medicine*, **4**, 432–444.

Chapter 12

The therapeutic relationship

Three patients with drinking problems talk about their care providers:

> I remember when I first met that doctor. She seemed friendly but when I tried to con her, she laughed and told me to get my priorities right. Typical alcoholic thinking – just told myself that she didn't understand, and I didn't bother to turn up for the next appointment. What happened next? I get a letter, not one of those form-letters that hospitals send out, but a personal letter from this doctor saying something like, "I know it's difficult. I don't want to push you into anything, but I'll be in the clinic on Friday afternoon if you want to talk about things further." So I went back to tell her she didn't understand!

> That social worker was the first guy in years who seemed to really believe in me, after all my screw ups and all my broken promises. At first I was able to stop drinking simply because I didn't want to let him down, didn't want to prove that he was wrong for having confidence in me. When I went back to the drink I was so ashamed that I could barely face him. But he didn't condemn me, he just said that we would figure out together how it happened and try to get back on track.

> I don't know why it didn't work, because everyone told me how smart a psychiatrist he was and they were right. He had more awards and degrees and books in his office than I have hairs on my head. But whenever I tried to tell him how I really felt, he either contradicted me or changed the subject. Even though I was drinking less, and I guess that's to his credit, I left most of our psychotherapy sessions feeling 2 inches tall. And then I stopped going. All I have now is my AA [Alcoholics Anonymous] sponsor, who didn't even go to university and isn't any smarter than I am. But he "gets me," and he treats me with respect, and that's what I need.

The previous chapters have described how to assess a patient, formulate the case, set a treatment goal, and conduct any needed detoxification. After all this preliminary work, the time has come for treatment to begin in earnest. Yet we cannot jump directly into specific clinical techniques without first discussing their essential context: the therapeutic relationship.

Human beings are not machines who passively allow repairs by a tool-wielding expert. They are active parties in the change process, which is pursued in alliance with a clinician who is also a human being. Attention should therefore be given to the subtle and important range of happenings that occur whenever patient and clinician interact – the what, when, and how of what is felt and said and done between them. Otherwise, we are at risk of throwing out as packaging an essential content of the parcel.

The characteristics of a high-quality therapeutic relationship

The relationship between patient and clinician is fundamental both to what can be achieved in any one therapeutic session and to what changes can be won over time (Luborsky et al., 1985). It begins to be built at the first moment of contact, is developed during the assessment interview (or interviews), is vital to the effectiveness of the initial counselling and goal-setting, and continues thereafter as an important component of treatment (Edwards, 1996). "What is said" matters, but it cannot be abstracted from the feelings between the two people who are doing the saying and the listening. Take, for instance, the following remarks by a clinician that might be necessary at a certain point in an individual's treatment:

> You know that I believe you can stop drinking and make sense of your life, but things can't usefully just drag on. You've been coming up here regularly to talk about your problems for the last 6 months, and we are both aware that you're now becoming badly caught up in this business of, "I'll start tomorrow ... the day after." Here's a challenge. Instead of us meeting next week as usual, I propose that you come back in a month's time and show me that by then you have stopped these binges and started instead to do some of those things with your family that you have been talking about. I want you to show yourself that you can succeed, and that will be a great feeling. It's time to make a start. You *can* make a start.

That same form of words may have three different types of impact. The impact may be negative, with the patient reinforced in their sense of hopelessness. The second alternative is for the patient in effect not to hear what is said because no words spoken within a meaningless relationship can matter: if they bother to come back in a month's time, it will be with nothing having changed. Last, there is the possibility that the challenge is taken and used as a turning point, but this outcome can only be expected when the relationship positively matters. At worst, the word "relationship" is devalued into a catch-phrase of professional jargon, and yet every now and then one senses again the intensely important reality of what is being talked about.

Working with drinking problems requires an awareness of how relationships are made and used, but there is little that is unique to alcohol problems in this regard (Levin & Weiss, 1994). Certain characteristics of clinicians account for between 10–50 percent of treatment outcome variance. More effective clinicians are empathic, supportive, and also goal-directed (Najavits & Weiss, 1994; Raistrick, Heather, & Godfrey, 2006). Being goal-directed bears special comment in that the successful professional is not the mushy stereotype of the clinician who approves of everything and sets no limits or change-targets in treatment. Rather, effective clinicians both take the work of change seriously while maintaining an attitude of respect and support toward the patient. The way in which clinicians interact with patients may be at least as important as the specific approach used (Carroll, 2001; Connors et al., 2000).

The qualities of the therapeutic relationship that should be aimed for are summarized in Table 12.1. All of them overlap to some degree but will be discussed separately because they each merit attention.

Table 12.1. Characteristics of a high-quality therapeutic relationship

- The clinician and patient are allied in pursuit of a common goal.
- The clinician shows empathy and the patient feels cared about and understood.
- Both clinician and patient take responsibility for their own behaviour.
- The patient finds the relationship motivating.

Alliance in pursuit of a common goal

Rivers of ink have been spilt in the psychotherapy literature regarding whether one theoretical orientation is superior to all others. Yet, regardless of whether treatment is psychodynamic, cognitive, or behavioural in nature, the strength of the alliance between the clinician and patient will be a significant determinant of success (Luborsky et al., 1985). To put it bluntly, *even the most skillfully applied treatment techniques will be ineffective if, fundamentally, the clinician and patient are working against each other.*

Clear formulation of the case, clearly articulated to the patient is critical for building the alliance from the start of treatment (see Chapter 11). So, too, is the negotiation of treatment goals. Some differences regarding goals is tolerable: for example, if the patient is 80 percent sure that a moderate drinking goal is best and the clinician is only 60 percent sure, they can proceed together toward that goal in good faith, with one or both potentially revising their view as treatment moves along. But if the clinician believes, for example, that treatment is about changing drinking behaviour and thereby improving the patient's marriage, whereas the patient believes treatment is about getting his or her spouse to stop complaining about the drinking – which will go on as before – treatment is quite possibly a lost cause from the start.

Empathy, caring, and trust

The therapeutic relationship is not a friendship such as both the patient and clinician may each have with other people outside of treatment. But it is a partnership with a purpose that will be aided by a warm tone and empathic understanding. Warmth cannot be invented, and a show of pretended warmth can backfire. When warmth is genuinely experienced, the clinician must still be actively conveyed in voice tone, gestures, and words in ways that are not cloying.

Across treatment approaches, empathy increases the likelihood of success (Moyers & Miller, 2013). Empathy does not necessarily imply liking the patient, but rather experiencing and demonstrating an understanding of their struggles, hopes, and life situation. Empathy can be built by the simplest of clinical techniques, including verbalizing recognition of the patient's emotions (e.g., "You seem very sad about losing your job") and paraphrasing the patient's words to communicate that he or she has been heard (e.g., "What I hear you saying is that while your father is trying to be supportive, he's not giving you the sort of support you really need. Is that right?").

Warmth and empathy held establish a sense of trust, which will be evidenced by the patient trusting the clinician sufficiently to become vulnerable. Novice clinicians are sometimes upset when a patient revises their story a few weeks into treatment, for example, by admitting to problems (e.g., needing a drink in the morning) that were denied in the initial assessment. But rather than castigate the patient for not being more forthcoming earlier, the clinician should note positively that trust has grown sufficiently for the patient to self-disclose more honestly.

Both the clinician and patient are responsible for their own behaviour

The clinician and patient clearly share responsibility for the progress of treatment, but they remain responsible – and should perceive themselves as responsible – for their own behaviour. The clinician must guard against taking up a "parental" position in which, for example, the patient can be ordered about like a child or that the clinician is at personal fault if the patient returns to drinking. Likewise, blaming patients for being unmotivated should not be used as an easy out for clinicians who do not invest time in building motivation for change.

For their part, patients must not behave like a surgical patient (i.e., expect to lie there as if anesthestized while the all-powerful doctor fixes them). Even in the most intensive treatments, the time spent with the clinician is but a small part of the patient's life. The only person with the patient all the time is the patient, and that means the patient must be an active participant in the change process rather than dump that existential responsibility onto the clinician. Every clinician will encounter and will need to intervene in situations where nurses, doctors, family members, and friends are all running around trying to help while the patient, in contrast, is doing very little to move the change process along.

Respectful, firm confrontation is sometimes needed to encourage human beings to act responsibly. This includes the situation in which a clinical supervisor must point out that a clinical staff member is blaming a patient unfairly and in which a clinician must call a patient on "phoning in" treatment participation rather than actively engaging. In such situations, it is important to remember a clinical reality: you can say almost anything to another human being if they know that you care about them. Thus, paradoxically, a habit of exuding warmth and empathy is the foundation that makes any needed confrontations effective and hearable rather than chastising and cold.

The therapeutic relationship as a source of motivation

Changing drinking behaviour is impossible without significant motivation on the part of the patient, and such motivation must be nurtured by the clinician before virtually any other therapeutic task. Even at its worst, problem drinking may include enjoyable elements that make patients ambivalent about change. Other patients may lack motivation simply because they feel defeated by alcohol or because the initial goals of treatment are too ambitious. Motivation is a topic to which skilled clinicians will return again and again (Gerdner & Holmberg, 2000).

CLINICIAN: Robert, when you started treatment you told me how much you wanted to be a better father, and that you could see your drinking was getting in the way of that. Do you remember when we talked about that?

ROBERT: Of course. It's the only reason I came in.

CLINICIAN: Well, you stopped drinking for a month, and I know you were proud of that. And you have every right to be. But since then you don't seem very engaged in our sessions together, and you have missed others besides. I would really like to help you, but it's really up to you if you want to change. So I am just wondering, do you still feel that this a change you want to make?

ROBERT: Kind of. Well, I am less sure than I used to be. It's so boring in the evenings without my friends at the pub that I feel like I'm climbing the walls.

CLINICIAN: I see. You're missing some of the things about drinking that you liked, which is understandable. What about the reason you came in, your children?

ROBERT: That is going better. I see my son looking at me differently, with respect.

CLINICIAN: What is that like?

ROBERT: I feel so puffed up that my buttons are going to burst off my shirt.

CLINICIAN: So you miss one aspect of drinking, but you have gained something from stopping that makes you feel wonderful. Since you can't have both things, this is a major choice for you. Tell me: what matters more to you?

This example illustrates a number of therapeutic tactics that foster motivation, including communication of support, giving credit for steps taken, not arguing about the benefits of drinking, and directing the conversation to the rewards of changing behaviour. The clinical snippet ends with underscoring a critical quality of the therapeutic relationship: namely, keeping the responsibility for change on the patient rather than trying to rescue him or force him to become sober.

Motivation to change can be enhanced by specific techniques (see Chapters 9 and 13), but it is important to remember that the quality of the therapeutic relationship also shapes it. Motivation prospers when the relationship is empathic, goal-directed, trusting, and honest. In contrast, a cold, distant, overly demanding or antagonistic therapeutic relationship is the enemy of motivation to change.

Importantly, motivation is not a spring that is wound up at the start of treatment and powers matters from then onward. Rather, motivation must be nurtured within the therapeutic relationship throughout treatment. Whenever the clinician, the patient, or both feel "stuck" in treatment, the first two questions on the table should generally be "What is the status of the therapeutic relationship?" and "Does the patient really want to make a change?" More often than not, the source of a stall in progress is found in one or both of those interrelated areas. Clinicians facing this challenge can usefully draw on the material in this book on motivational enhancement (Chapters 9 and 13) and values clarification (Chapter 14) techniques.

When does the therapeutic relationship end?

A specific duration of treatment may be proposed by the clinician but is effectively determined by the patient. There are patients who appear to have benefited from one or two sessions and who decide this is all they need, whereas, at the other extreme, are patients who want to maintain at least intermittent contact over years.

A fixed course of so many sessions over so many months cannot in reality meet the needs of an enormously varied patient population. Judgment needs to be made in terms of the patient's progress along a number of dimensions of recovery, the likelihood of further useful work, the timeliness of a move that further emphasizes the patient's ability to handle their own responsibilities, and negotiation on timing between clinician and patient. Rather than there being a "this is the end of your treatment – good bye forever" type of announcement, what is said might often be something like this:

> We've been meeting each month for the last 8 months, and you've achieved a great deal. What I would now suggest is that we reduce the frequency of our meetings to once every three weeks, and, if you are still doing well through the Christmas holidays, we would end treatment then. Even after discharge though, you would be free to come back anytime when you are not doing well or even if you feel you are on the edge of beginning to not do well. How does that sound to you?

As the prior chapters of this book make clear, drinking problems and the motivation to manage them can wax and wane over time. For this reason, there is usually value in stepping a successful patient down to lower level monitoring before terminating treatment entirely. This could be a reduced in-person visit schedule, but it could also include relying on a schedule of occasional brief phone calls or on a secure form of electronic reporting using text messages, email, or a smartphone app. When contact is finally broken, it is important to convey to the patient that the door remains open for further contact if the patient comes to feel it is necessary.

Finally, although a less pleasant task, one must acknowledge that not all treatment terminations will be triggered by the achievement of a good outcome. In situations in which the clinician has worked for months with a patient with little progress, the clinician has the responsibility to explore in a nonpunitive fashion whether the time has come for the patient to either try a different treatment provider (either elsewhere or within the same agency) or take a break from treatment entirely. As with successful cases, the door should be left open for a return to treatment if the patient wishes.

References

Carroll, K. M. (2001). Constrained, confounded and confused: Why we really know so little about therapists in treatment outcome research. *Addiction*, **96**, 203–206.

Connors, G. J., DiClimente, C. C., Dermen, K. H., Kadden, R., Carroll, K. M., & Frone, M. R. (2000). Predicting the therapeutic alliance in alcoholism treatment. *Journal of Studies on Alcohol*, **61**, 139–149.

Edwards, G. (1996). Addictive behaviours: The next clinic appointment. In G. Edwards & C. Dare (Eds.), *Psychotherapy, psychological treatments and the addictions* (pp. 94–109). Cambridge: Cambridge University Press.

Gerdner, A., & Holmberg, A. (2000). Factors affecting motivation to treatment in severely dependent alcoholics. *Journal of Studies on Alcohol*, **61**, 548–560.

Levin, J. D., & Weiss, R. H. (Eds.). (1994). *The dynamics and treatment of alcoholism: Essential papers*. Northvale, NJ: Jason Aronson.

Luborsky, L., McLellan, A. J., Woody, G. E., O'Brien, C. P., & Auerbach, A. (1985). Therapist success and its determinants. *Archives of General Psychiatry*, **42**, 602–611.

Moyers, T. B., & Miller, W. R. (2013). Is low therapist empathy toxic? *Psychology of Addictive Behaviors*, **27**, 878–884.

Najavits, L. M., & Weiss, R. D. (1994). Variations in therapist effectiveness in the treatment of patients with substance use disorders: An empirical review. *Addiction*, **89**, 679–688.

Raistrick, D., Heather, N., & Godfrey, C. (2006). *Review of the effectiveness of treatment for drinking problems*. London: National Treatment Agency for Substance Misuse.

Chapter 13

Specialist treatment of drinking problems

This chapter describes a range of psychosocial and pharmacological approaches to treating problem drinkers. Much of the evidence described in this chapter comes from studies of patients in specialty alcohol treatment settings. The term "specialist," however, should not deter the "nonspecialist" from reading on because the majority of approaches can be adapted to lower level drinking problems as well as to other health problems commonly encountered in generalist settings.

What treatments work?

A return to heavy drinking is common during and after treatment, consistent with the relapsing-remitting nature of alcohol dependence. Relapse should be seen as an opportunity for learning and for improving treatment planning rather than as a failure. At one time, it was common to consider any outcome of treatment other than lifelong abstinence as a failure. By this metric, only 25–40 percent of patients in any given setting would be considered to have benefited from treatment. However, no other treatments for chronic disorders are held to such a perfectionistic standard. Treatments for diabetes that dramatically reduce complications are considered effective, as are treatments for back pain that greatly reduce pain severity and treatments for hypertension that reduce blood pressure from extremely high to slightly above average. Treatments for drinking problems should be judged in the same fashion.

From that perspective, roughly two-thirds of patients appear to derive benefit from treatment, which compares well to other treatments for chronic disorders. Patients who benefit fall into two comparably sized groups. The first group attains abstinence or consistently moderate alcohol consumption and few or no further alcohol-related problems (Miller, Walters, & Bennett, 2001). The second group continues to have periods of heavy drinking, but less often and/or at lower consumption amounts (e.g., 10 pints an evening rather than 15). They still experience some alcohol-related health and social problems, but these problems are less numerous and less severe.

Obviously, the maths indicates that the remaining one-third of patients do not improve, and, in fact, 7–15 percent patients may even get worse (Moos, 2005). That said, there is every reason to be optimistic that treatment can help a given patient. Indeed, the odds are 2:1 in favour of that proposition.

Given that treatment has value in general, what specific treatment should be adopted in the particular? Treatment choices should, wherever possible, be research-based, although, at the same time, a spurious scientism should not be allowed to inhibit the efforts of the individual clinician who is trying to help the individual patient in difficult and unique

Table 13.1. Appraisal of research underpinning professionally provided specialist treatments for drinking problems

- *Motivational interventions* including motivational interviewing and motivational enhancement therapy (MET). Well-supported by research.
- *Cognitive-behavioural treatments* including coping and social skills training, the community reinforcement approach (CRA), contingency management, behavioural self-control training, and cue exposure. Well-supported by research.
- *Couples and family therapy.* Research support for a subset of approaches.
- *Twelve-step facilitation counselling and social behaviour and network therapy.* Positive results in major clinical trials.
- *Mindfulness training.* Emerging research support.
- *Psychodynamic/Insight-oriented psychotherapies.* Little or no research support: deploy with discrimination.
- *Group therapy.* Probably useful for basic support but efficacy as a treatment of choice not supported.
- *Pharmacotherapy.* A range of medication is available, including those that are aversive if alcohol is consumed (e.g., disulfiram) and those targeting brain mechanisms (e.g., acamprosate, naltrexone, nalmefene). All well-supported by research.

circumstances. Practically speaking, most services offer a variety of approaches in response to the needs of the patient, and this variety will expand further as interventions delivered via computer and smartphone are more widely adopted.

A wealth of scientific evidence is available to guide alcohol treatment. Table 13.1 highlights key features of the evidence base on professional treatment (peer-led mutual help organizations will be addressed in Chapter 14). Readers interested in comprehensive reviews are referred to reports prepared by national government agencies and professional bodies (Berglund, Thelander, & Jonsson, 2003; Haber, Lintzeris, Proude, & Lopatko, 2009; Lingford-Hughes, Welch, Peters, & Nutt, 2012; Management of Substance Use Disorders Workgroup, 2009; Miller, Wilbourne, & Hetema, 2003; National Institute for Health and Clinical Excellence, 2011; Raistrick, Heather, & Godfrey, 2006; Slattery et al., 2003).

Although this chapter discusses types of professional treatment individually, anyone working with people who have drinking problems will recognize that they are a heterogeneous population and that different combinations of approaches are needed for different patients. As described in Chapter 10, it is therefore best to carry out an individual assessment and, on the basis of this assessment, identify the type of treatment best suited to that person. Thus, a treatment "package" may usefully incorporate several different techniques tailored to the individual's need. These could include approaches focused on drinking as well as on related problems the individual may have (e.g., communication difficulties, poor coping skills, depression).

Motivational interventions

Brief motivational interviewing as a stand-alone intervention provided in nonspecialist settings was described in Chapter 9. Motivational interviewing techniques can be used at the beginning of specialist treatment, for example, to motivate entry into treatment and increase likelihood of retention. The tactics of motivational interviewing can also be incorporated into ongoing therapy, as described herein.

In motivational interviewing, the therapist does not assume an authoritarian role within the sessions but seeks to create a positive atmosphere conducive to change. The overall goal is to increase the intrinsic motivation of the patient, thus enabling them to take the responsibility for change themselves. The approach is underpinned by four broad principles: expressing empathy, developing discrepancy, rolling with resistance, and supporting self-efficacy (Miller & Rollnick, 2002). Rather than applying a confrontational stance, the therapist uses warmth and empathy to establish the therapeutic relationship. The patient is then helped to perceive a discrepancy between their present behaviour and where they want to be; this discrepancy is then amplified. The therapist seeks to be "gently persuasive" and does not oppose resistance. When resistance is encountered, the therapist shifts strategies and tries to use it to good advantage. Finally, the therapist aims to impart a sense of hope and potential for change, thus supporting self-efficacy.

In the first phase, the patient is encouraged to do most of the talking. The clinician asks open questions, affirms, listens reflectively, and summarizes. This will often include reflecting accurately and without judgment the patient's enjoyment of alcohol and ambivalence about change. Reflective listening is an active process on the part of the clinician, a way of checking out what the patient means. Summary statements are used to show the patient that the clinician has been listening, to link material that has been discussed, or to move things on (a transitional summary). These techniques help to facilitate "change talk." Change talk, in turn, develops discrepancy, and this helps to build intrinsic motivation.

The first phase of motivational interviewing may take much longer with some patients than with others. As patients come to the point where they are ready to change but have not yet made a firm commitment, a plan is negotiated. This can involve setting goals and considering options for change.

The style of motivational interviewing has particular relevance to changing alcohol consumption and risky behaviour in adolescent and young people. It can be challenging to engage them in treatment, few specialist services may be available, and psychiatric comorbidity is likely to be present (see National Institute for Health and Clinical Excellence, 2011). Motivational interviewing has been shown in a Cochrane meta-analysis to result in reduced frequency and quantity of drinking in adolescents, although the effects were not substantial or necessarily clinically meaningful (Foxcroft et al., 2014). Limited other benefits were found, such as on binge drinking and alcohol-related problems. A systematic review of motivational interviewing for young people in emergency care settings found that it was at least as effective as other brief interventions (e.g., education, giving contacts for local services) in reducing alcohol consumption, but it has to be said that this is not a high bar to clear (Kohler & Hofmann, 2015).

There are also some trials of motivational interviewing to reduce drinking or maintain abstinence in pregnant women. However, as with other educational and psychological approaches, there is little robust evidence that motivational interviewing reduces alcohol consumption in pregnancy or has a positive impact on birth outcomes (Haug, Duffy, & McCaul, 2014; Stade et al., 2009).

Motivational enhancement therapy (MET) is an adaptation of motivational interviewing that has been evaluated in two large multicentre trials, Project MATCH and the United Kingdom Alcohol Treatment Trial (UKATT). Project MATCH, the largest trial of alcohol treatment ever conducted, found that MET, delivered over four sessions, was as effective on most outcomes as cognitive behavioural therapy (CBT) and 12-step facilitation (TSF) delivered over 12 sessions. The exception was abstinence, which was consistently higher in the TSF condition. The improvements that occurred during the 12-week treatment period were still evident at 1- and 3-year follow-up (Project MATCH Research Group, 1997*a*, 1997*b*, 1998).

Another very large clinical trial, UKATT, compared three sessions of MET with eight sessions of social behaviour and network therapy (SBNT) (UKATT Research Team, 2005*a*, 2005*b*). Both groups of participants showed marked improvements at 3-month and 1-year follow-up, and there were no significant differences between the groups on alcohol-related measures. The evidence thus suggests that MET should be considered a valuable method of treatment.

Cognitive behavioural treatments

The cognitive behavioural approach to treatment assumes that problem drinking is a problem in itself, as opposed to the psychoanalytic view that the drinking is merely a symptom or symbol of an underlying psychodynamic conflict or neurosis. Implicit in this approach is the belief that problem drinking is mainly a learnt behaviour and that treatment involves replacing the maladaptive pattern of drinking behaviour with moderate drinking or abstinence. Cognitive behavioural psychology also highlights the roles of coping skills and of expectations about alcohol in the development of drinking and its consequences.

The cognitive behavioural approach can be useful in helping problem drinkers to address skills that they are lacking. Drinkers who use alcohol to cope with anxiety or anger or as a result of negative cognitions associated with low self-esteem and depression may benefit from techniques such as relaxation training, anger management, and cognitive restructuring. These approaches are not specific to alcohol problems, but find their application as treatments aimed at dealing with postulated psychological causes of excessive drinking. It also bears mentioning that, in addition to being a mainstay of the acute phase of many treatments, cognitive behavioural approaches are also employed in relapse prevention efforts with patients who have attained abstinence or moderate drinking (Marlatt & Gordon, 1985).

Coping and social skills training

Some patients with drinking problems are handicapped by an inability to function confidently in social situations and to manage everyday hassles. Coping skills training concentrates on developing interpersonal and communication skills and cognitive behavioural mood management (Monti et al., 1990; Monti, Rohsenhow, Colby, & Abrams, 1995). Social skills deficits are assessed, and patients are then taught how to initiate social interactions and express their thoughts and feelings. This is typically done in a group setting where role-play and other behavioural methods can be used. For instance, the patient who is not assertive may find it difficult to say "no" to an offered drink; one element in treatment may involve teaching him or her to rehearse saying "no."

Social skills training, which includes assertiveness training, is an extremely effective method of treatment for alcohol problems (Holder, Longabaugh, Miller, & Rubonis, 1991; Miller, Andrews, Wilbourne, & Bennett, 1998). It can be delivered on an individual or group basis and is particularly suited to individuals with moderate alcohol dependence. It requires a certain level of cognitive functioning, and patients with neuropsychological impairment/alcohol-related brain damage are unlikely to benefit from this approach. Project MATCH found positive effects for a form of CBT that was largely composed of coping skills training. Coping and social skills training is an effective treatment for those who are moderately dependent on alcohol (Haber et al., 2009; National Institute for Health and Clinical Excellence, 2011; Raistrick et al., 2006; Slattery et al., 2003).

The community reinforcement approach and contingency management

The community reinforcement approach (CRA) is based on the principles of instrumental learning, and the emphasis is on manipulation of real-life rewards in the patient's environment. It focuses on altering reinforcement contingencies in the home environment, involves significant others, and uses positive reinforcement. The family's positive reactions, aid with job-finding, membership in a social club, and other social rewards are presented to the patient as contingent on treatment success, and the clinical team accepts responsibility to ensure that such rewards are in fact on offer. This technique was developed for in-patients by Hunt and Azrin (1973) but has evolved over time and is now used in out-patient/community treatment programmes (Azrin, 1976; Meyers & Miller, 2001).

Treatment components include motivational counselling, drink-refusal training, communication skills training, problem-solving training, relapse prevention, and disulfiram with monitored compliance. The CRA retains its focus on drinking behaviours and family- and job-related problems. Early research found that married patients with family support did well using the stand-alone disulfiram component, whereas unmarried, unsupported patients only benefited from the full CRA package (Azrin, Sisson, Meyers, & Godley, 1982). Although CRA-based strategies are also effective when disulfiram is not used, particularly for drinkers with serious problems, it has never been widely adopted in clinical practice (Meyers & Miller, 2001).

More recently, one element of CRA, contingency management, has received attention for its effectiveness in treating stimulant dependence, and it is increasingly being studied for treating alcohol use disorders. Contingency management generally relies on four types of incentives – vouchers, prize, cash, or privileges. The resource required for the "positive reinforcement" may impede its clinical utilization in resource-poor settings. Because all the studies were undertaken in the United States, replication evidence from other nations would be highly desirable (National Institute for Health and Clinical Excellence, 2011).

Behavioural self-control training

Behavioural self-control training (BSCT) is particularly effective in helping individuals at the less severe end of the dependence spectrum to reduce their alcohol consumption. Initially, the therapist and client negotiate sensible limits of alcohol consumption, and the client keeps a drinking diary or fills out a self-monitoring card to record all drinks taken (this could also, of course, be done electronically). A craving diary or daily activity diary can also be helpful. Clients are then taught techniques for reducing the rate of drinking and are helped to identify triggers to drinking, in particular negative moods (boredom, anxiety, depression), positive moods (excitement, happiness), and external cues (meeting with friends, particular time of day, a particular place). The aim is to develop positive experiences with reduced drinking or abstinence alongside creating negative experiences of drinking to excess. Behavioural self-control training can be used in the individual or group setting, and self-help manuals are available (Hester, 1995; Jarvis, Tebbutt, Mattick, & Shand, 2005). It is an extremely effective treatment modality for individuals able to moderate their drinking (Haber et al., 2009; National Institute for Health and Clinical Excellence, 2011; Raistrick et al., 2006).

Cue exposure

This approach is based on the principles of classical conditioning and borrows from a treatment strategy developed for phobias, obsessive-compulsive disorder, and other anxiety disorders. Patients commonly cite cues as causing them difficulties, and therefore reducing their impact has appeal. The patient is exposed to conditioned stimuli or cues that have previously precipitated craving or excessive drinking and is encouraged either not to drink or not to drink excessively. For instance, they may be asked to carry around with them a bottle of whisky and sniff at it without drinking, the therapist may accompany them on outings to a bar, or they may be asked to take sufficient alcohol to activate craving and then desist from further drinking. Cue exposure reduces the likelihood that the stimulus will trigger a response in the future and improves the individual's self-efficacy. It can be combined with coping skills and communication skills (Monti et al., 1993; Rohsenhow et al., 2001) or incorporated into a relapse prevention programme (Drummond, Tiffany, Glautier, & Remington, 1995). Although it has shown promise as a treatment method, its clinical success in preventing relapse is limited (Conklin & Tiffany, 2002).

Couple and family therapies

As described in the opening chapters of this book, a problem drinker's loved ones can both affect and be affected by the course of drinking. From this, it follows that helping the drinker can be facilitated by engaging partners and/or other family members in treatment. This also provides a clinical opportunity to attend to the suffering of those in the problem drinker's life, which can be enormous.

Couples and family therapy can be conducted from a variety of theoretical standpoints, and, in general, the best approaches draw from the list of effective treatments for individuals just reviewed (e.g., cognitive behavioural therapy). A mixture of support and coping skills training for both the partner/family member and the problem drinker is commonly employed both to reduce potential conflict and to encourage the drinker to alter their drinking and enter treatment. Support may also come from organizations such as Al-Anon (see Chapter 14). Such a supportive approach has proved effective at helping loved ones cope better and motivating the alcohol dependent person to enter treatment (O'Farrell & Clements, 2012). Behavioural contracts may be used to underpin changes in drinking and improve the quality of the relationship by resolving conflicts and problems.

Once in treatment, behavioural couples therapy (BCT) has strong research support (National Institute for Health and Clinical Excellence, 2011). Older evidence comes from a time when the problem drinker was a man married to a non-problem drinking woman (e.g., O'Farrell et al., 1993), but, more recently, the approach has been evaluated with same-sex couples and in couples where a problem-drinking woman is married to a non-problem drinking man. Behavioural marital therapy then has been shown to improve drinking outcomes at 18 months and to maintain marital stability and satisfaction (O'Farrell et al.,

1993). Whether such an approach has merit if both partners have an alcohol problem is less clear.

BCT is now commonly structured and combines cognitive behaviour treatment strategies with addressing relationship issues arising from alcohol misuse as well as more general relationship problems (Haber et al., 2009; National Institute for Health and Clinical Excellence, 2011; O'Farrell & Clements, 2012; Raistrick et al., 2006; Slattery et al., 2003). Cognitive behavioural forms of family therapy are also widely used and effective (Berglund et al., 2003; Copello, Velleman, & Templeton, 2005; Shand, Gates, Fawcett, & Mattick, 2003). Although not everyone may have a partner and/or family member able or willing to engage in couples therapy or services able to offer the option, such an approach has been shown to be more effective than individual treatment (Haber et al., 2009; National Institute for Health and Clinical Excellence, 2011; O'Farrell & Clements, 2012). Therefore, it should be carefully considered by patients and services.

Family therapy is commonly considered when an adolescent has a drinking problem because adverse family dynamics may also be playing a crucial role in his or her problem drinking. However, a recent meta-analysis reported that although family interventions were effective, individual-only interventions had a greater impact (Tripodi, Bender, Litschge, & Vaughn, 2010).

Family and couples therapy can also be employed in situations where the problem drinker is unwilling to attend treatment. Crucially, however, even if the problem drinker does not want to engage, family interventions or support and information about organizations such as Al-Anon and Alateen should be available to "carers" (i.e., family, close friends etc.; see Chapter 14). In particular, the needs of any children should be considered. Although many parents declare that their child(ren) are not aware of their problem drinking, this is generally not the case. As well as supporting children, some approaches also address prevention to reduce the risk that these children also develop alcohol problems (Copello et al., 2005). A range of approaches involving carers has been studied, with self-help interventions providing equally effective reduction in stress and improvements in psychological functioning as more intensive psychological therapies (National Institute for Health and Clinical Excellence, 2011). For instance, the community reinforcement and family training (CRAFT) approach teaches behaviour change strategies and is an effective modality for engaging resistant drinkers into treatment (Meyers, Smith, Serna, & Belon, 2013). SBNT usually involves the wider network of family and friends but can be used with families alone (Copello et al., 2002).

Twelve-step facilitation therapy and social behaviour and network therapy

TSF therapy derives its philosophy from Alcoholics Anonymous (AA), which is described in detail in Chapter 14. Project MATCH and a recent Cochrane review of multiple clinical trials (Kelly, Humphreys, & Ferri, in press) indicates that the approach is as effective as other evidence-based psychotherapies (e.g., motivational and cognitive behavioural) for all outcomes other than abstinence, for which TSF is superior. Critical to its approach is introducing the patient to an enduring social network that will reinforce abstinence and other behaviour changes.

SBNT therapy was developed for the UK Alcohol Treatment Trial, where it was found effective (Copello et al., 2002; Copello, Hodgson, Tober, & Orford, 2009). It does not adopt the disease model philosophy of TSF therapy, but it does pursue the same goal of connecting the patient to enduring social networks that support change (which may or may not include AA meetings). Family members, friends, and others from the client's social network are offered support and, in turn, are facilitated to help the client engage in treatment and change their drinking behaviour. Put another way, the social network mobilizes positive social support to change the drinking behaviour. The therapist thinks in terms of the social network and introduces topics such as communication, coping skills, and the enhancing of the social support network. Nonjudgmental listening, provision of information, exploration of sources of support, and arrangement for other help if needed are all part of this very practical way of working with drinkers and their significant others.

Mindfulness training

Mindfulness meditation has its origins in Buddhist traditions and has been growing in popularity in the Western world. Its evidence base is still in its infancy with regard to treating substance use disorder (Witkiewitz et al., 2014). Mindfulness training aims to "maintain awareness moment by moment, disengaging oneself from strong attachment to beliefs, thoughts, or emotions, thereby developing a greater sense of emotional balance and well-being" (Ludwig & Kabat-Zinn, 2008). Unlike therapies that focus on mastering or controlling aversive emotional states, mindfulness emphasizes accepting them. The addition of mindfulness to relapse prevention is conceptualized to add to awareness of internal and external cues to relapse. Mindfulness training has been shown to reduce anxiety and depression and also has some evidence for reducing heavy drinking itself (Bowen et al., 2014).

Psychodynamic/insight-oriented psychotherapy

Neither individual or group insight-oriented or psychodynamic psychotherapy is now thought to be an effective treatment for alcohol problems. However, once abstinence or stable moderate drinking has been achieved, insight-oriented psychotherapy has something to offer the carefully selected patient and may, on occasion, be essential to that improvement in the quality of recovery. What should particularly be cautioned against is the danger of forgetting that suitability for psychotherapy does indeed have to be determined by careful assessment. The enthusiasm of those not specially trained in general psychotherapeutic work may lead to the prescription of psychotherapy for a patient whom no experienced psychotherapist would regard as a suitable patient for such engagement. Many clinicians will make the offer of psychotherapy actually conditional on the patient achieving a stable period of sobriety or other life changes.

Group therapy

Group therapy has been widely employed in the treatment of drinking problems, even to the extent of sometimes being viewed as the intervention of choice. Unstructured group chat and psychoeducation have no evidence of benefit, but well-defined therapies with good research behind them (cognitive behavioural treatment and relapse prevention) can be delivered in structured, well-managed therapeutic groups (Najavits, Weiss, & Liese, 1996).

Group work often has a place within the therapeutic structure of a treatment centre. Such groups tend to have an open rather than a closed membership as patients are admitted and discharged. At the other extreme, one may find practitioners who will work with closed groups of, say, 8–10 patients selected for their homogeneity (all women, for instance) and who will run these groups in terms of orthodox group-therapy principles.

One can identify variations on some general themes as to the type of the work likely to be accomplished in groups. In *educational* groups, patients may learn about the nature of dependence. A second important and general theme is *problem solving*: this may relate to such reality issues as how to find a job or deal with debts, or it may focus on interpersonal and dynamic issues. Rehearsal of relapse prevention strategies is often a useful part of group work as patients share ideas with each other on how sobriety can be consolidated and relapse avoided. Cohesion of group sentiment can assist in the definition of goals, in overcoming resistance, and in the strengthening of motivation. Last, the fellowship of the group and the opportunity to share problems may very generally contribute to support and help to overcome feelings of isolation.

The clinician should be willing to take responsibility for excluding any patient who comes to a group when intoxicated. Having anyone who has been drinking participate in a group usually causes such anxiety and anger as to rule out the possibility of constructive work.

Pharmacotherapy

Pharmacotherapy in alcohol dependence has been available for many years, and its use recommended by all evidence-based guidelines (e.g., Jonas et al., 2014; Maisel et al., 2013; Management of Substance Use Disorders Workgroup, 2009; National Institute for Health and Clinical Excellence, 2011). Pharmacotherapy should not generally be used in isolation but in conjunction with psychosocial treatments. It should be considered for all alcohol dependent patients. Currently, the evidence does not support the use of medication in individuals who are not alcohol dependent (i.e., in those with harmful drinking [ICD-10] or mild alcohol use disorder [DSM-5]).

Despite its potential to improve recovery, pharmacotherapy is not considered for the majority of patients, with only 5–10 percent receiving medication. This low level of prescribing is likely to be due to lack of awareness and training; concerns about cost; and lack of belief by clinician, service, and/or patient in "providing drugs to addicts." This section of this chapter should make clear that this underutilization represents a serious problem for the field.

As with the psychosocial treatments just reviewed, this chapter highlights key findings regarding pharmacotherapy rather than providing a comprehensive review of each medication and how to best use it. In addition, pharmacotherapeutic strategies to treat alcohol dependence in the presence of comorbid psychiatric disorders will also be outlined. The clinician should supplement this chapter with the practice guidelines cited earlier, alongside adequate training about how to achieve optimal prescribing. In all cases, whenever medication is being considered, the patient should have a physical examination and routine blood tests such as liver and renal function and a full blood count.

Since disulfiram was first employed in treatment in the 1950s, other medications such as acamprosate and naltrexone were licensed in 1990s, followed by nalmefene in the past few years. Although these medications may be described as "anti-craving" drugs, clinical trials and experience has not necessarily supported this, and their mechanism of action may not be exclusively tied to altering craving but rather to modulating other important mechanisms, such as impulsivity and stress. In addition, some medications used "off-licence/off-label," such as baclofen and topiramate, also show efficacy. This so-called repurposing of medication with licenses for other indications is likely to increase as our understanding of the neurobiology of alcohol dependence improves, thus providing more targets for therapy.

Disulfiram

Since its introduction more than 50 years ago (see Box 13.1), disulfiram (Antabuse) has been used very widely in the treatment of alcohol problems. Disulfiram blocks the breakdown of alcohol at the acetaldehyde stage by inhibiting the hepatic enzyme aldehyde dehydrogenase (ALDH; see Chapter 2). This leads to an accumulation of acetaldehyde in

BOX 13.1 From the pages of history: The discovery of disulfiram

> The laborers working with these chemicals, especially the ones who grind the finished products, find that they cannot drink alcohol in any form. Even beer will cause a flushing of the face and hands, with rapid pulse, and some of the men describe palpitations and a terrible fullness in the face, eyes and head.

This text appeared 80 years ago in a letter to the *Journal of the American Medical Association* (Williams, 1937). The author was the physician at a factory that prepared chemicals used to accelerate the vulcanization of rubber. Similar stories had emerged from the rubber boot industry in Sweden. This serendipitous discovery led to the development of disulfiram, modern medicine's first drug approved for the treatment of alcohol dependence.

Disulfiram's history begins in 1881, when a German chemist synthesized this new compound from thiocarbamide (Kragh, 2008). By the early 20th century, the compound was being employed in the emerging rubber industry, with unpleasant side effects for labourers who tried to enjoy a drink after work. Its initial medical applications, however, were to the treatment of scabies and intestinal worms. This changed in 1947 in Denmark, when two scientists who had been studying disulfiram (Erik Jacobsen and Jens Hald) began collaborating with Oluf Martensen-Larsen, a physician engaged in the treatment of alcohol dependence. Their commitment was impressive: Jacobsen experimented on himself, documenting carefully the unpleasant subjective effects caused by disulfiram's ability to retard the metabolization of ethanol.

Molecular Structure of Disulfiram

In 1952, the Danish team patented disulfiram as "antabus," which was Anglicized to "Antabuse" in the coming years. Americans learnt of it from an article on "Drug for Drunks" in *Time* magazine (Kragh, 2008). Although the medication was greeted with enthusiasm in the 1950s, it became a core feature of treatment in only a few countries. It did, however, have a central role in the maturation of addiction research in the United States.

Multisite clinical trials are often viewed as the crown jewel of medical research, and, in the United States, the most common site for the largest of such trials has been the Department of Veterans Affairs (VA) Cooperative Studies Program. Richard Fuller, a physician researcher who went on to become an important figure at the National Institute of Alcohol Abuse and Alcoholism, persuaded the VA to mount what was then probably the most expensive and sophisticated multisite trial ever done of addiction treatment. In this study of disulfiram, published like the 1937 letter in the prestigious *Journal of the American Medical Association* (Fuller et al., 1986) patients who took a placebo version of Antabuse were as likely to achieve total abstinence as those taking the actual medication.

However, the negative result in the high-profile trial had no apparent influence on the drug's popularity. More recently, its applications have expanded to include use as an implanted version and as a possible treatment for co-occurring alcohol and cocaine dependence – a remarkable evolution of an accidental discovery made by rubber industry workers.

the body and to the aversive disulfiram–ethanol reaction (DER), characterized by flushing of the face and upper trunk, throbbing headache, palpitations, an increased heart rate, nausea, vomiting, and general distress. The practice of exposing patients to a challenge dose of alcohol to experience such effects as a therapeutic test is not justified and no longer undertaken. The rationale of treatment with disulfiram is therefore that a patient cannot drink pleasurably while under the protective cover of the drug, and they will therefore only have to make a daily decision to take the medication rather than have to resist the sudden temptation to drink at any moment. Disulfiram also has effects on the central nervous system, inhibiting dopamine beta-hydroxylase and increasing concentrations of dopamine in the mesolimbic system, although it is not clear if this effect contributes to effectiveness. Patients taking disulfiram have reported a reduction in desire for alcohol.

Ethanol levels as low as 5–10 mg/100 mL (5–10 mg%) can cause a reaction in patients taking disulfiram. Patients should therefore be advised to avoid products with an ethanol concentration of greater than 5 mg%, which may include cough mixtures, mouthwash, perfumes, aftershaves, deodorants, and other similar over-the-counter preparations. Patients should also check whether alcohol is present in any foodstuffs. If a large amount of alcohol is consumed with disulfiram, there is a risk of cardiac arrhythmia, hypotension, and collapse. The reaction usually starts within 10–30 minutes of drinking and can last for several hours, with the peak effect occurring within 8–12 hours. Reactions have been reported up to 2 weeks after stopping disulfiram, although generally avoiding alcohol for next 7 days is advised. The severity of the DER varies greatly: it may be so slight that the patient "drinks through it" or so severe as to be life-threatening. The severity of the reaction has been reported to be proportional both to the amount of alcohol consumed and to the dose of the drug, although there is individual variability. Severe reactions are more likely to be seen with disulfiram as part of an overdose (intentional or accidental) rather than with daily dosing up to 250 mg per day. If a reaction is suspected, urgent medical attention should be sought for possible treatment to stabilize pulse and increase blood pressure, for convulsions, and methaemoglobinaemia. Patients prescribed disulfiram should carry a medical card with emergency instructions.

There are several contraindications and cautions about using disulfiram. Contradictions include cardiac failure, coronary artery disease, history of cerebrovascular accident, hypertension, severe personality disorder, and suicide risk, as well as pregnancy and breast-feeding. Although psychosis has historically been considered a contraindication, recent trials have shown disulfiram can be safely prescribed to individuals with a psychotic disorder (Petrakis et al., 2005). Caution is advised with hepatic or renal impairment, respiratory disease, diabetes, or epilepsy.

Disulfiram should be used with discretion, and its dangers should not be underestimated. Doctors instituting treatment should advise patients of the side effects and set up arrangements for regular reviews. Disulfiram is usually given in a daily dose of 100–250 mg, although it can be given in larger doses. It is absorbed slowly, and therefore must be taken for a few days to build up an effective blood level. Possible side effects include initial lethargy and fatigue, vomiting, an unpleasant taste in the mouth and halitosis, impotence, and unexplained breathlessness. Other less common side effects include psychosis (usually accompanied by delirium; likely linked to increased dopamine levels in brain), allergic dermatitis, optic and peripheral neuropathy, and hepatic cell damage. Disulfiram interacts with other drugs, enhancing the effect of warfarin and inhibiting the metabolism of tricyclic antidepressants, phenytoin, and benzodiazepines. Patients should be told not to take any more medication if they feel unwell and to seek urgent medical review (National Institute for Health and Clinical Excellence, 2011). Due to its potential in altering dopamine levels in the brain, disulfiram may also be useful in the treatment of individuals with co-occurring alcohol and cocaine use disorder (Carroll et al., 2004; see Chapter 7). Caution is needed here because disulfiram has been reported to increase plasma levels and reduce the clearance of both intranasal and intravenous cocaine (Baker, Jatlow, & McCance-Katz, 2007).

Many patients have found disulfiram helpful, especially in the early stages of abstinence. Some prefer to take a low maintenance dose over many years whereas others use it intermittently to cover high-risk periods.

Although reviews of clinical trials of disulfiram have concluded that it is not significantly better than placebo in preventing return to drinking or improvement in alcohol-related outcomes (Jonas et al., 2014; National Institute for Health and Clinical Excellence, 2011; Slattery et al., 2003), some trials have shown superiority. Due to its interaction with alcohol, true blinded studies with disulfiram are not possible – the patient must know they could be on disulfiram due to the potential seriousness of the interaction with alcohol, and it is easy for them to test whether they have been given a placebo. A meta-analysis of open-label studies supports disulfiram's efficacy (Skinner, Lahmek, Pham, & Aubin, 2014), and, compared with naltrexone or acamprosate, disulfiram has been shown to result in better drinking outcomes (De Sousa & De Sousa, 2004, 2005; Laaksonen et al., 2008).

Disulfiram is also available in a long-acting implant form, but evaluation studies are methodologically weak and suggest that the implant does not give patients a pharmacologically active concentration of disulfiram (Garbutt et al., 1999). Court-mandated disulfiram also has also been proposed to have a role in treatment, but this is not a widely applied or necessarily accepted approach (Martin et al., 2003).

In the light of present evidence, disulfiram has a lesser role in the treatment of alcohol dependence than other medications and is generally considered only after acamprosate or naltrexone, or if the patient wants it (Hughes & Cook, 1997, National Institute for Health and Clinical Excellence, 2011). The best results are likely to be seen when one or both of the following conditions are fulfilled. First, the use of the drug should be explained to and negotiated with the patient so that the taking of these tablets becomes not only acceptable but wanted; the patient is not being muzzled or surrendering autonomy but making a free decision to engage in this type of treatment. Second, an acceptable degree of supervision or witnessing should be set up – for instance, the tablet taken in the doctor's office, in the medical room at work, or in the presence of a supportive family member or friend – or a contingency management plan or therapeutic contract established.

Drugs that modulate brain function

Unlike disulfiram, the medications described herein do not result in an aversive reaction if alcohol is consumed. Instead, their mechanisms involve modulating brain circuits involved in alcohol dependence such as reward, motivation, and stress (see Chapter 2). Unlike with disulfiram, these medications carry no risk if the patient consumes alcohol.

Naltrexone

Naltrexone is an opioid receptor antagonist. Alcohol is thought to be reinforcing because it stimulates release of endorphin (an endogenous opioid) in the brain, which leads to activation of the dopaminergic "pleasure-reward-motivation" pathway (see Chapter 2). Naltrexone blocks this activation, which is hypothesized to explain its clinical effectiveness. In addition, other mechanisms, such as reducing impulsivity and modulation of the HPA axis and stress system, have also been proposed to be involved in mediating naltrexone's effects.

First approved for the treatment of alcohol dependence in 1994 by the U.S. Food and Drug Administration, naltrexone has been subject to numerous randomized and controlled clinical trials in which small to medium effect sizes have been reported (Jonas et al., 2014; Maisel et al., 2013; Rösner, Leucht, Lehert, & Soyka, 2008). It is now licensed in many countries in Europe, including the UK, as well as in Australia. At the dose commonly used, 50 mg daily, naltrexone has been shown to reduce relapse rates in alcohol dependent patients in combination with psychosocial treatment (for references, see Donoghue et al., 2015; Jonas et al., 2014; Lingford-Hughes et al., 2012; Maisel et al., 2013; National Institute for Health and Clinical Excellence, 2011). For this effect, the number needed to treat (NNT) has been calculated at about 12 (Jonas et al., 2014). However, naltrexone does not appear as effective in maintaining abstinence, with an NNT of 20. Therefore, naltrexone may be better used in those patients who have the occasional drink or lapse to prevent a full-blown relapse rather than to sustain abstinence (Maisel et al., 2013). Naltrexone has also been shown to reduce the euphoria or pleasure associated with alcohol intake and, in some studies, to reduce craving. No single psychosocial approach has shown a particular advantage over another when combined with naltrexone.

In relapse prevention trials, naltrexone is started once someone has stopped drinking. Treatment is usually for 3–6 months in the first instance, but should be reassessed as to whether to continue if the patient has relapsed. Although earlier studies suggested that the beneficial effects of naltrexone may not persist, later studies such as COMBINE reported continued benefit persisting for up to a year (Donovan et al., 2008). Although not everyone benefits from naltrexone, no robust predictors have been identified to guide clinical decision-making, although some studies have found potential indicators worthy of replication studies (Bogenschutz, Scott Tonigan, & Pettinati, 2009). Although a functional polymorphism, Asp40 allele, of the mu opioid receptor gene had been shown to predict naltrexone treatment response in a range of studies (e.g., COMBINE; Anton et al., 2006), a more recent prospective trial did not find such an effect (Oslin et al., 2015).

Naltrexone is generally a well-tolerated and safe medication. Side effects include nausea, vomiting and abdominal pain, headache, reduced energy, joint and muscle pain, and sleeping difficulty. Loss of appetite, diarrhea, constipation, increased thirst, chest pain, increased sweating, increased energy, irritability, chills, delayed ejaculation, and decreased potency are less frequent side effects. Although concerns about hepatic toxicity have been raised, this occurred with much higher doses (>300 mg/d) than the dose generally used to treat alcohol dependence (50 mg/d). Indeed, liver function test improvement is often seen in trials of naltrexone as alcohol consumption reduces. Nevertheless, naltrexone should not be used in those with acute liver failure and should be used cautiously when serum aminotransferases are four to five times above normal. It should not be prescribed to women who are pregnant or breast-feeding.

Most people tolerate the daily 50 mg dose, although it may be sensible to take a lower dose (25 mg) for the first 3–4 days of treatment to minimize side effects, particularly nausea in women. More recent trials of naltrexone have used 100 mg/d rather than 50 mg/d, but this higher dose has not been shown to be clearly more effective and may incur more side effects (Jonas et al., 2014). Naltrexone can be safely taken with many other medications but, as an opioid antagonist, it cannot be taken by those requiring opioid analgesia. Careful assessment of whether the patient is taking prescribed or over-the-counter opioid medications is therefore essential. If in an emergency analgesia is required, nonopioid medication will have to be used because blockade due to naltrexone may last up to 72 hours. Patients should be encouraged to carry a card stating that they are taking naltrexone in case of such an emergency.

Patients do not have to be abstinent before they commence naltrexone, but outcomes are better when they are (Maisel et al., 2013). Unlike for disulfiram, it is safe to drink with naltrexone. Indeed, it has been suggested that due to naltrexone's hypothesized mechanism of action in reducing the pleasurable effects of alcohol, naltrexone may be beneficial in reducing consumption in those who are still drinking. The few studies of naltrexone in those who are less dependent or who are "heavy drinkers" have shown some benefit, including recently in younger drinkers (e.g., Heinälä et al., 2001; Kranzler et al., 2009; O'Malley et al., 2015), although the evidence is insufficient to justify widespread clinical use.

Naltrexone has also recently become available in a long-term injected formulation. Due to the once-a-month dosing, this approach may improve treatment compliance, thus helping the patient whose motivation to stop drinking waxes and wanes frequently. An early trial was positive and was also associated with improvements in quality of life, but a large amount of clinical experience has not yet accumulated (Garbutt et al., 2005; Pettinati et al., 2009). Because injectable naltrexone has shown impressive benefits when used with heroin dependent patients, its use should be considered for any problem-drinking patients who are also dependent on opioids (Krupitsky et al., 2012).

Nalmefene

Nalmefene is also an opioid antagonist whose first trial as a treatment for alcoholism took place in the 1990s. But it has only recently been licensed for this indication in several countries in Europe, including the UK. Whereas naltrexone is an antagonist at mu and kappa receptors, nalmefene is an antagonist at the mu opiate receptor and a partial agonist at the kappa receptor. The impact of this on the clinical efficacy of nalmefene is not clear, but preclinical data show a greater role for kappa compared with mu receptors in reducing consumption in dependent animals (Walker, Zorrilla, & Koob, 2011). No clinical trials have compared nalmefene with naltrexone.

In two European trials, nalmefene reduced heavy drinking days and total alcohol consumption in alcohol dependent patients at 6 months (Gual et al., 2013; Mann, Bladström, et al., 2013). The psychosocial intervention used combined motivational and adherence-enhancing elements to support behaviour change. Alcohol dependent patients did not have to be sober before entering the trial and also were instructed to take nalmefene "as-needed" (i.e., when they perceived there was a risk of drinking). Most patients took it at least 4 days per week. Further analyses of these trials showed that the effect of nalmefene was not evident in those who had reduced their drinking levels between screening and randomization. Thus, nalmefene benefited those who were still drinking at a high risk level (>60 g/d for a man; >40 g/d for a woman) (van den Brink et al., 2013). Nalmefene is therefore licensed to reduce alcohol consumption in alcohol dependent patients "who continue to have a high drinking risk level two weeks after initial assessment, without physical withdrawal symptoms and who do not require immediate detoxification."

Greater adverse effects such as nausea, dizziness, insomnia, and fatigue were also reported for nalmefene than placebo. These side effects were generally mild to moderate and present only for first 1–2 days, but nonetheless contributed to treatment dropout.

Acamprosate

Acamprosate (calcium bis-acetyl homotaurinate), a simple derivative of the amino acid taurine, has been used in the treatment of alcohol dependence in Europe for more than 20 years and more recently became available in the United States. Its target in the brain is uncertain; however, it does modulate glutamatergic *N*-methyl-D-aspartic acid (NMDA) receptor transmission, probably involving metabotropic glutamate receptor subtype 5 (mGluR5) antagonism. Acamprosate may have indirect effects on gamma-aminobutyric acid ($GABA_A$) receptor activity as well (Kalk & Lingford-Hughes, 2014). It is thought to modulate alcohol withdrawal effects and limit any aversiveness associated with the cessation of drinking.

Numerous clinical trials of acamprosate in combination with a psychosocial intervention have been conducted throughout the world, with a particular concentration in Europe. Meta-analyses have shown acamprosate significantly improves abstinent rates, with a NNT of around 12 to prevent return to any drinking (Donoghue et al., 2015; Jonas et al., 2014; National Institute for Health and Clinical Excellence, 2011; Rosner et al., 2010). Acamprosate's ability to reduce quantity and frequency of drinking is less certain. Therefore, acamprosate's main effect is to maintain abstinence rather than prevent a lapse becoming a relapse, which is thus the opposite of naltrexone's (Maisel et al., 2013). Acamprosate tablets (333 mg each) are taken in doses of either 1,998 mg or 1,332 mg daily, depending on the patient's weight. The number and size of pills may present challenges with adherence for some patients.

Like naltrexone, in clinical trials, acamprosate is started once the person is abstinent. U.S. (COMBINE) and UK trials have suggested that poorer outcomes are seen with longer periods of abstinence before starting acamprosate (Chick, Howlett, Morgan, & Ritson, 2000; Gueorguieva et al., 2015). Given the potential neuroprotective effect of acamprosate and that it can be given safely along with medication for detoxification (see Chapter 11), acamprosate could be started before or during detoxification rather than after (Lingford-Hughes et al., 2012). Treatment with acamprosate is generally recommended for up to

6 months, although license suggests 1 year, and its beneficial effects may persist after stopping (Rosner et al., 2010). If abstinence is not maintained and drinking behaviour is not changing after 4–6 weeks, it is wise to consider whether acamprosate should be continued (National Institute for Health and Clinical Excellence, 2011). Although earlier reports suggested that those with anxiety or more severe dependence were more likely to respond to acamprosate, this was not found in reviews (e.g., National Institute for Health and Clinical Excellence, 2011; Verheul et al., 2005).

Acamprosate is generally a well-tolerated and safe medication. Its main side effects are related to the gastrointestinal system such as nausea and diarrhoea. Acamprosate should not be prescribed to individuals with significant renal impairment or hepatic failure, nor to women who are pregnant or breast-feeding. It does not interact with alcohol or diazepam, appears to have no addictive potential itself, and can be used safely with a wide range of medications, including antidepressants.

Naltrexone versus Acamprosate

Most clinical studies compare active medication with placebo, but some have directly compared acamprosate and naltrexone. A European study found that naltrexone (50 mg/d) was superior to acamprosate (1,998 mg/d) or placebo (Kiefer et al., 2003). but an Australian study using the same doses found that neither were superior to placebo (Morley et al., 2006). Combined naltrexone and acamprosate has been shown to improve drinking outcomes compared with acamprosate alone but not to naltrexone alone (Kiefer et al., 2003). One of the largest studies ever conducted in alcohol dependence, COMBINE, a nine-arm U.S. study, compared acamprosate (3 g; i.e., a larger dose than is now licensed) with naltrexone (100 mg) individually or together in addition to standard "medical management" or more intensive combined behavioural intervention (CBI) (Anton et al., 2006). Naltrexone with medical management alone or in combination with CBI resulted in greater improvements than placebo or medical management alone, whereas acamprosate showed no evidence of additional efficacy in any combination. Combined acamprosate and naltrexone conferred no benefit. Modeled on COMBINE, PREDICT was a German study that found neither medication was superior to placebo (Mann, Lemenager, et al., 2013). Meta-analysis of all these studies found no difference in global effectiveness between acamprosate and naltrexone (Jonas et al., 2014). However, another meta-analysis of clinical trials reported that effect sizes for naltrexone tend to be larger than those for acamprosate when the outcome is reduced heavy drinking and craving, but acamprosate has larger effect sizes when the measured outcome is abstinence (Maisel et al., 2013).

What contributes to these disparate findings of whether naltrexone or acamprosate are effective, and does it inform clinical decision-making? There are more trials of naltrexone conducted in the United States than elsewhere, whereas most trials of acamprosate are conducted in Europe. Indeed the few U.S.-based studies did not find acamprosate efficacious, whereas European trials did find naltrexone efficacious. There has been extensive discussion of these different results from U.S. and European trials (Donoghue et al., 2015). In European trials, participants are typically recruited from in-patient programmes and treatment services, whereas U.S.-based trials usually advertise for participants who have to be able to be sober for 3 days. U.S. participants are therefore less likely to be severely dependent, and this, along with the differences in healthcare settings, is likely to contribute the variability in outcomes seen.

Other pharmacotherapies

A number of other medications have been evaluated and continue to be studied for their efficacy in improving outcomes in alcohol dependence. It is not advised to use any of these medications for alcohol dependence in patients who are pregnant or breast-feeding.

Baclofen

Baclofen is a $GABA_B$ receptor agonist licensed to treat muscle spasms in disorders such as multiple sclerosis. Evidence is accruing to support a role for baclofen in treating alcohol dependence, with trials in Italy and Germany reporting reduced craving, anxiety, and relapse rates (Addolorato et al., 2007; Müller et al., 2015). A U.S. study failed to find superiority of baclofen over placebo, but, as discussed earlier, this was likely due to differences in participants (Garbutt et al., 2010). In the U.S. study, patients were less severely alcohol dependent and the majority did not desire abstinence, unlike in the two European trials.

Baclofen is started after detoxification and is titrated up from 5 mg three times a day. The optimal dose of baclofen is unknown; some alcohol dependent participants require 10 times the dose used in the first trial (i.e., 300 mg/d vs. 30 mg/d). Although some appear to tolerate such large doses, side effects such as sedation and withdrawal seizures become more likely over time. Larger doses have been investigated in recent studies, with one allowing up to 270 mg, although only a third of patients reached this amount (Müller et al., 2015). Other studies are due to report shortly to help inform clinicians about the optimal dose of baclofen, as well as its use in other substance dependencies such as nicotine or cocaine alone and when comorbid with alcoholism.

Topiramate

Topiramate is an anticonvulsant affecting many systems in the brain including glutamate, GABA, and dopamine. A meta-analysis of trials reported that topiramate reduced heavy drinking and increased abstinence (Blodgett, Del Re, Maisel, & Finney, 2014). Notably, in some of these trials, topiramate was started while the patient was still drinking rather than after detoxification.

Side effects reported included paresthesia/numbness, nausea/vomiting, and cognitive impairment, particularly at higher doses and without slow enough titration. More research on dosing regimes is clearly needed. Topiramate is also being investigated as a treatment for stimulant use disorders.

Pregabalin and gabapentin

Despite their names, pregabalin (Lyrica) and gabapentin (Neurontin) do not directly target the GABA system but instead are calcium channel modulators. They are licensed for treating a range of disorders such as seizures, neuropathic pain, and generalized anxiety disorder (pregabalin only). These medications are being evaluated as possible treatments for alcohol and other substance dependence. Both medications have been studied for treating alcohol withdrawal, but the evidence is not promising (Guglielmo, Martinotti, Clerici, & Janiri, 2012; Leung et al., 2015). However, some studies suggest that gabapentin and pregabalin could aid in relapse prevention, although the evidence is insufficient to recommend them for routine use over other medications (Pani, Trogu, Pacini, & Maremanni,

2014). There are concerns about the abuse liability of these medications and also their safety in combination with other central depressants such as alcohol and opioids. Trials thus far have reported, however, that these medications are well-tolerated and have a favourable safety profile.

Pharmacotherapy for alcohol patients with psychiatric comorbidities

Treating alcohol dependence alongside another psychiatric disorder is likely to be the norm (see Chapter 6). Only a small number of pharmacotherapy studies, most with small samples and short follow-up periods, have focused on such dually diagnosed patients. Much of the evidence thus does not reach the standard required by national guidelines. However, given how common psychiatric comorbidities are, the clinician should be familiar with these studies and keep abreast of developments in this active area of investigation.

Depression

Three meta-analyses of trials of antidepressants in treating comorbidity all suggest that antidepressants may reduce depressive symptoms but not necessarily alcohol consumption in depressed alcohol dependent patients (Iovieno et al., 2011; Nunes & Levin, 2004; Torrens, Fonseca, Mateu, & Farré, 2005). Mixed serotonin-noradrenergic antidepressants appear superior to serotonin reuptake inhibitors (SSRIs). There are no placebo-controlled trials of the newer antidepressants. Meta-analytic reviews indicate that antidepressants are less effective in treating depression when the patient is still drinking and that stopping or considerably reducing drinking generally leads to a substantial improvement in mood. It is therefore better to assess the need for an antidepressant once abstinence (or, failing that, significantly reduced consumption) is achieved.

Concerning relapse prevention medication, in one of the largest trials in comorbidity, disulfiram and naltrexone alone and in combination were compared with placebo in patients with a psychiatric comorbidity that included depressive, anxiety, and psychotic disorders (Petrakis et al., 2005). A secondary analysis comparing those with and without depression concluded that naltrexone and disulfiram can be used safely in depressed alcohol dependent patients with comparable efficacy to those not depressed (Petrakis et al., 2007). A recent study comparing naltrexone (100 mg) or sertraline (200 mg) alone or in combination found that only the combination improved drinking outcomes and mood (Pettinati et al., 2010).

The reviews and trials support the commonly given clinical advice to not start an antidepressant in a patient while they continue to drink heavily and to assess their depression and need for antidepressant once abstinent, ideally for at least 2–3 weeks (Lingford-Hughes et al., 2012; National Institute for Health and Clinical Excellence, 2011). There is also support for using relapse prevention medication, with the most evidence available for naltrexone, although an adverse impact on outcome has not been seen for any such medication.

Anxiety disorder

Careful assessment is required to establish whether a comorbid anxiety disorder is present because, if left untreated, reducing alcohol consumption is less likely. As with depression, because treatments have limited impact on the anxiety disorder with continued drinking, abstinence should be encouraged (Lingford-Hughes et al., 2012; National Institute for

Health and Clinical Excellence, 2011). In post-traumatic stress disorder (PTSD), naltrexone or disulfiram alone or in combination have been shown to result in greater improvements in alcohol consumption than placebo (Petrakis et al., 2006*b*). A later study of combat veterans with PTSD, however, did not show any additional benefit of naltrexone when combined with either desipramine or paroxetine (Petrakis et al., 2012).

Bipolar disorder

There is limited evidence to suggest the optimal mood stabilizer regimen for patients with drinking problems and bipolar disorder (Lingford-Hughes et al., 2012). Concerning relapse prevention medication, preliminary reports suggest no particular benefit with acamprosate although also no worsening in mental state. A secondary analysis of Petrakis's study of naltrexone and disulfiram compared those with a psychotic disorder, of which the majority (73 percent) had bipolar disorder, to participants without a psychotic disorder and reported that medication was superior to placebo (Petrakis, Nich, & Ralevski, 2006*a*). Given the potential of disulfiram to increase psychotic symptoms, naltrexone is easier and safer to use in bipolar disorder.

Schizophrenia

The few studies of relapse prevention medication in schizophrenia identified no adverse impact on mental state but no particular benefit to drinking outcomes either. Although disulfiram has been safely used in schizophrenia, it is however best used in a specialist setting once other options have been exhausted. The limited evidence available suggests there is no benefit from the second- over the first-generation antipsychotics (Lingford-Hughes et al., 2012; Petrakis et al., 2006*a*). Although there are no prospective trials, some evidence suggests that clozapine improves drinking outcomes. Given its beneficial effect in improving treatment-resistant schizophrenia, clozapine should be considered in those patients with problem drinking and whose schizophrenia persists despite adequate antipsychotic medication.

Delivering evidence-based treatments in the real world

Clinicians have a professional responsibility to incorporate evidence-based treatment methods into their repertoire and to follow the continuing evolution of treatment research. But this need not imply a rigid or mechanical effort to replicate precisely the manualized treatment featured in the latest, most sophisticated clinical trial. What can be accomplished in frontline care is always shaped by the nature of the patient population, the quality and quantity of the staff, and the larger organizational and financial environment of the care system. It is thus common, and indeed entirely appropriate, for clinicians to improvise and innovate as they find ways to implement evidence-based treatments in their particular setting. As it is often said of politics, frontline clinical care is "the art of the possible."

Due to the diversity of patients with drinking problems, there is no one single pathway to recovery, nor even, for that matter, one single destination. If a clinician finds that the evidence-based treatment that well serves the majority of patients is remarkably ineffective with a particular subgroup (or indeed a particular patient), then the clinician should set that approach aside. The proper use of the treatment research base reviewed in this chapter is to inform and guide the judgment of the clinician, never to replace it.

References

Addolorato, G., Leggio, L., Ferrulli, A., Cardone, S., Vonghia, L., Mirijello, A., … Gasbarrini, G. (2007). Effectiveness and safety of baclofen for maintenance of alcohol abstinence in alcohol-dependent patients with liver cirrhosis: Randomised, double-blind controlled study. *Lancet*, **370**(9603), 1915–1922.

Anton, R. F., O'Malley, S. S., Ciraulo, D. A., Cisler, R.A., Couper, D., Donovan, D.M., … COMBINE Study Research Group. (2006). Combined pharmacotherapies and behavioural interventions for alcohol dependence. *Journal of the American Medical Association*, **295**, 2003–2017.

Azrin, N. H. (1976). Improvements in the community-reinforcement approach to alcoholism. *Behaviour Research and Therapy*, **14**, 339–348.

Azrin, N. H., Sisson, R. W., Meyers, R., & Godley, M. (1982). Alcoholism treatment by disulfiram and community reinforcement therapy. *Journal of Behaviour Therapy and Experimental Psychiatry*, **13**, 105–112.

Baker, J. R., Jatlow, P. M., & McCance-Katz, E. F. (2007), Disulfiram effects on responses to intravenous cocaine administration. *Drug and Alcohol Dependence*, **87**, 202–209.

Berglund, M., Thelander, S., & Jonsson, E. (2003). *Treating alcohol and drug abuse: An evidence-based review.* Weinheim, Germany: Wiley-VCH.

Blodgett, J. C., Del Re, A. C., Maisel, N. C., & Finney, J. W. (2014). A meta-analysis of topiramate's effects for individuals with alcohol use disorders. *Alcoholism: Clinical and Experimental Research*, **38**(6), 1481–1488.

Bogenschutz, M. P., Scott Tonigan, J., & Pettinati, H. M. (2009). Effects of alcoholism typology on response to naltrexone in the COMBINE study. *Alcoholism: Clinical and Experimental Research*, **33**(1), 10–18.

Bowen, S., Witkiewitz, K., Clifasefi, S. L., Grow, J., Chawla, N., Hsu, S. H., … Larimer, M. E. (2014). Relative efficacy of mindfulness-based relapse prevention, standard relapse prevention, and treatment as usual for substance use disorders: A randomized clinical trial. *JAMA Psychiatry*, **71**(5), 547–556.

Carroll, K. M., Nich, C., Ball, S. A., McCance, E., Frankforter, T. L., & Rounsaville, B. J. (2000). One-year follow-up of disulfiram and psychotherapy for cocaine-alcohol users: Sustained effects of treatment. *Addiction*, **95**, 1335–1349.

Chick, J., Howlett, H., Morgan, M. Y., & Ritson, B. (2000). United Kingdom Multicentre Acamprosate Study (UKMAS): A 6-month prospective study of acamprosate versus placebo in preventing relapse after withdrawal from alcohol. *Alcohol and Alcoholism*, **35**(2), 176–187.

Conklin, C. A., & Tiffany, S. T. (2002). Applying extinction research and theory to cue-exposure addiction treatments. *Addiction*, **97**(2), 155–67.

Copello, A., Orford, J., Hodgson, R., Tober, G., & Barrett, C. (2002). Social behaviour and network therapy: Basic principles and early experiences. *Addictive Behaviours*, **27**, 354–366.

Copello, A. G., Hodgson, R., Tober, G., & Orford, J. (2009). *Social behaviour and network therapy for alcohol problems.* London: Routledge.

Copello, A. G., Velleman, R. D., & Templeton, L. (2005). Family interventions in the treatment of alcohol and drug problems. *Drug and Alcohol Review*, **24**, 369–385.

De Sousa, A., & De Sousa, A. (2004). A one-year pragmatic trial of naltrexone vs disulfiram in the treatment of alcohol dependence. *Alcohol and Alcoholism*, **39**(6), 528–531.

De Sousa, A., & De Sousa, A. (2005). An open randomized study comparing disulfiram and acamprosate in the treatment of alcohol dependence. *Alcohol and Alcoholism*, **40**(6), 545–548.

Donoghue, K., Elzerbi, C., Saunders, R., Whittington, C., Pilling, S., & Drummond, C. (2015). The efficacy of acamprosate and naltrexone in the treatment of alcohol dependence, Europe versus the rest of the world: A meta-analysis. *Addiction*, **110**(6), 920–930.

Donovan, D. M., Anton, R. F., Miller, W. R., Longabaugh, R., Hosking, J. D., Youngblood, M., & COMBINE Study Research Group. (2008). Combined pharmacotherapies and behavioral interventions for alcohol dependence (The COMBINE Study): Examination of posttreatment drinking outcomes. *Journal of Studies on Alcohol and Drugs*, **69**(1), 5–13.

Drummond, D. C., Tiffany, S. T., Glautier, S., & Remington, B. (1995). *Addictive behaviour: Cue exposure, theory and practice*. Chichester, UK: John Wiley & Sons.

Foxcroft, D. R., Coombes, L., Wood, S., Allen, D., & Almeida Santimano, N. M. (2014). Motivational interviewing for alcohol misuse in young adults. *Cochrane Database of Systematic Reviews*, CD007025.

Fuller, R. K., Branchley, L., Brightwell, D. R., Derman, R. M., Emrick, C. D., Iber, F. L., ... Shaw, S. (1986). Disulfiram treatment of alcoholism: A Veterans Administration cooperative study. *Journal of the American Medical Association*, **256**, 1449–1455.

Garbutt, J. C., Kampov-Polevoy, A. B., Gallop, R., Kalka-Juhl, L., & Flannery, B. A. (2010). Efficacy and safety of baclofen for alcohol dependence: A randomized, double-blind, placebo-controlled trial. *Alcoholism: Clinical and Experimental Research*, **34**(11), 1849–1857.

Garbutt, J. C., Kranzler, H. R., O'Malley, S. S., Gastfriend, D. R., Pettinati, H. M., Silverman, B. L., ... Vivitrex Study Group. (2005). Efficacy and tolerability of long-acting injectable naltrexone for alcohol dependence: A randomized controlled trial. *Journal of the American Medical Association*, **293**, 1617–1625.

Garbutt, J. C., West, S. L., Carey, T. S., Lohr, K. N., & Crews, F. T. (1999). Pharmacological treatment of alcohol dependence: A review of the evidence. *Journal of the American Medical Association*, **281**, 1318–1325.

Gual, A., He, Y., Torup, L., van den Brink, W., Mann, K., & ESENSE 2 Study Group. (2013). A randomised, double-blind, placebo-controlled, efficacy study of nalmefene, as-needed use, in patients with alcohol dependence. *European Neuropsychopharmacology*, **23**(11), 1432–1442.

Gueorguieva, R., Wu, R., Tsai, W. M., O'Connor, P. G., Fucito, L., Zhang, H., & O'Malley, S. S. (2015). An analysis of moderators in the COMBINE study: Identifying subgroups of patients who benefit from acamprosate. *European Neuropsychopharmacology*. Advance online publication. http://dx.doi.org/10.1016/j.euroneuro.2015.06.006

Guglielmo, R., Martinotti, G., Clerici, M., & Janiri, L. (2012). Pregabalin for alcohol dependence: A critical review of the literature. *Advances in Therapy*, **29**(11), 947–957.

Haber, P., Lintzeris, N., Proude, E., & Lopatko, O. (2009). *Guidelines for the treatment of alcohol problems*. Sydney: Australian Government Department of Health and Ageing.

Haug, N. A., Duffy, M., & McCaul, M. E. (2014). Substance abuse treatment services for pregnant women: Psychosocial and behavioral approaches. *Obstetrics and Gynecology Clinics of North America*, **41**(2), 267–296.

Heinälä, P., Alho, H., Kiianmaa, K., Lönnqvist, J., Kuoppasalmi, K., & Sinclair, J. D. (2001). Targeted use of naltrexone without prior detoxification in the treatment of alcohol dependence: A factorial double-blind, placebo-controlled trial. *Journal of Clinical Psychopharmacology*, **21**(3), 287–292.

Hester, R. K. (1995). Behavioural self control training. In R. K. Hester & W. R. Miller (Eds.), *Handbook of alcoholism treatment approaches: Effective alternatives* (2nd ed., pp. 148–159). Needham Heights, MS: Allyn and Bacon.

Holder, H., Longabaugh, R., Miller, W. R., & Rubonis, A. V. (1991). The cost effectiveness of treatment for alcoholism: A first approximation. *Journal of Studies on Alcohol*, **52**, 517–540.

Hughes, J. L., & Cook, C. C. H. (1997). The efficacy of disulfiram: A review of outcome studies. *Addiction*, **92**, 381–396.

Hunt, G. M., & Azrin, N. H. (1973). A community-reinforcement approach to alcoholism. *Behaviour Research and Therapy*, **11**, 91–104.

Iovieno, N., Tedeschini, E., Bentley, K. H., Evins, A. E., & Papakostas, G. I. (2011). Antidepressants for major depressive disorder and dysthymic disorder in patients with comorbid alcohol use disorders: A meta-analysis of placebo-controlled randomized trials. *Journal of Clinical Psychiatry*, **72**(8), 1144–1151.

Jarvis, T. J., Tebbutt, J., Mattick, R. P., & Shand, F. (2005). *Treatment approaches for alcohol and drug dependence: An introductory guide* (2nd ed.). Chichester, UK: John Wiley & Sons.

Jonas, D. E., Amick, H. R., Feltner, C., Bobashev, G., Thomas, K., Wines, R., ... Garbutt, J. C. (2014). Pharmacotherapy for adults with alcohol use disorders in outpatient settings: A systematic review and meta-analysis. *Journal of the American Medical Association*, **311**(18), 1889–1900.

Kalk, N. J., & Lingford-Hughes, A. R. (2014). The clinical pharmacology of acamprosate. *British Journal of Clinical Pharmacology*, **77**(2), 315–323.

Kelly, J. F., Humphreys, K., & Ferri, M. (in press). Alcoholics Anonymous and twelve-step treatments for alcohol use disorder. *Cochrane Database of Systematic Reviews.*

Kiefer, F., Jahn, H., Tarnaske, T., Helwig, H., Briken, P., Holzbach, R., … Wiedemann, K. (2003). Comparing and combining naltrexone and acamprosate in relapse prevention of alcoholism: A double-blind, placebo-controlled study. *Archives of General Psychiatry*, **60**(1), 92–99.

Kohler, S., & Hofmann, A. (2015). Can motivational interviewing in emergency care reduce alcohol consumption in young people? A systematic review and meta-analysis. *Alcohol and Alcoholism*, **50**(2), 107–117.

Kragh, H. (2008). From disulfiram to antabuse: The invention of a drug. *Bulletin for the History of Chemistry*, **33**, 82–88.

Kranzler, H. R., Tennen, H., Armeli, S., Chan, G., Covault, J., Arias, A., & Oncken, C. (2009). Targeted naltrexone for problem drinkers. *Journal of Clinical Psychopharmacology*, **29**(4), 350.

Krupitsky, E., Zvartau, E., Blokhina, E., Verbitskaya, E., Wahlgren, V., Tsoy-Podosenin, M., … Woody, G. E. (2012). Randomized trial of long-acting sustained-release naltrexone implant vs oral naltrexone or placebo for preventing relapse to opioid dependence. *Archives of General Psychiatry*, **69**(9), 973–981.

Laaksonen, E., Koski-Jännes, A., Salaspuro, M., Ahtinen, H., & Alho, H. (2008). A randomized, multicentre, open-label, comparative trial of disulfiram, naltrexone and acamprosate in the treatment of alcohol dependence. *Alcohol and Alcoholism*, **43**(1), 53–61.

Leung, J. G., Hall-Flavin, D., Nelson, S., Schmidt, K. A., & Schak, K. M. (2015). The role of gabapentin in the management of alcohol withdrawal and dependence. *Annals of Pharmacotherapy*. Advance online publication. doi:10.1177/1060028015585849

Lingford-Hughes, A. R., Welch, S., Peters, L., & Nutt, D. J. (2012). BAP updated guidelines: Evidence-based guidelines for the pharmacological management of substance abuse, harmful use, addiction and comorbidity: Recommendations from BAP. *Journal of Psychopharmacology*, **26**(7), 899–952.

Ludwig, D. S., & Kabat-Zinn, J. (2008). Mindfulness in medicine. *Journal of the American Medical Association*, **300**(11), 1350–1352.

Maisel, N. C., Blodgett, J., Wilbourne, P. L., Humphreys, K., & Finney, J. W. (2013). Meta-analysis of naltrexone and acamprosate for treating alcohol dependence: When and for what are these medications most helpful? *Addiction*, **108**, 275–293.

Management of Substance Use Disorders Workgroup. (2009). *VA/DOD clinical practice guideline for the management of substance abuse disorders.* Washington, DC: Departments of Defense and Veterans Affairs.

Mann, K., Bladström, A., Torup, L., Gual, A., & van den Brink, W. (2013). Extending the treatment options in alcohol dependence: A randomized controlled study of as-needed nalmefene. *Biological Psychiatry*, **73**(8), 706–713.

Mann, K., Lemenager, T., Hoffmann, S., Reinhard, I., Hermann, D., Batra, A., … PREDICT Study Team (2013). Results of a double-blind, placebo-controlled pharmacotherapy trial in alcoholism conducted in Germany and comparison with the US COMBINE study. *Addiction Biology*, **18**(6), 937–946.

Marlatt, G. A., & Gordon, J. R. (1985). *Relapse prevention.* New York: Guilford.

Martin, B., Clapp, L., Bialkowski, D., Bridgeford, D., Amponsah, A., Lyons, L., & Beresford, T. P. (2003). Compliance to supervised disulfiram therapy: A comparison of voluntary and court-ordered patients. *American Journal of Addictions*, **12**, 137–143.

Meyers, R. J., & Miller, W. R. (2001). *A community reinforcement approach to addiction treatment.* Cambridge, UK: Cambridge University Press.

Meyers, R. J., Smith, J. E., Serna, B., & Belon, K. E. (2013). Community reinforcement approaches: CRA and CRAFT. In P. Miller (Ed.), *Interventions for addiction: Comprehensive addictive behaviors and disorders* (pp. 47–56). San Diego, CA: Academic Press.

Miller, W. R., Andrews, N. R., Wilbourne, P., & Bennett, M. E. (1998). A wealth of alternatives: Effective treatments for alcohol problems. In W. R. Miller & N. Heather, eds., *Treating Addictive Behaviours* (2nd ed., pp. 203–216). New York: Plenum.

Miller, W. R., & Rollnick, S. (2002). *Motivational interviewing: Preparing people for change.* New York: Guilford.

Miller, W. R., Walters, S. T., & Bennett, M. E. (2001). How effective is alcoholism treatment in the United States. *Journal of Studies on Alcohol*, **62**, 211–220.

Miller, W. R., Wilbourne, P. D., & Hetema, J. E. (2003). What works? A summary of alcohol treatment outcome research. In R. K. Hester & W. R. Miller (Eds.), *Handbook of alcoholism treatment approaches: Effective alternatives* (3rd ed, pp. 13–63). Boston, MA: Allyn and Bacon.

Monti, P. M., Abrams, D. B., Binkoff, J. A., Zwick, W. R., Liepman, M. R., Nirenberg, T. D., & Rohsenow, D. J. (1990). Communication skills training, communication skills training with family and cognitive behavioural mood management training for alcoholics. *Journal of Studies on Alcohol*, **51**, 263–270.

Monti, P. M., Rohsenhow, D. J., Colby, S. M., & Abrams, D. B. (1995). Coping and social skills training. In R. K. Hester & W. R. Miller (Eds.), *Handbook of alcoholism treatment approaches: Effective alternatives* (2nd ed., pp. 221–241). Needham Heights, MS: Allyn and Bacon.

Monti, P. M., Rohsenhow, D. J., Rubonis, A. V., Niaura, R. S., Sirota, A. D., Colby, S. M., … Abrams, D. B. (1993). Cue exposure with coping skills treatment for male alcoholics: A preliminary investigation. *Journal of Consulting and Clinical Psychology*, **61**, 1011–1019.

Moos, R. H. (2005). Iatrogenic effects of psychosocial interventions for substance use disorder: Prevalence, predictors, prevention. *Addiction*, **100**, 595–604.

Morley, K. C., Teesson, M., Reid, S. C., Sannibale, C., Thomson, C., Phung, N., … Haber, P. S. (2006). Naltrexone versus acamprosate in the treatment of alcohol dependence: A multi-centre, randomized, double-blind, placebo-controlled trial. *Addiction*, **101**(10), 1451–1462.

Müller, C. A., Geisel, O., Pelz, P., Higl, V., Krüger, J., Stickel, A., … Heinz, A. (2015). High-dose baclofen for the treatment of alcohol dependence (BACLAD study): A randomized, placebo-controlled trial. *European Neuropsychopharmacology*, **25**,1167–1177.

Najavits, L. M., Weiss, R. D., & Liese, B. S. (1996). Group cognitive behavioural therapy for women with PTSD and substance use disorder. *Journal of Substance Abuse Treatment*, **13**, 13–22.

National Institute for Health and Clinical Excellence. (2011). *Alcohol dependence and harmful alcohol use* (NICE Clinical Guideline 115). London: National Institute for Health and Clinical Excellence.

Nunes, E. V., & Levin, F. R. (2004). Treatment of depression in patients with alcohol or other drug dependence: A meta-analysis. *JAMA*, **291**(15), 1887–1896.

O'Farrell, T. J., Choquette, K. A., Cutter, H. S. G., Brown, E. D., & McCourt, W. F. (1993). Behavioural marital therapy with and without additional couples relapse prevention sessions for alcoholics and their wives. *Journal of Studies on Alcohol*, **54**, 652–666.

O'Farrell, T. J., & Clements, K. (2012). Review of outcome research on marital and family therapy in treatment for alcoholism. *Journal of Marital and Family Therapy*, **38**(1), 122–144.

O'Malley, S. S., Corbin, W. R., Leeman, R. F., DeMartini, K. S., Fucito, L. M., Ikomi, J., … Kranzler, H. R. (2015). Reduction of alcohol drinking in young adults by naltrexone: A double-blind, placebo-controlled, randomized clinical trial of efficacy and safety. *Journal of Clinical Psychiatry*, **76**(2), e207–e213.

Oslin, D. W., Leong, S. H., Lynch, K. G., Berrettini, W., O'Brien, C. P., Gordon, A. J., & Rukstalis, M. (2015). Naltrexone vs placebo for the treatment of alcohol dependence: A randomized clinical trial. *JAMA Psychiatry*, **72**(5), 430–437.

Pani, P. P., Trogu, E., Pacini, M., & Maremmani, I. (2014). Anticonvulsants for alcohol dependence. *Cochrane Database of Systematic Reviews*, CD008544.

Petrakis, I. L., Nich, C., & Ralevski, E. (2006a). Psychotic spectrum disorders and alcohol abuse: A review of pharmacotherapeutic strategies and a report on the effectiveness of naltrexone and disulfiram. *Schizophrenia Bulletin*, **32**(4), 644–654.

Petrakis, I. L., Poling, J., Levinson, C., Nich, C., Carroll, K., Rounsaville, B., & VA New England VISN I MIRECC Study Group. (2005). Naltrexone and disulfiram in patients with alcohol dependence and comorbid psychiatric disorders. *Biological Psychiatry*, **57**(10), 1128–1137.

Petrakis, I. L., Poling, J., Levinson, C., Nich, C., Carroll, K., Ralevski, E., & Rounsaville, B. (2006b). Naltrexone and disulfiram in patients with alcohol dependence and comorbid post-traumatic stress disorder. *Biological Psychiatry*, **60**(7), 777–783.

Petrakis, I. L., Ralevski, E., Desai, N., Trevisan, L., Gueorguieva, R., Rounsaville, B., & Krystal, J. H. (2012). Noradrenergic vs serotonergic antidepressant with or without naltrexone for veterans with PTSD and comorbid alcohol dependence. *Neuropsychopharmacology*, **37**(4), 996–1004.

Petrakis, I., Ralevski, E., Nich, C., Levinson, C., Carroll, K., Poling, J., … VA VISN I MIRECC Study Group. (2007). Naltrexone and disulfiram in patients with alcohol dependence and current depression. *Journal of Clinical Psychopharmacology*, **27**(2), 160–165.

Pettinati, H. M., Gastfriend, D. R., Dong, Q., Kranzler, H. R., & O'Malley, S. S. (2009). Effect of extended-release naltrexone (XR-NTX) on quality of life in alcohol dependent patients. *Alcoholism: Clinical and Experimental Research*, **33**, 350–356.

Pettinati, H. M., Oslin, D. W., Kampman, K. M., Dundon, W. D., Xie, H., Gallis, T. L., Dackis, C. A., & O'Brien, C. P. (2010). A double-blind, placebo-controlled trial combining sertraline and naltrexone for treating co-occurring depression and alcohol dependence. *American Journal of Psychiatry*, **167**(6), 668–675.

Project MATCH Research Group. (1997*a*). Matching alcoholism treatments to client heterogeneity: Project MATCH post-treatment drinking outcomes. *Journal of Studies on Alcohol*, **58**, 7–29.

Project MATCH Research Group. (1997*b*). Project MATCH secondary a priori hypothesis. *Addiction*, **92**, 1671–1698.

Project MATCH Research Group. (1998). Matching alcoholism treatments to client heterogeneity: Treatment main effects and matching effects on drinking during treatment. *Journal of Studies on Alcohol*, **59**, 631–639.

Raistrick, D., Heather, N., & Godfrey, C. (2006). *Review of the effectiveness of treatment for alcohol problems*. London: National Treatment Agency for Substance Misuse.

Rogers, C. R. (1957). The necessary and sufficient conditions for therapeutic personality change. *Journal of Consulting Psychology*, **21**, 95–103.

Rohsenhow, D. J., Monti, P., Rubonis, D., Gulliver, S. B., Colby, S. M., Binkoff, J. A., & Abrams, D. B. (2001). Cue exposure with coping skills training and communication skills training for alcohol dependence: 6- and 12-month outcomes. *Addiction*, **96**, 1161–1174.

Rösner, S., Leucht, S., Lehert, P., & Soyka, M. (2008). Acamprosate supports abstinence, naltrexone prevents excessive drinking: Evidence from a meta-analysis with unreported outcomes. *Journal of Psychopharmacology*, **22**(1), 11–23.

Rösner, S., Hackl-Herrwerth, A., Leucht, S., Lehert, P., Vecchi, S., & Soyka, M. (2010). Acamprosate for alcohol dependence. *Cochrane Database Syst ematic Reviews* (**9**):CD004332.

Shand, F., Gates, J., Fawcett, J., & Mattick, R. (2003). *The treatment of alcohol problems: A review of the evidence*. Canberra, Australia: Commonwealth Department of Health and Ageing.

Skinner, M. D., Lahmek, P., Pham, H., & Aubin, H. J. (2014). Disulfiram efficacy in the treatment of alcohol dependence: A meta-analysis. *PloS One*, **9**(2), e87366.

Slattery, J., Chick, J., Cochrane, M., Craig, J., Godfrey, C., Macpherson, K.,. & Parrott, S. (2003). *Prevention of relapse in alcohol dependence*. Glasgow: Health Technology Board for Scotland.

Stade, B. C., Bailey, C., Dzendoletas, D., Sgro, M., Dowswell, T., & Bennett, D. (2009). Psychological and/or educational interventions for reducing alcohol consumption in pregnant women and women planning pregnancy. *Cochrane Database of Systematic Reviews*, CD004228.

Torrens, M., Fonseca, F., Mateu, G., & Farré, M. (2005). Efficacy of antidepressants in substance use disorders with and without comorbid depression: A systematic review and meta-analysis. *Drug and Alcohol Dependence*, **78**(1), 1–22.

Tripodi, S. J., Bender, K., Litschge, C., & Vaughn, M. G. (2010). Interventions for reducing adolescent alcohol abuse: A meta-analytic review. *Archives of Pediatrics & Adolescent Medicine*, **164**(1), 85–91.

UKATT Research Team. (2005*a*). Effectiveness of treatment for alcohol problems: Findings of the randomised UK Alcohol Treatment Trial (UKATT). *British Medical Journal*, **331**, 541–544.

UKATT Research Team. (2005*b*). Cost effectiveness of treatment for alcohol problems: Findings of the randomised UK Alcohol Treatment Trial (UKATT). *British Medical Journal*, **331**, 544–547.

van den Brink, W., Aubin, H. J., Bladström, A., Torup, L., Gual, A., & Mann, K. (2013). Efficacy of as-needed nalmefene in alcohol-dependent patients with at least a high drinking risk level: Results from a subgroup analysis of two randomized controlled 6-month studies. *Alcohol and Alcoholism*, **48**(5), 570–578.

Verheul, R., Lehert, P., Geerlings, P. J., Koeter, M. W., & van den Brink, W. (2005). Predictors of acamprosate efficacy: Results from a pooled analysis of seven European trials including 1485 alcohol-dependent patients. *Psychopharmacology*, **178**(2–3), 167–173.

Walker, B. M., Zorrilla, E. P., & Koob, G. F. (2011). Systemic κ-opioid receptor antagonism by nor-binaltorphimine reduces dependence-induced excessive alcohol self-administration in rats. *Addiction Biology*, **16**(1), 116–119.

Williams, E. E. (1937). Effects of alcohol on workers with Carbon Disulfide. *Journal of the American Medical Association*, **109**, 1472–1473.

Witkiewitz, K., Bowen, S., Harrop, E. N., Douglas, H., Enkema, M., & Sedgwick, C. (2014). Mindfulness-based treatment to prevent addictive behavior relapse: Theoretical models and hypothesized mechanisms of change. *Substance Use & Misuse*, **49**(5), 513–524.

Chapter 14

Alcoholics Anonymous and other mutual-help organizations

Alcoholics Anonymous (AA) is an ubiquitous yet at the same time widely misunderstood presence in the addiction treatment field. Although it includes members of all faiths and of no faith, some clinicians regard it as a Christians-only club. Its groups vary widely in composition, process, and atmosphere, but some problem drinkers think that if they've seen one AA group, they've seen them all. Although AA's system of one-on-one sponsorship offers individualized attention, some outsiders imagine that it is an impersonal organization whose main business is conducted in cavernous rooms crammed with meeting goers. This chapter "busts the myths" about the AA fellowship and guides clinicians in how to help their patients make best use of AA and other mutual-help organizations that focus on drinking problems.

> I crawled into Alcoholics Anonymous, physically, mentally, and spiritually bankrupt, to find an amazing bunch of men and women who had suffered the same physical and mental agony as myself.
>
> At last there were people who thought like me. Dear God – I was no longer alone. And, slowly, slowly, the fog has started to clear. Today, nearly 4 years later, I have not had a drink and am happy and contented for the first time in nearly 50 years of existing. Now I am really starting to Live with a capital "L" – and it's just great. I never knew that life could be such fun without booze.

This quotation by a long-time AA member reflects the sense of gratitude that countless successful affiliates have experienced over the past 80 years. Founded in the town of Akron, Ohio, in 1935 (Wilson, 1994), the AA organization has grown dramatically to comprise more than 60,000 face-to-face groups in its country of origin alone. By the end of the 1940s, AA had diffused throughout North America and spread to other countries as well (Eisenbach-Stangl & Rosenqvist, 1998), in part due to the increased contact between military personnel of different nations during and after World War II. As of 2014, the AA World Service Office is aware of more than 100,000 face-to-face groups in more than 170 countries worldwide, and these numbers do not include nations and individuals who access AA solely via the Internet. The precise worldwide membership of AA today is unknown, but epidemiologic research suggests that the fellowship comprises about 5 million people (Humphreys, 2004).

AA has helped countless individuals (often when professional intervention has failed); is a repository of astonishing experience and subtle, often humorously conveyed, wisdom; and has helped humanize social attitudes toward people with drinking problems. Clinicians should regard AA as a potential resource for their patients and should not deflect patients from AA by negative statements born of ignorance, misunderstanding, or professional preciousness (e.g., "I think you would find it all too religious" or "Let's leave your treatment to trained professionals").

The clinician must be willing to find out how AA operates, what its beliefs and practices are, and how to help patients get the most out of the fellowship. This chapter provides an introduction to these issues, but the best professional education would also include personal visits to several "open" AA meetings, which welcome all interested persons (closed meetings, in contrast, are restricted to individuals "with a sincere desire to stop drinking").

The definition of a mutual-help organisation

Mutual-help organisations (sometimes termed "self-help organisations") are peer-created and -operated social networks whose members share some problem or status, such as having breast cancer, being the parent of a child with a disability, or suffering from an anxiety disorder. The range of concerns addressed by mutual-help organisations is vast, but drug and alcohol problems seem particularly prominent, being the focus of the world's largest mutual-help organization (AA), as well as of many other organisations including The Links (Sweden), Danshukai (Japan), Women for Sobriety (United States), and Narcotics Anonymous (worldwide).

Although mutual-help organisations are sometimes lumped conceptually into the category of "treatment," they differ from professionally provided interventions in multiple respects. First, they are not formally licensed, supervised, or manualised, meaning that different groups of the same organisation may vary widely in style, norms, and composition. Second, unlike professional treatment services in which there are designated helpers and helpees, reciprocal helping is normative in mutual help organisations, such that a member might give support and advice at one moment and receive it the next. Third, attendance at mutual help organisations is either free of charge or paid for with a small, "pass the hat" contribution.

AA activities

The central work of the AA organisation occurs in the meeting of its groups. Groups have a unique atmosphere, marked by a seeming informality but with an underlying and purposeful method of working. The number of people at a meeting will vary from group to group, but it is typically around 10–20. Larger meetings tend to sit classroom style, whereas smaller groups typically sit facing each other around a table. Some of those present will have been attending AA for years, whereas the person sitting in the back may have just walked hesitantly through the door for the first time. The leadership of each group rotates, and "elections," such as they are, are usually quick and informal (e.g., "I led us for October … Margaret, do you mind leading the meetings for November?"). As within the higher levels of the organisation, leaders aren't invested with significant power to govern. Rather, they function as "trusted servants" who take care of essential tasks.

The most common sort of meeting is organised around a chosen speaker's story of alcoholism and recovery; others may focus on an AA reading taken from one of the AA books or pamphlets. Another type of meeting focuses on discussion of the first step (see Table 14.1) and is geared toward newcomers. In some areas, AA meetings have a tradition of making the focus of any meeting where newcomers are present a "first-step" meeting.

Finally, some meetings focus on discussion of a particular topic or topics (e.g., shame, sponsorship, gratitude, spirituality, criticism, honesty, cravings) suggested on the spot by those present.

The meeting will start with the leader saying, "My name is …" (only first names are used), "I am an alcoholic." These words carry immense implications: the speaker is not ashamed of being alcoholic but without reservation acknowledges the condition as an inalienable fact. Note also that the speaker is making a statement about essential identity rather than a disorder per se (i.e., not, "I have the disease of alcoholism" as one might have cancer or a cold). The starting point of the evening is thus one individual's reaffirmation, for all present, of what in AA terms must be the starting point of recovery for every individual – namely, the admission that he or she is "powerless over alcohol."

The chairman (who may be male or female) will then greet the assembled attendees, potentially asking any newcomers to raise their hands, and specifically extending a welcome to them. This serves the additional function of cueing experienced members to which attendees might appreciate an added greeting, shared cup of coffee, or words of encouragement after the meeting ends. The meeting might then be opened with a reading from one or several AA-related books.

With these preliminaries out of the way, the substance of the meeting begins. The starter will normally be a speaker who has agreed to relate his or her story of "What I was like, what happened, and what I am like now." He (or she) will speak for perhaps 20–30 minutes without interruption, giving an account of their personal background and then going on to describe the development of their drinking problem, the sufferings they endured and inflicted on others, the deceptions and prevarications of their drinking days, and then often some turning point or "rock bottom" experience. They will go on to describe their introduction to AA, their recovery within the fellowship, and their evolving understanding of the meaning of AA as a way of life. Within this biographical format, different speakers each develop their own approach, and the ability of the person who has never given a public speech in any other setting to make a personal statement that is both moving and convincing is no doubt related to the unwritten guidelines, which propose that a personal story should be given, rather than a prepared speech or abstract lecture. A story told in unadorned manner by the person with fairly recent experience of recovery is often better received than the highly polished performance of the old hand who has told his or her story many times, but who is by now rather distanced from the acuteness of the experience. Stories that deal with practical strategies for attaining recovery and describe its rewards usually draw more audience attention and smiles than do drawn-out accounts of drinking days ("drunkalogues").

These life stories are followed by briefer comments and personal statements from the floor. This typically centres on finding commonalities and "identifying" with the speaker or "looking for the similarities and not the differences." Throughout this process, unlike in typical professional group therapy, "cross talk" – meaning interruptions or critiques of someone who is speaking or dialogues between members – is deeply frowned on. Rather, members talk about *their own*: experience, strength and hope." Themes raised by prior speakers may, however, be caught up and explored by subsequent speakers, who often stress their similarities with the speaker's story – "That happened to me too. …"

Despite the emotionally heavy topics engaged at AA meetings, many include moments of wit and even unrestrained laughter. Humor is a treasured aspect of the

AA community, not least because replacing the often convivial social surround of drinking with an atmosphere of unrelentingly grim earnestness is unlikely to entice many newcomers (Humphreys, 2000). The particular type of humor employed is often self-puncturing and therefore consistent with AA's characterization of alcoholics as individuals who lack self-awareness of their problematic relationship to alcohol (e.g., "My drinking was destroying my career and I knew I had to make a change. So I quit my job," "I dreamt last night that I went into a magical store and the owner offered me a beer bottle that never runs out no matter how much you drink from it. So I asked him 'how much for a case?").

The formal proceedings end with a closing ritual, which might be a reading, a group recitation of a slogan, or a prayer. A common one, which embodies some useful advice on coping with life's challenges, is the Serenity Prayer:

> God grant me the serenity
> To accept the things I cannot change
> The courage to change the things I can
> And the wisdom to know the difference.

The members then chat and exchange news over tea or coffee, and subtle but positive effort will likely be made to put the newcomer at their ease and draw them into contact. Smaller groups of members often break off and continue their discussions elsewhere after the meeting has formally ended.

In addition to the meetings themselves, much else is potentially on offer. Members may start to visit each other at home, go out to meals together, or share other social activities. In some localities, AA also arranges sober dances, country walks, retreats, and other outings. Drinking mates are dropped, and new friends found who think and talk AA. In some localities, routine meetings will be supplemented by study groups and AA literature shared and passed around. Weekend retreats and regional and national AA conventions may be attended, and the more experienced member may help with prison or hospital groups or offer availability as a speaker at meetings of community organizations.

The other key activity of AA is sponsorship, a tradition that evolved organically over time despite not being mentioned in the organisation's original writings. A sponsor is an experienced AA member who offers a newer member personal advice and a special degree of availability – a phone number to call or text, an arrangement to meet in the evening to attend an AA meeting, and so on. The sponsor is also a role model and a coach in the member's work on the 12 steps. For example, a classic question of sponsors to sponsees who bemoan how many problems they have yet to solve is, "Did you drink today?" If the sponsee says, "No," the sponsor will say something encouraging like, 'That was the most important thing you had to do today, and you accomplished it.'"

Unlike in meetings where the no crosstalk norm is in force, sponsors can and do speak directly to their sponsees (e.g., "Instead of blaming your wife for everything, you should face up to how you also contribute to the unhappiness in your marriage.") Sponsors vary substantially in their style, and their effectiveness depends in part on their interpersonal match with a sponsee (Whelan, Marshall, Ball, & Humphreys, 2009). The newcomer who is grandiose or bullying in manner may benefit from a bluntly spoken sponsor with a lot of attitude, whereas a more emotionally fragile, self-doubting member may prosper with a gentle, reassuring sponsor.

BOX 14.1 From the pages of history: The spectacular rise and fall of the Washingtonians

> We whose names are annexed, desirous of forming a society for our mutual benefit, and to guard against a pernicious practice which is injurious to our health, standing, and families, do pledge ourselves as gentlemen that we will not drink any spirituous or malt liquors, wine or cider.
>
> *–From the Pledge of the Washingtonians (Maxwell, 1950)*

On April 5, 1840, six heavy-drinking Baltimoreans wrote and signed this pledge, thereby founding a society that they named in honor of their country's first President, George Washington. Although the Washingtonian Society drew on the cultural popularity of the Temperance Movement, it was qualitatively different in its focus on the individual "drunkard" rather than on societal change. Its meetings, which quickly became wildly popular, bore similarity to Evangelical Christian Revivals. Moving stories of personal destruction and redemption were told, and lost souls were invited to come forward and promise to transform their lives. Members also conducted their daily work in Evangelical fashion, energetically spreading the word to problem drinkers and recruiting them to meetings to hear the society's message of hope.

The Washingtonians opened membership not only to those with serious drinking problems, but also to any man who simply wished to sign a pledge of abstinence. This open-door policy, as well as the emotionally riveting nature of its meetings, led to an astonishing boom in attendance. Within a year of its founding, thousands of Americans had joined. By 1842, the organizations had hundreds of thousands of members and was sufficiently high-profile and credible to merit a visit and speech from an up and coming politician: future President Abraham Lincoln.

Yet, by the end of the decade, the fad had passed and the organization dissipated. Historian William White (1998) attributed the Washingtonians' startling change in fortune to

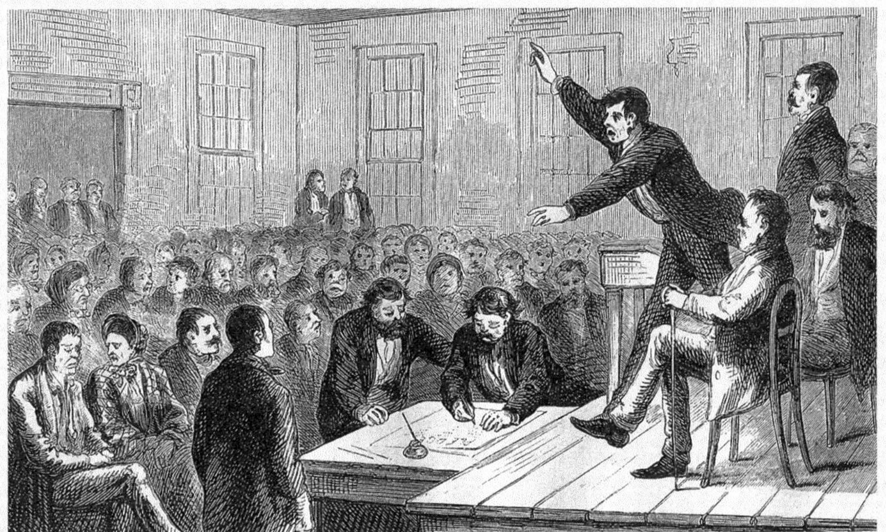

Figure 14.1: A meeting of the Washingtonians. Courtesy Illinois Addiction Study Archives.

their engagement in conflicts with outside entities (e.g., prohibition advocates, religious organizations, the Temperance movement), inability to constrain self-seeking leaders, and lack of a workable organizational structure and coherent therapeutic approach, among other problems. It would not be for almost a century before a different voluntary association – Alcoholics Anonymous – found a way to solve these problems and become a more sustainable fellowship for sobriety.

Table 14.1. The Twelve Steps of Alcoholics Anonymous (AA, 1977)

1 We admitted we were powerless over alcohol – that our lives had become unmanageable.
2 Came to believe that a Power greater than ourselves could restore us to sanity.
3 Made a decision to turn our will and our lives over to the care of God as we understood Him.
4 Made a searching and fearless moral inventory of ourselves.
5 Admitted to God, to ourselves, and to another human being the exact nature of our wrongs.
6 Were entirely ready to have God remove all these defects of character.
7 Humbly asked Him to remove our shortcomings.
8 Made a list of all persons we had harmed and became willing to make amends to them all.
9 Made direct amends to such people wherever possible, except when to do so would injure them or others.
10 Continued to take personal inventory, and when we were wrong, promptly admitted it.
11 Sought through prayer and meditation to improve our conscious contact with God as we understood Him, praying only for knowledge of His will for us and the power to carry that out.
12 Having had a spiritual awakening as the result of these steps, we tried to carry this message to alcoholics and to practice these principles in all our affairs.

Change processes

What are the essential processes through which AA helps members change? Although the answer to this question surely varies across individuals, the following dimensions are typically important.

A sobriety-focussed action programme

AA recommends – although it does not mandate – that members make efforts to change in ways captured in various slogans and in the 12 steps (see Table 14.1). The goal of this action programme is not simply abstinence, but "sobriety," which AA defines as a fulfilling, responsible, generous, and serene way of life. The importance of these broader changes is implicit in the construction of the 12 steps. Although Step 1 is of paramount importance, it is also the only mention of alcohol in the 12 steps.

The steps are central to AA literature, are referred to by speakers in meetings, and are often specifically "worked" with sponsors (e.g., Step 5). In early recovery, members are typically advised to focus solely on taking Step 1 seriously (e.g., "Don't drink. Go to meetings. Ask for help"). They will be advised to take things "one day at a time" and to work for short-term goals. The stories and discussions they listen to at AA meetings and the guidance from their sponsor will provide them with many hints on coping and problem-solving. Their first priority is to deal with their drinking, but the 12 step programme will also cue them to examine psychological problems such as self-centredness, chronic dishonesty, and pervasive resentment. Step 4, in which one catalogues honestly one's shortcomings, is a key part of this process of self-examination and may relieve years of accumulated shame and guilt.

The steps also comprise recommendations to repair relationships that have been scarred by the member's drinking. This includes both atoning for past transgressions (Steps 8 and 9) and conducting oneself more forthrightly and kindly when interacting with others in the future (Step 10).

AA is "a selfish programme" and each individual is working for sobriety for his or her own sake and not to please anyone else, and he or she thus gives no hostages to fortune. If members relapse, they are not rejected but may return any number of times to try again. When stable sobriety is achieved, the programme will finally include "twelfth-stepping," but, by then, members should have learnt that in the process of helping other people they will help themselves and confirm their own strength. That said, members are expected to proselytize, "pull people down lamp posts" or put their own sobriety at risk.

As mentioned, the steps are supplemented by numerous slogans: "fake it until you make it," "put some gratitude in your attitude," "keep it simple, stupid (KISS)," "easy does it, but do it," "first things first" It is easy, but wrong-headed, for educated professionals to poke fun at AA's many slogans and seemingly simplistic advice. Most of the practical advice offered by AA members directly parallels that which a scientifically informed cognitive behavioural psychologist would offer, albeit in different words. Two of many possible examples make the point. "Avoid slippery people, places, and things" contains the same wisdom as, "Let's examine what stimuli lead you to drink and then make a plan to avoid those relapse triggers." "Watch your stinking thinking" is but a more pithy way of emphasizing how automatic cognitive distortions can shape substance use behaviour.

Coherent, flexible ideas

In *Persuasion and Healing*, a classic text of psychiatry and anthropology, Jerome Frank (1973) noted that, across cultures, healers offer a philosophy or narrative that explains why the sufferer is ill and how the pain can be relieved. AA fits this characterization, providing a coherent yet flexible philosophy that makes members feel understood and gives meaning to their experience. They are suffering from "the disease of alcoholism," which is pictured as metaphorically akin to an "allergy to alcohol." Their constitution is such that they will react to this drug differently from other people. They can never be "cured," but the disease will be "arrested" if they never drink again.

Yet AA's definition of disease is broader than that of traditional medicine, comprising emotional and spiritual elements as well as physical ones. This broad conception allows members more "latch-on points" with the AA programme than would a purely biological view, in that most alcoholics have problems in addition to drinking to which AA's philosophy can speak. Through a process of continually telling and retelling the story of their own experience of alcoholism, AA members integrate AA's narrative about alcoholism into their own life story (Humphreys, 2000). It can also serve to "keep the memories green" so that motivation for recovery can continue.

The flexible nature of AA philosophy is evident in its "spiritual rather than religious" posture (Kurtz, 1991). The 12 steps unambiguously talk about God as a Higher Power essential to recovery, and yet there are geographic areas (e.g., Sweden) where most AA members are atheist or agnostic (Mäkelä et al., 1996). Relatedly, though the founders of AA were Protestants, it claims among its members countless Catholics, as well as Jews, Muslims, and Buddhists (Humphreys, 2004). In the mind of some members, their Higher Power is the AA fellowship itself, a stance captured in the equation "G.O.D. = Group Of Drunks." We will give extensive attention to spiritual issues in Chapter 15. Here, suffice it to say that AA's conception of "God as we understand Him" is broad enough to cover almost any interpretation of a Higher Power that a member wishes to employ.

The influence of the fellowship

Individuals trained in psychotherapeutic techniques are inclined to think of change in terms of individual behaviours, thoughts, emotions and insights. As described, all of these are implicated in AA's change process, but this should not lead observers to overlook the reality that, unlike psychotherapy, AA is a living, breathing social network that an individual may join for a lifetime. Indeed, although the 12 steps and spiritual framework of AA are important, sophisticated research has established that the most consistent mediators of AA's benefits are social in nature (Kelly, Hoeppner, Stout, & Pagano, 2011).

The AA fellowship gives members new friends, introduces them to a social network that does not centre on drinking, relieves their loneliness, helps them to structure and employ their time, and lessens the social stigma of having a drinking problem. This network also provides social reinforcement and encouragement, which is particularly important in the early stages of recovery when members are often struggling to build a new life and tempted to return to their old ways.

The fellowship is also a key way for AA to instil an essential ingredient of change: hope. The network of experienced, sober role models makes recovery seem possible to even the most disillusioned drinker. AA does not work through an abstract set of ideas but through those ideas being found persuasive and possible by the individual. The most apt theoretical definition of the disorder and the pathways to recovery would remain useless if AA did not have the ability to convince newcomers that AA can meet their particular problems and show them personally the way ahead. AA can carry this conviction because the experienced members of the fellowship so evidently know what they are talking about; they, too, have been through it all and know every stratagem of deceit and denial while at the same time bearing tangible witness to the possibility of success.

Professional facilitation of AA affiliation

Which patients are likely to affiliate with AA? Like professional treatment, AA is not a panacea. Its membership is primarily composed of people who have suffered from at least moderate and typically severe alcohol dependence, and group cohesion is therefore built around total acceptance of the abstinence goal. A person with a low-severity drinking problem who is pursuing a controlled drinking goal is highly unlikely to find AA compatible. The founders of AA fully accepted that some problem drinkers could return to "drinking like a gent," but that was not the population they created their organisation to help.

Beyond that universal feature of AA, meetings are so variable in composition and process that predicting a priori who is a good match for "AA writ large" is a nearly meaningless exercise. Rather, the question for a clinician and patient to explore is whether a comfortable niche can be found in a particular kind of AA meeting. In any referral to AA, the clinician should emphasize the diversity of the organisation's groups, which cannot be appreciated in a single visit to a single meeting. The location and time of day a meeting is held may lead it to draw members from particular social strata. The Wednesday evening AA meeting in the spare room above the petrol station or in the basement of a local church will feature a different cast of characters than the lunchtime meeting in the financial district. Some chapters have standing rules of serving a particular subpopulation, for example men, women, gays and lesbians, nonsmokers, barristers, or physicians. Some groups will emphasise the spiritual aspect of AA much more than others. Some meetings have such large attendance (e.g., 100 people) that a newcomer can slip quietly into the back row unnoticed, whereas others are small affairs where everyone knows each other, and a newcomer will always be noticed and specifically welcomed.

Rather than exhaust the patient by relating all the potential variants of AA, the clinician can convey the simple message that it may take some time and perseverance to find the group that most suits the patient's needs. Clinicians can increase the likelihood that AA will "stick" by helping the patient talk through important decisions about a "home group" and a sponsor. This is particularly important for patients who have a history of poor interpersonal relationships. It can be useful for the clinician to inquire, for example, whom the patient is considering asking to be a sponsor and what about the person makes them worthy of such trust. Likewise, the clinician can help the patient to explore why a particular meeting felt safe and comfortable whilst another was anxiety-producing.

The clinician's attitude about trying AA should be optimistic but not dogmatic. Most patients understandably dislike having AA "rammed down their throat." Indeed, an oppositional subset may resist AA not because it wouldn't help them but because they want to show the therapist who is the captain of their ship. If a sincere effort at AA affiliation is not productive during the current treatment or if the patient has had consistently negative experiences with AA in the past, the clinician should not scold the patient; rather, the task becomes finding other sources of support for sustaining change in drinking behaviour.

In making referrals, clinicians should be aware that simply mentioning AA and providing a brochure or phone number yields low rates of uptake. In contrast, explaining the basic workings of AA meetings, addressing anxieties about attendance, and providing a direct introduction to a trusted, experienced AA member all dramatically increase the chances that a patient will give AA a try (Timko, DeBenedetti, & Billow, 2006). Clinicians who occasionally attend open AA meetings will enhance their credibility as informants and build up valuable contacts with local groups. Other strategies for facilitating AA attendance and creating synergies between treatment and AA are available free of charge in the *Twelve Step Facilitation Handbook* produced by the U.S. National Institute on Alcohol Abuse and Alcoholism (NIAAA; Nowinski, Baker, & Carroll, 1999, downloadable at http://pubs.niaaa.nih.gov/publications/ProjectMatch/match01.pdf).

In making referrals, the clinician should remain alert for two patient concerns. First, occasionally an errant AA member will tell a newcomer that the organisation forbids the taking of psychiatric medication. The clinician can provide patients concerned about this issue AA's statement on medications, which enjoins members from "playing doctor" (free of charge on the Internet at http://www.alcoholics-anonymous.org/en_pdfs/p-11_aamembers.pdf). Second, because many people are uncomfortable speaking in front of groups, the clinician should offer reassurance that speaking in meetings is not a requirement of membership. New members may simply sit and listen for months on end if they wish. In the case of a patient whose discomfort about these matters approaches a phobia, the therapist could suggest exploration of online AA meetings (directory available at http://www.aa-intergroup.org/directory.php).

Research on AA's effectiveness

For many years, claims that AA was effective were based on popularity, personal testimony, and perceived subjective benefit rather than scientific proof (Edwards, 1995). But, in recent decades, rigorous longitudinal research has vindicated the faith of AA members in the healing power of their fellowship.

Timko and colleagues conducted a randomized trial with 345 out-patients being treated for alcohol and/or illegal drug dependence (Timko et al., 2006). Half received a standard referral to AA and other 12-step organizations (i.e., a list of meetings and encouragement to attend), whereas the other half received a more intensive referral, including being linked to an experienced AA member known to the treatment programme. The intensive referral produced higher rates of 12-step group attendance and greater improvement in alcohol and drug problems at 6-month follow-up.

Timko and colleagues' study was conducted in a sample composed mainly of male racial minorities who were being treated in a facility serving military veterans. It thus bears mentioning that other clinical trials using markedly different samples reinforce her central finding that AA is effective (Humphreys, Blodgett, & Wagner, 2014).

A detailed analysis of research on AA is beyond the scope of this book, but the interested reader should consult the recently updated Cochrane Collaboration review (Kelly, Humphreys, & Ferri, in press).

Other 12-step fellowships

Since AA's founding, countless other organizations have applied the 12 steps to problems as diverse as chronic indebtedness, gambling, smoking, and schizophrenia. We adumbrate here the subset of these organizations that are most likely to interest patients with drinking problems and their families.

Al-Anon is an organization that is independent of, but allied with, AA. Al-Anon caters to "anyone who loves an alcoholic." Most Al-Anon members are spouses (or romantic partners), but designated chapters are available for offspring who are teenagers (Alateen), as well as those who have grown to adulthood (Adult Children of Alcoholics). Al-Anon has its own 12 steps, which it adapted from AA's. Quite often, an AA meeting will be going on in one room and an Al-Anon meeting in the next room, with everyone getting together afterwards over the tea and biscuits. Alcohol problems often cluster in families and can persist for generations, making it common to encounter individuals who attend AA and Al-Anon at the same time.

The functioning of Al-Anon will not be discussed here in detail because its principles and methods of working have much in common with AA. That Al-Anon can fulfil an extremely important function does, however, need to be emphasised, and the clinician should again be able knowledgeably to point the way. Al-Anon may give immediate relief to the husband or wife who has been struggling by every stratagem to stop a spouse from drinking and who has in the process been experiencing stress and frustration. Al-Anon will teach "loving detachment" to help such individuals stop trying the impossible task of controlling their mate's behaviour. Instead, the member will be encouraged to examine his or her own behaviour, both in terms of restraining destructive habits and increasing (often long-neglected) self-care. The small but solid research base available on Al-Anon indicates that participation tends to reduce members' resentment, anxiety, depression, and anger (Humphreys, 2004).

Twelve-step organizations focused on drugs other than alcohol (e.g., Marijuana Anonymous, Cocaine Anonymous) may be useful to those alcohol dependent patients who have other drug problems as well. The largest is Narcotics Anonymous, which, contrary to its name welcomes individuals with problems with any drug, narcotic, or otherwise (including alcohol). Narcotics Anonymous is widely available in more than 100 countries and in most respects is similar to AA in its philosophy and meeting process.

Alternative alcohol mutual-help organizations

Other organizations have deliberately set out to take a different approach to AA. Secular Organizations for Sobriety and LifeRing Secular Recovery offer a network of groups and a philosophy that contains no inherent spiritual component (Connors & Dermen, 1996; Humphreys, 2004). SMART Recovery also includes no spiritual content and draws its change strategies explicitly from scientifically supported cognitive behavioural principles. Women for Sobriety is an all-female alternative to AA that focuses on enhancing the self-worth of members (Kaskutas, 1996). Moderation Management (MM) stands apart from all other options in providing group support for moderation of drinking rather than total abstinence (Kishline, 1995). MM members tend to have higher social capital and less severe drinking problems than do affiliates of AA (Klaw, Luft, & Humphreys, 2003).

Face-to-face meetings of these five alternatives to AA can mainly be found in selected parts of the United States and Canada and, to a lesser extent, in Australia and the British Isles. No other mutual-help organization for people with drinking problems is even remotely as international or as readily accessible as AA. The main challenge to helping patients take advantage of alternatives to AA is, therefore, difficulty in locating nearby groups to attend. This problem can be ameliorated by accessing the Internet-based fora of these organizations. But, in the long term, expansion of face-to-face groups is likely essential to increasing the range of persons who recover with the aid of a mutual-help organization. Clinicians and professional agencies who make efforts to establish new chapters of alternative organizations may see gratifying benefits among some of their alcohol dependent patients who simply do not mesh well with AA.

References

Alcoholics Anonymous. (1977). *Twelve steps and twelve traditions*. New York: Alcoholics Anonymous World Services.

Connors, G. J., & Dermen, K. H. (1996). Characteristics of participants in Secular Organizations for Sobriety (SOS). *American Journal of Drug and Alcohol Abuse*, **22**, 281–295.

Edwards, G. (1995). Alcoholics Anonymous as mirror held up to nature. In G. Edwards & C. Dare (Eds.), *Psychotherapy, psychological treatments, and the addictions* (pp. 220–239). Cambridge: Cambridge University Press,.

Eisenbach-Stangl, I., & Rosenqvist, P. (1998). *Diversity in unity: Studies of Alcoholics Anonymous in eight societies*. Helsinki, Finland: Nordic Council for Alcohol and Drug Research.

Frank, J. D. (1973). *Persuasion and healing: A comparative study of psychotherapy*. Baltimore, MD: Johns Hopkins University Press.

Humphreys, K. (2000). Community narratives and personal stories in Alcoholics Anonymous. *Journal of Community Psychology*, **28**, 495–506.

Humphreys, K. (2004). *Circles of recovery: Self-help organisations for addictions.* Cambridge: Cambridge University Press.

Humphreys, K., Blodgett, J. C., & Wagner, T. H. (2014). Estimating the efficacy of Alcoholics Anonymous without self-selection bias: An instrumental variables re-analysis of randomized clinical trials. *Alcoholism: Clinical and Experimental Research*, **11**, 2688–2694.

Kaskutas, L. A. (1996). A road less travelled: Choosing the Women for Sobriety Program. *Journal of Drug Issues*, **26**, 77–94.

Kelly, J. F., Hoeppner, B., Stout, R. L., & Pagano, M. (2011). Determining the relative importance of the mechanisms of behaviour change within Alcoholics Anonymous: A multiple mediator analysis. *Addiction*, **107**, 289–299.

Kelly, J. F., Humphreys, K., & Ferri, M. (in press). Alcoholics Anonymous and twelve-step treatments for alcohol use disorder. *Cochrane Database of Systematic Reviews.*

Kishline, A. (1995). *Moderate drinking: The Moderation Management (TM) guide for people who want to reduce their drinking.* New York: Three Rivers.

Klaw, E., Luft, S., & Humphreys, K. (2003). Characteristics and motives of problem drinkers seeking help from Moderation Management self-help groups. *Cognitive and Behavioral Practice*, **10**, 385–390.

Kurtz, E. (1991). *Not-god: A history of Alcoholics Anonymous.* Center City, MN: Hazelden.

Mäkelä, K., Arminen, I., Bloomfield, K., Eisenbach-Stangl, I., Helmersson Bergmark, K., … Zielinski, A. (1996). *Alcoholics Anonymous as a mutual-help movement: A study in eight societies.* Madison: University of Wisconsin Press.

Maxwell, M. (1950). The Washingtonian Movement. *Quarterly Journal of Studies on Alcohol*, **11**, 410–452.

Nowinski, J., Baker, S., & Carroll, K. (1999). *Twelve-step facilitation therapy manual.* Washington, DC: National Institute on Alcohol Abuse and Alcoholism.

Timko, C., DeBenedetti, A., & Billow, R. (2006). Intensive referral to 12-step self-help groups and 6-month substance use disorder outcomes. *Addiction*, **101**, 678–688.

Whelan, P. J., Marshall, E. J., Ball, D. M., & Humphreys, K. (2009). The role of AA sponsors: A pilot study. *Alcohol and Alcoholism*, **44**, 416–422.

White, W. L. (1998). *Slaying the dragon: The history of addiction treatment and recovery in America.* Bloomington, IL: Chestnut Health Systems.

Wilson, W. (1994). The society of Alcoholics Anonymous. *American Journal of Psychiatry*, **151**, 259–262.

Chapter 15

Religion, spirituality, and values in treatment

> I stopped drinking the day my son was born. Ariel's labor was really, really difficult and she was dead asleep. Mark was in the nursery, and I was standing at the window, marveling at this beautiful creature. Yet I found myself thinking that I could nip off down to the pub I had seen on a way to the hospital for some celebratory pints because, you know, the staff could watch over Ariel and Mark. At that moment, in what I consider a gift from God, I caught my own reflection in the glass and thought *"Who is this terrible person who would leave the people he loves the most when they need him the most just so that he could go get pissed?"* I felt like I was looking at the image of a monster, and I just couldn't stand the fact that the monster was me.

Religious, spiritual, and values issues can arise in many domains of healthcare (Koenig, 1998), including palliative treatment of terminal illness and decision-making about sex and pregnancy. But in few areas do these issues arise as consistently as they do in the care of people with drinking problems, for two reasons. First, the major religions have long taken a particular interest in drinking problems, both in terms of trying to explain them and in supporting organizations that are intended to help people who suffer from them. Second, unlike people with health conditions such as diabetes, hypertension, asthma, and cancer, people with drinking problems often engage in behaviour that violates their own moral values: putting others at risk through drink driving; making a drunken, clumsy pass at a co-worker; saying cruel things to friends and family; spending money meant for family essentials on drink; failing to follow through on promises; and the like. Irrespective of whether the drinker's moral values are religiously derived or not, such transgressions against his or her deeply felt sense of right and wrong can induce shame and guilt that becomes a problem in itself and must therefore be addressed in the treatment process.

After defining its terms, this chapter walks the reader through the antecedents and consequences of religious and spiritual understandings of drinking problems. It also discusses the role of moral values in the treatment of drinking problems; these values can arise from a patient's religious and spiritual views but can also be entirely independent of them.

Definitions

To define *religion* is often to start an argument because every definition has trouble accounting for at least some cases. Here, we adapt Smith's (1963) definition of religions as organisations as those that have (1) a dogma (in the nonpejorative sense of the word), meaning a set of shared beliefs that are taken on faith; and (2) a set of cumulative traditions, such as sacred writings and pictures, rituals, apologues, and buildings. By these two criteria, Christianity, Islam, and Hinduism are religions. In contrast, Alcoholics Anonymous (AA), despite its spiritual content, is not a religion because it does not define membership as requiring specific beliefs.

Spirituality is another much-debated term, although one with a shorter history than *religion* (Cook, 2004). Although emerging within the Christian tradition, it has come to be applied not only to all faith traditions, but also to an ineffable aspect of human nature. The following definition – although as arguable as any other – has been widely adopted in writings on spirituality and mental health:

> Spirituality is a distinctive, potentially creative and universal dimension of human experience arising both within the inner subjective awareness of individuals and within communities, social groups and traditions. It may be experienced as relationship with that which is intimately "inner," immanent and personal, within the self and others, and/or as relationship with that which is wholly "other," transcendent and beyond the self. It is experienced as being of fundamental or ultimate importance and is thus concerned with matters of meaning and purpose in life, truth and values. (Cook, 2004, pp. 548–549)

Some individuals experience and develop their spiritual life in a religious context, but the connection is not essential. An atheist or agnostic could do so in an entirely nonreligious fashion.

Finally, *values* are clusters of interrelated goals (Kanfer & Schefft, 1988), and *moral values* are the subset of values that have an ethical weight to the person concerned. They are the things that people invoke when describing their sense of right and wrong or "the kind of person that I believe I should be." Moral values go well beyond strictly health-related goals and could, for example, include being a good citizen or loyal friend, showing compassion in the face of suffering, and striving to seek and tell the truth. Values may be religiously derived directly by those in a faith tradition and indirectly through cultural norms that reflect religious influence (i.e., even secular societies such as the UK incorporate once explicitly religious values into their laws and norms). Moral values can also arise independently of any direct or indirect religious influence.

Religious and spiritual influences on the understanding of drinking problems

Up until the late 18th century, drinking problems (then known as "chronic inebriety") were largely understood within Europe and North America as being a matter of morality. This was not necessarily the popularly understood moral model that is now so often denounced (i.e., that such people are morally bad in a category apart from other people). It rather reflected a Judeo-Christian understanding of drunkenness as being among a range of sins to which all human beings were more or less subject, all of which were primarily spiritual/religious concerns rather than medical ones. All of this changed in the 19th century under a progressive medicalization of the concept of inebriety.

The 19th-century Temperance Movement understood inebriety as a "disease of the will," a disease caused by alcohol. However, in the 20th century, with the repeal of Prohibition in the United States and the waning of the Temperance Movement in Europe and North America, a new disease model arose. Associated particularly with the spiritual but not religious organization AA (see Chapter 14), this disease model identified certain individuals – "alcoholics" – as suffering from a disease that made them unable to control their drinking.

In Europe and North America, the Temperance Movement did more than simply change attitudes to drinking and drunkenness. It spawned a variety of projects aimed at "reclaiming the drunkard," or, as we would now say, offering treatment for drinking problems. Many of these projects found inspiration and motivation in the Christian tradition. Perhaps most famously, the Salvation Army devoted itself (among other concerns) to helping those whose lives had been destroyed by alcohol, but it was not alone. Alongside the secular spirituality that emerged from AA, various Christian groups in Europe and North America continued to concern themselves with rescuing those whose lives were ruined by alcohol, and they did so in explicitly Christian ways.

Today, there continue to be numerous projects around the world that offer rehabilitation from addiction within a Christian framework. Differences of approach may be identified between more liberal and more conservative traditions. Typically, the latter are likely to define a sharper boundary with secular practice (although this is not always or necessarily the case). For example, Teen Challenge provides an example of an approach within which the concept of addiction is understood as more or less coterminous with the theological concept of sin. In this paradigm, recovery from addiction is more or less identical with the process of conversion and Christian growth that is expected in this tradition of all Christians. Less conservative Christians, in contrast, might be expected to rely on medical and other secular treatments, or else on a programme like AA, which is not explicitly linked to any particular faith or denomination.

For Christianity, concern for those whose lives have been shackled by bonds of addiction has been a part of a broader tradition of concern with social and spiritual bonds from which people need to be set free. Elsewhere in the world, and increasingly also in the West, treatment programmes are integrated with, inspired by, and motivated by other faith traditions, including Islam, Buddhism, and Native American religion (Abdel-Mawgoud, Fateem, & Al-Sharif, 1995; Barrett, 1997; Garrett & Carroll, 2000). These traditions each find their own distinctive point of contact with problems related to alcohol and other drugs.

Buddhism recognizes that all human beings have a tendency to develop attachments to things, which causes suffering. What might otherwise be identified as "addiction" is but one manifestation of this universal problem. Treatments founded on basic tenets of Buddhism (and which are not dissimilar to forms of cognitive behavioural therapy) thus lend themselves readily to the treatment of alcohol dependence (Marlatt & Kristeller, 1999).

In Islam, alcohol use is *haram:* forbidden on the basis of texts in the Quran. The response of this tradition to drinking problems has thus emphasized prevention (in the form of injunction to total abstinence) rather than treatment. Yet, as with any such injunction, adherence is not universal. UK-based Muslims are significantly less likely to drink than other Britons, but a plurality nonetheless at least occasionally consume alcohol (Valentine, Holloway, & Jayne, 2010). This population includes some problem drinkers whose personal and family shame may reduce the likelihood of seeking treatment, as well as others who seek treatment but find it poorly matched to their cultural and religious values. Fortunately, culturally tailored addiction treatment programmes and mutual help organizations that incorporate Islamic spiritual practices are emerging (Abdel-Mawgoud et al., 1995; Millati Islami World Services, 2015).

Native American religion deserves attention here because of the extremely high rates of alcohol-related problems that Native American peoples have experienced since beverage alcohol was introduced by European settlers. Although this might still leave its importance limited to North America, it also provides an example of the way in which spirituality and religious practices of a faith tradition may be woven into the fabric of treatment programmes based upon the 12 steps of AA or other models. Native American religion understands spiritual reality as more "real" than the visible order of the world, but addiction represents a closing down of connection with this reality. Treatment is therefore about reconnecting to this reality, and various treatment programmes now integrate traditional Native American practices such as talking circles, sweat lodges, tribal music, and pow wows in support of recovery from alcohol dependence.

Treatment programmes based explicitly on other faith traditions are relatively unusual in Western countries. However, scattered findings suggest that similar principles are at play regarding the treatment of drinking problems in these faith communities. For example, Morjaria and Orford found that South Asian men in the UK undergoing counselling for drinking problems experienced a reaffirmation of existing beliefs (Hindu or Sikh) during recovery. This contrasted with members of AA who underwent a "conversion" experience (Morjaria & Orford, 2002). However, both groups found a deeper sense of connectedness with God, and it is this spiritual dynamic of recovery, understood within the particular spiritual or religious tradition of the individual concerned, which seems to be of general importance in the treatment of drinking problems (and other forms of substance misuse).

Religion, spirituality, and moral values in the treatment of drinking problems

Harold Koenig (2005), writing about the relationship between religious organizations and the delivery of mental health services, identifies five categories of faith-based organizations:

1. Local churches, synagogues, mosques, etc., that provide services
2. Networking and advocacy organizations
3. Groups that provide largely secular services for religious reasons
4. Trained counsellors who utilize a mixture of secular and religious methods
5. Groups and counsellors who provide largely faith-based therapies

Examples of each of these categories could probably be identified in respect of projects and individuals working with people with drinking problems, but the nature and range of provision varies from country to country. For example, in the UK, the Salvation Army might be identified as working under each of these headings – although probably more under 1 and 3 than the others. Christian charities with an evangelical tradition providing residential rehabilitation might most frequently be found under 5.

For some Christians, the choice between secular and religious approaches is a difficult one. Anxieties about compromising Christian belief have been expressed in movements that have sought to re-express the 12 steps in more explicitly Christian terms (e.g., Overcomers Outreach). On the other hand, other Christians have written first-hand accounts of how AA does not require any compromise of faith and in fact can be helpful both to the process of recovery and to growth in faith (K. D., 2002).

Spiritual approaches can be integrated within completely secular treatment programmes, such as those provided by the National Health Service in the UK (Jackson & Cook, 2005). This is not simply a question of the provision of chaplaincy services, which are a part of all healthcare provision within the UK, but rather a matter of recognizing the spiritual needs of all health service users and recognizing spirituality as a component of all truly comprehensive assessments and treatment programmes.

Working with the individual

What does all of this mean when working with an individual person with drinking problems?

The first and most important lesson is that spirituality and faith are matters that can be discussed in the counselling room or clinic. It takes only a few seconds to ask one or two simple questions about whether someone has any spiritual or religious beliefs that are important to them. After making it clear in this way that such things can be discussed, it usually becomes clear whether the conversation needs to be taken further and, if so, in which direction.

Second, the context of a faith community and a spiritual or religious belief system can be important in planning treatment. This might be at a very explicit level of referral to a faith-based organization offering services for people with drinking problems, or it might be a matter of allaying fears that AA is either "too religious" or else not a suitable place for a Christian, Muslim, Jew, or other faith adherent. Or, it might be at a much more implicit level of acknowledging that there are spiritual aspects to all treatment programmes and to most (if not all) kinds of drinking problems. Clinicians well versed in and practicing a particular religious tradition may also use religious metaphors and language with patients of similar faith to help them understand the change process. For example, the experience of struggling with urges to drink despite wishes not to may be experienced as an acutely painful inner division of self. This experience of inner conflict is well-described in many religions, including Christianity (Cook, 2006), and pointing this out can help validate the suffering of an individual who practices the relevant faith.

Third, health professionals, religious or not, should do their homework. We cannot all be experts on comparative religion, and those who come to us for help do not expect this. They are, after all, the experts on what they believe – which may in any case not be exactly according to what the orthodoxy of their tradition would expect. However, when working in a given locality, it is important to know what is available. Where are the pastoral counsellors in the community who take on addicted individuals? Are there any faith-based organizations locally working in this field? Where might someone with a strong sense of belonging to a particular faith tradition most feel at home? How might questions about the compatibility of (say) the Christian faith and AA be handled?

Fourth, a patient's moral values, religiously derived or not, can be powerful motivators. Frequently, they are the answer to the question "*Why* should I change?" A patient who is not put off by the risk of liver cirrhosis or auto accident may nonetheless respond powerfully when a clinician gently points out a contradiction between drinking behaviour and a cherished moral value (e.g., being a devoted parent). The following questions, adapted and expanded from Kanfer and Schefft (1988), can help stimulate a patient to articulate those values:

- For whom or for what would you be willing to sacrifice something you value?
- What kinds of things make your proud of yourself and ashamed of yourself even when you no one but you knows about them?
- If you were given a 60-second television spot that would be seen by billions of people all over the world, what message would you most want to convey?

- If I were to visit you in 5 years, what kind of person would you most hope I would encounter?
- If you had a year to live, how would you spend the time?
- After you are dead, what do you hope people will say about the kind of person that you were?

Fifth, professionals should not use the treatment process to impose a particular religious viewpoint. Sometimes it will be easier working with someone from a different faith tradition or spiritual perspective than one's own – sometimes it will be more difficult. However, the relationship between helping professional and patient should never be misused as a place for proselytizing, whether to a particular tradition or to a position of agnosticism or unbelief. Only in exceptional circumstances (e.g., when working with those who have survived involvement with cults) is it appropriate to engage someone in questioning the validity of the tradition to which they have belonged. Even then, it may be very important (where appropriate) to involve family or members of a healthy faith community in the process of recovery.

In closing, we wish to imply that being able to skillfully explore a patient's spirituality typically requires that one has explored one's own spirituality and is not afraid to grapple with the same kinds of questions that the patient is grappling with. In fact, spirituality is a great antidote for the so-called moral model. Spirituality reminds us that we are all spiritual beings, struggling within ourselves over various desires and motives that draw us in different directions. People afflicted with drinking problems are not morally weak – they are simply human. Those of us who work with them will best be able to help them when we have recognized this common humanity within ourselves as well.

References

Abdel-Mawgoud, M., Fateem, L., & Al-Sharif, A. I. (1995). Development of a comprehensive treatment program for chemical dependency at Al Amal Hospital, Damman. *Journal of Substance Abuse Treatment*, **12**, 369–376.

Barrett, M. E. (1997). Wat Thamkrabok: A Buddhist drug rehabilitation program in Thailand. *Substance Use and Misuse*, **32**, 435–459.

Cook, C. C. H. (2004). Addiction and spirituality. *Addiction*, **99**, 539–551.

Cook, C. C. H. (2006). *Alcohol, Addiction and Christian Ethics*. Cambridge: Cambridge University Press.

Garrett, M. T., & Carroll, J. J. (2000). Mending the broken circle: treatment of substance dependence among Native Americans. *Journal of Counseling and Development*, **78**, 379–388.

Jackson, P., & Cook, C. C. H. (2005). Introduction of a spirituality group in a community service for people with drinking problems. *Journal of Substance Use*, **10**, 375–383.

Kanfer, F. H., & Schefft, B. K. (1988). *Guiding the process of therapeutic change*. Champaign, IL: Research Press.

K. D. (2002). *Twelve steps with Jesus*. Luton, UK: New Life.

Koenig, H. G. (1998). *Handbook of religion and mental health*. San Diego, CA: Academic Press.

Koenig, H. G. (2005). *Faith and mental health*. Philadelphia, PA: Templeton Foundation Press.

Marlatt, G. A., & Kristeller, J. L. (1999). Mindfulness and meditation. In W. R. Miller (Ed.), *Integrating spirituality into treatment: Resources for practitioners* (pp. 67–84). Washington DC: American Psychological Association.

Millati Islami. (2015). What is Millati Islami? Retrieved from http://www.millatiislami.org/

Morjaria, A., & Orford, J. (2002). The role of religion and spirituality in recovery from drink problems: a qualitative study of Alcoholics Anonymous members and South Asian men. *Addiction Research & Theory*, **10**, 225–256.

Smith, W. C. (1963). *The meaning and end of religion: A new approach to the religious traditions of mankind*. New York: MacMillan.

Valentine, G., Holloway, S. L., & Jayne, M. (2010). Contemporary cultures of abstinence and the nighttime economy: Muslim attitudes toward alcohol and the implications for social cohesion. *Environment and Planning A*, **42**, 8–22.

Chapter 16

Pursuing treatment outcomes other than abstinence

For much of the 1960s and into the 1980s, the alcohol treatment field was riven by the "controlled drinking controversy" (Roizen, 1987). One side argued that any treatment goal short of abstinence was a death sentence for problem-drinking patients, and the other responded that refusing to acknowledge the possibility of a return to controlled drinking turned some problem drinkers away from treatment and thereby created significant damage of its own. In retrospect, the combatants were to some extent talking past each other because they were focusing on different subgroups within the diverse population of people with drinking problems. Eventually, it became clear that it was not a question of which treatment goal was correct in an absolute sense, but which was best for which individual drinker. Ironically enough, this was the position of the founders of Alcoholics Anonymous (AA), who, although often cited during the controlled drinking controversy as supporting abstinence for all problem drinkers, in fact specifically acknowledged that some could return to moderate drinking (Humphreys, 2003).

This chapter helps clinicians and patients navigate the difficult decision of whether a problem drinker is a good candidate for a return to non-problem drinking and also provides advice on how to help such individuals achieve their goal. It also attends to other nonabstinence outcomes that, although not as beneficial as establishment of lifelong abstinence or moderate drinking, can nonetheless be considered successes within particular clinical contexts.

Table 16.1 summarizes the key considerations for determining whether a moderate drinking goal may be appropriate for a given patient. The table takes an abstinence goal as the default choice because that will be the case in most clinical settings. For clinicians working in specialty treatment settings (e.g., in-patient alcoholism units), the column on the right of the table may seem like a fantasy, but it must be remembered that the treatment of drinking problems occurs in a broad range of locations, including some (e.g., college counselling centres, primary care settings) where the left side of the table will describe a significant proportion of help seekers.

Degree of dependence

No single factor is completely definitive when judging whether a moderate drinking goal is reasonable, but degree of dependence is certainly a useful indicator (Edwards et al., 1983; Rosenberg, 1993). Simply put, the more a patient has experienced shakes, sweats, convulsions, blackouts, morning drinking, and the like, the less likely they are to succeed at a moderate drinking goal.

Table 16.1. Factors relevant to the choice of a moderate drinking goal

Factors unfavourable to a moderate drinking goal	Favourable factors in support of a moderate drinking goal
Severe dependence	Mild or absent signs of dependence
Previous failures at controlled drinking	Recent sustained controlled drinking
Strong preference of the drinker for abstinence	Strong preference of the drinker for moderate drinking
Poorly developed capacity for self-control in other areas	Evidence of strong self-control in other areas of life
Co-occurring addictive or psychiatric disorder	Good mental health
Severe alcohol-related physical illness	Mild or no physical complications of alcohol misuse
Heavy drinking family, friends, and co-workers	Abstemious social network

Experience with recent efforts at sustained controlled drinking

A useful question for patients regarding their drinking is "Who has control, you or the alcohol?" Being able to gut out a week or two of abstinence is not control, particularly not when this dry period is followed by a weekend-long bender. Rather, control means being able to drink and not to drink when one wants and to maintain control of drinking once alcohol consumption has begun.

If within the last couple of years the patient has been able to drink in a relaxed and controlled manner continuously for 3 months or more, this may indicate that they retain a capacity for a normal style of drinking and that this capacity may now, with due care, be strengthened and extended. The evidence must, however, be approached warily. Careful questioning may reveal that this previous period of "sustained controlled drinking" was less sustained and less "controlled" than the patient at first suggested, and it may have been only a slide toward reinstatement of dependence.

Respecting a patient's realistic preference

Most patients with drinking problem would like to return to moderate drinking more than they would like to abstain. But it would be irresponsible for clinicians to agree to such an arrangement in cases where the odds of success seem low. Indeed, the clinician may justly be accused of conniving in a delusion. However, when success at moderate drinking is a realistic possibility, the preference of the patient for that goal or abstinence should be given significant weight. The golden rule for the clinician when talking through these patient choices is to be open-minded but not gullible. The clinician should also bear in mind that patient preferences can change over the course of treatment, and there is value in keeping the patient engaged in care even if the clinician harbors some modest doubts about the likelihood about the current drinking goal being achieved.

Capacity for self-control

The determined person who is good at exercising self-control in other areas of life (e.g., weight management, finances) is more likely to possess the psychological resources to succeed in drinking normally. In contrast, the individual whose life revolves around impulsive choices and is littered with half-completed projects is a poor candidate for a moderate drinking goal.

Co-occurring addictive and/or psychiatric disorders

The patient who is suffering from a psychiatric disorder – particularly a serious one – is not typically in a good position to attempt moderate drinking. Concurrent drug dependence that has not been dealt with successfully also rules out a return to safe use of alcohol. Pathological gambling may threaten maintenance of control over drinking. The euphoria of the win, the depression of the loss, or the tension associated with continuous gambling all rather easily invite a return to the heavy use of alcohol. In contrast, an individual whose sole struggle with addiction occurs in the alcohol realm and who is in generally good psychological health has a greater chance of returning to moderate drinking.

Alcohol-related physical illness

The decision in this instance must be made in relation to the actual type and degree of illness. Alcohol-related physical illness usually suggests that the patient would be wise to avoid any further drinking (permanently or at least long enough to recover) and risk of progressive tissue damage.

Drinking patterns of the social network

It is generally easier to return to moderate drinking when the individuals in one's life also drink moderately (or do not drink) than when they have a norm of heavy use. This reality should be discussed with the patient considering a moderate drinking goal, as should the eluctability of heavy drinkers in the social network; some friends, family members, and co-workers are easier to avoid than others.

Further considerations before committing to a moderate drinking goal

If a moderation goal seems a possible north star for treatment, a few other matters should be attended to before a mutual commitment is made. Each will make the process safer for the patient whether things go well or poorly.

Acknowledge the risk involved

To attempt a moderate drinking goal is to try to integrate into the patient's life a drug that has a history of being destructive and difficult to control. Furthermore, moderate drinking outcomes in problem drinkers tend to be less stable over time than does abstinence (Miller at al., 1992). Both the clinician and patient are thus taking on some risk in the venture. As in other areas of life, risks to well-being need not rule out attempting something challenging, but, for ethical reasons and for the sake of setting reasonable expectations, they should be explicitly acknowledged in advance by the parties concerned.

Adopt an experimental, honest attitude

The clinician and patient should agree up front that they will continue to evaluate the reasonableness of a moderate drinking goal as treatment progresses, becoming more or less confident in its value depending on the evidence from the patient's life. This approach is superior to committing absolutely to a moderate drinking goal up front, which may lead the patient who is unable to attain it to feel like a failure or to lie about the extent of drinking.

Consider an interval of initial abstinence

There is no evidence-based rule for whether a patient will be more likely to succeed at moderate drinking if he or she takes a few weeks off from drinking first, but the clinician and patient should always discuss this as a possible approach. For some patients, normal drinking emerges directly out of more chaotic drinking. Suddenly or gradually, the new pattern supersedes the old. Alternatively, the story may be of a shorter or longer initial period of abstinence followed by a tentative move toward moderate drinking. When drinking follows a period of sobriety, the clinician has the responsibility of working out with the patient whether this is a sadly familiar story of unguardedness and self-deception foreshadowing major relapse or whether this is indeed the evolution of re-established control.

Techniques for establishing and maintaining control

Patients are themselves often very inventive in designing ways to keep their drinking within a limit, and it is always useful to explore and encourage these personal strategies. The paragraphs that follow describe a variety of methods that may be employed (Alden, 1988; Connors, 1993; Marlatt & Gordon, 1985; Saunders, 1994).

Setting a clear, measurable goal for treatment

Almost everyone understand the term "abstinence" in the same way, but interpretations can vary across persons regarding what exactly constitutes "moderate," "normal," or "controlled" drinking. The clinician must therefore initiate a conversation about what precisely is being attempted and how treatment will support it (e.g., the patient will never drink two days in a row and will limit consumption to three drinks on drinking days; Sanchez-Craig, Wilkinson, & Davila, 1995). Such a process of careful goal-setting in itself can strengthen the therapeutic alliance and patient motivation at the same time (Kanfer & Schefft, 1988).

Limiting the type of beverage

Shifting from one type of alcoholic drink to another is often dismissed as the typical strategy of the drinker who refuses to face up to the fact that their problem lies not in the specific drink but in their relationship with any sort of alcohol – the whisky drinker who believes that "beer will be safe" is classically warned that alcohol is simply alcohol, whatever the label on the bottle. The clinician has to distinguish between self-delusion and sound strategy, but the patient who is going to effect a successful return to moderate drinking may often spontaneously discover that a change of beverage is helpful. They choose what they may term a "social drink" – beer instead of wine perhaps, or wine instead of beer, but in any case a beverage free of old associations.

Limiting the quantity and frequency of intake

The importance of strictly defining with each patient what is to count as "normal" has already been mentioned. If the patient is making their definition in terms of "a single of . . .," "a glass of . . .," or other such familiar but often rather vague measures (a "single" is a very uncertain quantity of alcohol if the patient is pouring their own drink), then properly objective measures have to be agreed.

Speed of drinking

A patient may learn to pace their drinking. This may be in terms either of not drinking faster than a slow-drinking companion or of pacing against the clock. It can also be a useful discipline to drink at least one nonalcoholic beverage between each serving of alcohol.

Motivations for drinking

The patient may discover that it is unwise for them to drink in response to mood: for instance, when they are sleep-deprived, peckish, angry, bored, or lonely. Many patients do better drinking only when they do not "need" a drink.

Circumstances and company

Just as going on a diet requires eating, becoming a moderate drinker requires alcohol consumption. In selecting where and with whom to drink, the patient should aim for those in which control has been easier to exercise in the past. For instance, the patient may decide that they will drink with their spouse on Tuesdays in the pub at the corner but will avoid the Saturday night crowd. They will stop by the pub for a quick drink with coworkers one night a week but not plant themselves alone at a hotel bar on a business trip away from home. When guests come to dinner, they will pass on pre-dinner drinks and instead wait until the meal is on the table.

Identifying "competing activities"

The client may usefully identify activities that can immediately be engaged in to prevent the risk of uncontrolled drinking. For instance, a retiree may find and plan activities that occupy otherwise lonely afternoons in which the temptation to drink heavily is strong. The retiree may decide on a simple strategy like scheduling shopping trips, visits to the grandchildren, and volunteer work to occur in the afternoon. If the dangerous circumstances that particularly invite uncontrolled drinking can thus be neutralized by a competing activity, practice in normal drinking can then be restricted to occasions when the chances of success are more real.

Individual behavioural analysis

The previous sections provide ideas about the kinds of strategies that might be suggested for any patient. Essentially, what is being learnt is self-control. It may in addition be useful to carry out an individual and more detailed behavioural analysis of the patient's drinking. The aim is to identify the circumstances in which a particular patient tends to drink excessively using recent instances and the experiences that evolve during treatment. General statements such as, "I drink when I am bored" are not to be discounted but are usually of far less value to the planning of treatment than minute analysis of the immediate antecedents and circumstances of, say, last Friday's drinking binge. The analysis identifies the *cues* that are related to excessive drinking, both in internal (mood) and external (event and situation) terms. It is necessary to form an idea of how such cues interact rather than seeing them only in isolation and to understand the sort of *pathway* that the individual is apt to move along when they indulge in excessive drinking. Such material is then used in planning the package of strategies that go to make up the individual drinking programme.

Formal cognitive behavioural treatment protocols

Heather and colleagues have described the content of moderation-oriented cue exposure and behavioural self-control training, which they found were comparably efficacious (Heather et al., 2000). As a general rule, most of the bread and butter of cognitive behavioural therapy techniques that are used to pursue a goal of abstinence are also of use when the goal is moderate drinking.

How testing should the programme be?

The patient must identify risky situations (Marlatt & Gordon, 1985), although it may then be difficult for them to avoid many of these. They may, for instance, occasionally have unusually stressful periods at a work site where heavy drinking is common among the employees. However, not only may exposure to such a risky situation be unavoidable but, for the real effectiveness of treatment, such exposure to temptation may be highly desirable. The patient should not make impossible demands on their own self-control, but the essence of treatment is that they should experience some sense of struggle, of temptation, and perhaps of craving to drink excessively, *and that temptation and craving should then be successfully resisted.* The repeated exposure to the relevant cues and the repeated resistance to an excessive drinking response extinguishes the potency of those cues. Without experience of craving there can be no long-term extinction of craving. In terms of a familiar analogy, a child who is afraid of dogs is unlikely to overcome that fear simply by avoiding all dogs. Such a normal fear is dealt with in terms of ordinary family wisdom by introducing a dog to the child and then, by praise and close support, persuading the child on this occasion to tolerate the transient anxiety and not run away.

In similar fashion, the patient who only avoids risk will probably only achieve behavioural compliance. Their drinking will be objectively within acceptable social limits, but it will still be associated with subjective unease and will be at risk of spiraling out of control if the patient gets into a situation where the old cues cannot be avoided. Subjective recovery comes about when there has been repeated exposure to cues and repeated resistance to an excessive drinking response. Treatment will, on the other hand, suffer a reverse if on too many occasions the patient does in fact drink excessively; the potency of the risky cue is confirmed rather than extinguished.

Using medications

Although alcohol-related medications are commonly thought of as supports for abstinence, those with opioid antagonist properties (see Chapter 13) may aid a return to moderate drinking when coupled with psychosocial intervention. As with the strategies just described, the goal is to use extinction to therapeutic advantage: the opiate antagonist makes alcohol consumption less rewarding, leading the patient to drink less. The UK National Institute for

Health and Care Excellence (2014) recently endorsed the use of nalmefene as a method of reducing consumption by dependent drinkers who did not need to abstain immediately; oral or injected naltrexone could serve a similar function.

Involving the partner

If the drinker has a partner, that person can support the patient's work on their problem. Partners are often accepted as a direct and useful restraining influence and – presuming the partner does not have a drinking problem – as the person within whose company normal drinking may most safely be attempted. If, however, their help is effectively to be enlisted their views should be taken into account. Treatment will be handicapped if any reservations the partner has about the patient's moderate drinking goal have not been discussed.

Seeing it through

The patient who is aiming at moderate drinking is likely to need close support and careful monitoring over some months. Technology makes this easier than it once was; patients can, for example, keep a record of daily drinking (or nondrinking) on their smartphone and/or text their clinic daily with the number of units consumed. Monitoring of progress should also involve the patient's own objective and subjective report in person at follow-up treatment sessions, and these sessions should probably be at not less than 2-week intervals. Feedback of repeat laboratory test results may be helpful with gamma-glutamyl transferase (GGT) and mean corpuscular volume (MCV) hopefully moving toward normal (see Chapter 8).

One of two alternative decisions will then at some point have to be made in the light of progress and monitoring:

Termination of successful treatment. A successful outcome may be assumed when, over the course of about 12 months, the patient has achieved both objective and subjective normality in their drinking. Judgment of success is, as ever, provisional, but at some point treatment and frequency of visits should be wound down. The patient may be left with an open invitation to return if they encounter further difficulties, or it may be wise to offer widely spaced (say 6-month) follow-up appointments and booster discussions over the next year or two. Where feasible, this could be supplemented with electronic reporting, preferably on a daily basis (e.g., over a secure website or by text).

Re-evaluation when treatment is not successful. The patient who is not making progress should not immediately and without review be told to abandon the normal drinking goal. Lack of progress is to be taken in the first instance as a matter for careful analysis of the causes of the difficulty, and, on that basis, some planned shift in the strategy may be possible. But if the patient still does not manage to progress toward their goal, there comes a moment when there is no profit in encouraging them in a frustrating and perhaps damaging pursuit of moderate drinking. They may now be persuaded by experience that it is better to opt instead for an abstinence goal, either as the short- or longer-term solution. If the clinician becomes convinced that moderate drinking efforts are failing, the reasons for this judgment and a recommendation to transition to an abstinence goal should be communicated, even if the patient would prefer to keep attempting moderate drinking.

Are outcomes other than abstinence or moderate drinking acceptable?

One common way of dividing up outcomes in the treatment of drinking problems is to use a three-category system: abstinence, return to moderate drinking, and failure. However, consider the following cases:

> Carrie is a 25-year-old single mother who was referred to an alcohol treatment programme after she presented grossly intoxicated and severely injured at the emergency room. At the time, she claimed to have fallen down a flight of stairs while drinking. In alcohol counselling, she revealed that while she indeed had a severe drinking problem, she had in fact been thrown down a flight of stairs by her violent live-in boyfriend, who had repeatedly assaulted her as well as her 5-year-old son. Her boyfriend had previously served time in prison for attempted murder and was known to police as a violent sociopath. A survivor of childhood sexual abuse, Carrie was both terrified of her boyfriend and at the same time felt unworthy of anything better in life. For the sake of Carrie and her child, the alcohol counsellor devoted himself entirely to shoring up Carrie's confidence to the point that she could move to another city with her son. She continued to drink as she had before, but she and her little boy were no longer at imminent risk of violence and death.
>
> Rinha is a 60-year-old, severely dependent store clerk who drinks a pint of vodka seven nights a week and sometimes chases it with prescription pain pills. Despite repeated, earnest efforts over a year of treatment, he is not able to string together more than 2 weeks of abstinence. But his psychiatrist continues to see him because their work together has led Rinha never to use pain pills and alcohol on the same day (thus reducing overdose risk) and has reduced Rinha's alcohol consumption to two-thirds of what it was at the beginning of treatment.
>
> Franklin is a 42-year-old man with schizophrenia and a long-established drinking problem. A social worker has repeatedly assisted him in becoming enrolled in alcohol-free recovery homes. On each occasion, he was abstinent from alcohol and actively engaged in care for his schizophrenia for 6–12 months but ultimately began drinking when his psychotic symptoms became severe, thereby leading to his ejection from the house. Yet each time she encounters Franklin in a homeless shelter, the social worker arranges another placement because she knows that while he will likely never be abstinent or free of psychiatric illness, giving up on him would likely lead to his premature death on the streets.

All three of these individuals would be better off if they became abstinent or returned to moderate drinking. Some clinicians would advocate insisting that they indeed did so as a condition of treatment, but the authors of this book would not. Sometimes there are people like Carrie and her child who face imminent, severe risks that trump the importance of trying to alter the course of drinking. Sometimes an individual simply cannot have an excellent treatment outcome but can have, like Rinha, a partial success. Sometimes an individual is so impaired that treatment becomes, as in Franklin's case, more palliative than curative in intent. Clinicians should always be wary of setting the bar for treatment success too low and thus sabotaging a patient or colluding in a patient's desire to ignore the problematic nature of his or her drinking. At the same time, when half a loaf is truly all that is available, the compassionate clinician will not be content to walk away with nothing.

References

Alden, L. (1988). Behavioral self-management: Controlled drinking strategies in a context of secondary prevention. *Journal of Consulting and Clinical Psychology*, **56**, 280–286.

Connors, G. J. (1993). Drinking moderation training as a contemporary therapeutic approach. In G. J. Connors (Ed.), *Innovations in alcoholism treatment: State of the art reviews and their implications for clinical practice* (pp. 117–134). New York: Haworth.

Edwards, G., Duckett, A., Oppenheimer, E., Sheehan, M., & Taylor, C. (1983). What happens to alcoholics? *Lancet*, **2**, 269–271.

Heather, N., Brodie, J., Wale, S., Wilkinson, G., Luce, A., Webb, E., & McCarthy, S. (2000). A randomized controlled trial of moderation-oriented cue exposure. *Journal of Studies on Alcohol*, **61**, 561–570.

Humphreys, K. (2003). A research-based analysis of the moderation management controversy. *Psychiatric Services*, **54**, 621–622.

Kanfer, F. H., & Schefft, B. K. (1988). *Guiding the process of therapeutic change*. Champaign, IL: Research Press.

Marlatt, G., & Gordon, J. (1985). *Relapse prevention*. New York: Guilford.

Miller, W. R., Leckman, A. L., Delaney, H., & Tinkcom, M. (1992). Long-term follow-up of behavioral self-control training. *Journal of Studies on Alcohol*, **53**, 249–261.

National Institute for Health and Care Excellence. (2014). *Nalmefene for reducing alcohol consumption in people with alcohol dependence* (NICE Technology Appraisal Guidance 325). London: National Institute for Health and Care Excellence.

Roizen, R. (1987). The great controlled-drinking controversy. In M. Galanter (Ed.), *Recent developments in alcoholism* (pp. 245–279). New York: Plenum.

Rosenberg, H. (1993). Prediction of controlled drinking by alcoholics and problem drinkers. *Psychological Bulletin*, **113**, 129–139.

Sanchez-Craig, M., Wilkinson, A., & Davila, R. (1995). Empirically based guidelines for moderate drinking: 1-year results from three studies with problem drinkers. *American Journal of Public Health*, **85**, 823–828.

Saunders, B. (1994). The cognitive-behavioural approach to the management of addictive behaviour. In J. Chick & R. Cantweel (Eds.), *Seminars on alcohol and drug misuse* (pp. 154–173). London: Gaskell.

Chapter 17

Managing setbacks and challenges in treatment

A novice clinician can get a false impression of how the treatment of drinking problems typically proceeds. Clinical case conferences, published case studies, and therapeutic gurus on television chat shows all tend to focus on remarkable successes rather than abject failures. This can be intimidating to inexperienced clinicians: the performance standard may seem to be a therapeutic record of unending triumphs as each patient responds beautifully to wise and well-delivered interventions.

This chapter is designed to explode such unrealistic and potentially damaging expectations. Specifically, it describes common reasons why setbacks are encountered as well as particular types of patients who pose unusual challenges in treatment (see Table 17.1). Throughout, the focus will be on how things can be put right when treatment goes wrong.

One cannot treat drinking problems without occasionally experiencing setbacks. The essence of treatment is very commonly a series of trials and errors rather than a straight-line advance. To acknowledge frankly that the best-laid treatment plans can fall apart is not a licence for complacency. Rather, it challenges clinicians to be alert to such situations and make immediate efforts to put them right.

When an effort to treat a patient with a drinking problems goes awry, clinicians must manage both the objective demands of the situation and their own subjective emotional reactions to it. This includes having the humility to seek consultation from colleagues and to accept that not everything that goes wrong in treatment can be blamed on patients: even highly skilled, highly experienced clinicians sometimes make a hash of things. A key professional development task for clinicians is to not be discouraged or defeated by clinical

Table 17.1. Setbacks and challenges in treatment

Losing the balance:

- Emphasizing the drinking/emphasizing all else
- Too ambitious/too unambitious goals
- Too indulgent/too demanding

Challenging patient types:

- The rebellious patient
- The patient from a different cultural background
- The aggressive/violent patient
- The "very important patient"
- The patient with a hidden agenda

reversals. Instead, treatment setbacks should be turned so far as possible to good therapeutic advantage and, just as importantly, should be understood as learning opportunities.

This chapter does not attempt a consideration of all possible eventualities. Anyone who has experience of this field will see ways in which the list might be extended, and a personal listing of cases where treatment was unproductive (a list kept, as it were, on mental file) is a valuable working tool.

Three common ways of losing the balance

Much of treatment is a matter of finding balances among clinical approaches, goals, and directions. Treatment can go off course when it veers toward either end of the following dimensions.

Emphasizing the drinking/emphasizing all else

In the life of a human being who has a drinking problem, alcohol is neither everything nor nothing. Accordingly, treatment should not become so exclusively focused on a patient's drinking that the complex human being doing that drinking in a multifaceted environment is overlooked, nor should sensitive awareness of a patient's total life situation result in a destructively pervasive drinking problem being minimized. Finding this balance can be difficult.

At a certain stage of learning and experience, many soft-hearted, open-minded clinicians fall into the trap of underestimating the seriousness of the drinking problem. But the admirable desire to see the whole person and to respect the complexities of that individual's life should not be put in opposition to awareness of the true threat of the drinking:

> A 44-year old man had experienced a deprived and troubled childhood. However, he reported that his adult life had been much happier, mainly due to what he described as a loving, stable marriage of 16 years. Then his wife had an affair, and his world fell to pieces. All his fearful beliefs as to the inevitability of rejection were proved to be well founded. His feelings towards his wife were unforgiving. He determined that an unhappy episode should be the occasion for catastrophe and he divorced, threw in his job, sold his house, gave up his friends, and moved to a new city. A couple of years later, he went through an emergency detoxification during a drinking bout and consequently came under the care of a psychotherapist who treated him for a year, exploring his problems relating to his mother. He frequently turned up drunk at therapy sessions, which was duly interpreted as understandable self-medication of his underlying psychodynamic conflicts. He was then admitted to a hospital after a nearly successful serious suicidal attempt. The psychiatrist who saw him on the medical ward the following morning diagnosed a severe and untreated depressive illness and started him on an antidepressant. He noted that the patient had "recently engaged in some secondary relief drinking." The evening following the first dose of the antidepressant, the patient developed an acute confusional state. One of the night nurses made the correct diagnosis of delirium tremens.

Both the psychotherapist and the psychiatrist had focused only on those aspects of this man's condition that fit comfortably within their own clinical predilections. Neither had bothered to take a drinking history. The patient never actively covered up the seriousness of his drinking because he never had to: both clinicians turned a deaf ear whenever he mentioned his alcohol use. A careful reconstruction of the history later identified a drinking problem going back to the early days of marriage. The marriage had been much affected by the husband's heavy alcohol consumption, and his wife had finally moved out because she could no longer tolerate the drinking and attendant violence. Had the drinking problem been taken more seriously by the genuinely compassionate clinicians who treated him, the patient may well have avoided significant suffering.

Clinicians can also commit the reverse error: seeing the patient as just "an alcoholic" whose every problem can be understood and treated within that definition alone. A short extract from another case history illustrates how this can occur:

> A 33-year-old construction worker had been admitted to an alcohol treatment unit, where a diagnosis of alcoholic hallucinosis was made. It was noted that he had previously been admitted to another hospital, but the other hospital's case notes were not requested because the correct diagnosis seemed obvious. The patient was put into the ward therapeutic group but seemed to spend more time listening to imaginary voices than participating. After 3 weeks, he was discharged to a hostel for people with drinking problems, which was run on intensive therapeutic community lines. He was put into a challenging group therapy session on the evening of his arrival and shortly thereafter again developed florid psychotic symptoms. This occasioned readmission to the first hospital rather than to the alcohol unit. Their case notes recorded the onset of a schizophrenic illness at the age of 17 years and many emergency readmissions since. He has since done fairly well provided he was not too stressed and could find a supportive environment. On an opportunistic basis, he engaged in binge drinking a few times a year, but otherwise rarely consumed alcohol.

The staff of the alcohol treatment unit had so specialized a perspective that when a case of schizophrenia presented to them they reacted in terms of a predetermined cognitive set. The consequent diagnosis led to a package of group therapy and confrontation for a man whose needs were quite otherwise.

These two rather extreme cases illustrate the poles of imbalance that can occur. The errors are usually on a smaller scale and more subtle. Perhaps the mass of general practitioners tend to underrate the importance of the drinking, whereas alcohol specialists sometimes overcompensate by being too alcohol-focused.

Too ambitious/too unambitious goals

Sometimes patients (or the clinician) become frustrated because they have unrealistic expectations of what changes may be achieved and at what pace. This dilemma can occur at any stage of treatment. The mistake may be that too great a therapeutic pace is being set, which can readily force the patient into breaking contact, but, equally, the problem may be in the direction of inertia:

> A 60-year-old man stopped drinking but continued to treat his wife in a curmudgeonly fashion, was at cross purposes with his grown-up children, and had no leisure activities other than watching television and grumbling about the quality of the entertainment provided. At the end of a further year, he was still sober and still regarding the world with unrelenting enmity.

What is the community psychiatric nurse to do the next time she or he calls round on this family and the man purposely turns up the volume on the television while otherwise angrily staring ahead and not acknowledging the caller's presence? The wife offers a cup of tea in the kitchen and says: "He's always been that way and I suppose he won't change – a real old misery I call him." What is the right balance of treatment ambition?

The reality may indeed be that a man of 60 who has for most of his existence defined the world as antagonistic and who has built up his self-image largely in terms of afflicted righteousness is unlikely to change his ways radically. His wife's assessment of the situation may be just about right, and she does not seem too put out by his ill-grace. Her father was much like that anyhow, and her husband's behaviour is in accord with what she expects of men. She is happy enough that he is no longer running her short of money.

Yet it seems sad to leave it at that. There is the lingering feeling that the goal is being set too low, that more happiness for two people should be possible than is seen here. The answer is perhaps to try setting a moderately more ambitious goal on a trial basis. The goal had better be expressed concretely, and the starting point must be the identification of something that patient and wife themselves at least half hint at being wanted. In this particular instance, the wife let drop, "and he never takes me on holiday of course." The "of course" was an important part of the statement; it was clear that the wife's communication with her husband often carried the implication that she expected his response to be negative. A modestly realistic goal in these circumstances was to see if this couple could go away for a week's holiday together and come home with the feeling that they had enjoyed themselves. Working at first through the wife and suggesting that she might for once expect the answer "yes" from her husband, the holiday was booked. The couple went for a week to the coast, and although the holiday provided much cause for grumbling, in sum, the week provided a real sense of shared reward. Beyond the immediate happening, a small shake-up had occurred in negative patterns of interaction, and the basis was established for the possibility of further small changes.

Clinicians can also set the bar too high for patients. Even when driven by compassion and optimism, this can have destructive effects on the therapeutic relationship:

> A 26-year old war veteran with chronic lower back pain, symptoms of post-traumatic stress disorder, and low self-esteem was treated at a veterans' medical facility for misuse of alcohol and prescribed medications (e.g., opioids and benzodiazepines). She had recently escaped homelessness but was unhappy with her shared accommodations because both of her flat mates were heavy users of alcohol and other drugs. Her counsellor, a fellow veteran and a successful Alcoholics Anonymous (AA) affiliate, urged her to commit to attending 90 AA meetings in 90 days and to giving up alcohol forever. Not wanting to disappoint her counsellor, whom she liked and respected, the patient threw herself into the endeavor, managing to stay sober for 10 days before joining in on late night drinking session with her flat mates. She woke up the next day with her confidence in her ability to recover shattered. Because she felt humiliated at the thought of having to acknowledge her drinking to her counsellor, she skipped her remaining scheduled appointments and broke off all contact with the treatment programme.

The counsellor was correct in thinking that the patient's life would have been improved by lifetime abstinence, but he established with little consultation that this would be the first goal of treatment. He was well-intended, yet set his patient up for failure. A smaller initial goal, for example, finding a place to live that would not result in constant temptations to drink or ceasing to use the potentially lethal combination of alcohol, opioids, and benzodiazepines on the same days would have been more attainable. Furthermore, such a smaller success would likely have strengthened the patient's battered self-confidence and the therapeutic alliance, both of which could become the foundation from which to pursue more ambitious goals as treatment progressed.

Too indulgent/too demanding

In the therapeutic relationship, clinicians must find a balance between being, on the one hand, supportive and nonjudgmental and, on the other, being tough-minded and confronting the patient with manifestly unpleasant realities. To put the matter in terms of absolutes and contradictions is an oversimplification, but consider two contrasting examples. First, imbalance in the direction of indulgence:

> A social worker of rather little professional experience became highly committed to helping a struggling family. The 30-year-old man was not alcohol dependent, but seemed to use drink to enhance his passivity and incompetence. He seldom worked. He borrowed, pawned, and stole. The wife, who was faced with this chronically difficult situation, tried to prop up the family as best she could. When the social worker arrived on the scene, she soon became no more than a provider of gifts, and she protected the man from the consequence of his having cheated on welfare payments. She found him good second-hand clothes so that he could go for a job interview, and when he sold the clothes and did not go to the interview she treated him as an amusingly naughty child.

The social worker was operating on the hypothesis that this patient was deprived and was testing out her "goodness"; she believed that she "must not reject him." Where she may have gone wrong is in her assumption that the opposite to rejection is indulgence.

The following case of an "unmotivated" patient illustrates the other extreme of the indulgent versus demanding continuum:

> A man with a serious drinking problem was to be discharged from prison and it had been agreed in principle that he should then be admitted to an alcohol rehabilitation unit. In the event, the Consultant in charge of the treatment unit decided that, "as a test of sincerity," the man would first be required to find himself lodgings and gainful employment. Coming out of prison after 4 years, the man was anxious, disoriented, and lacking any meaningful familial attachments. He made his way to old friends and resumed drinking within hours of his release. A few days later, he was arrested for drunk and disorderly conduct. The Consultant expressed to her staff the hope that they, too, would someday acquire her talent for being able to sense when a potential patient "just wasn't ready to change."

Five specific types of patients who pose challenges for clinicians

The preceding discussion of balancing emphases in treatment applies to all patients. We now turn to specific types of patients who challenge clinicians to manage treatment with particular care.

The rebellious patient

CLINICIAN: So, how did this week go?

PATIENT (SMILING): You will be happy to know that I didn't get pissed on Wednesday. That was the exception to the rule this week. Sorry doc!

CLINICIAN: I'm disappointed to hear that. I thought I had been pretty clear about the effect drinking is having on your family.

PATIENT: Well, I have other things to worry about.

CLINICIAN: Your family is understandably very concerned about you. What can we do to make this next week your first week of sobriety?

PATIENT (LOOKS AT DEGREE ON WALL): Did they train you to say that at Michigan State University?

CLINICIAN: It's an excellent university.

PATIENT: Yeah, I can just feel myself getting better every time I see you.

The dynamics of this unpleasant exchange may resonate with parents of adolescents. In the treatment of alcohol problems, adolescents come in all ages. For rebellious patients, treatment is a power struggle in which they demonstrate their autonomy by continuing to drink or otherwise violate agreements made with the clinician. Some rebellious patients go further, for example, by degrading the clinician's authority, blaming the clinician for their own decisions, and otherwise trying to "get the clinician's goat."

As described in Chapter 14, AA teaches that its members are powerless over alcohol, a difficult message for many to accept. For their part, clinicians must accept a different sort of powerlessness: fundamentally, they cannot control the lives of their patients. When patients make efforts to show the clinician who is ultimately in charge, the clinician should refuse the offer of a power struggle and instead agree that treatment cannot progress if the patient doesn't wish it to. The clinician is a partner in the change process, but the fundamental responsibility for the patient must always rest with the patient. Clinicians should neither fight to take that responsibility away nor accept it if the patient tries to throw that existential burden onto them. From this sensibility, the same interaction is handled not as a contest of wills but as an immediate, nondefensive acknowledgement of the limits of therapeutic control.

CLINICIAN: So, how did this week go?

PATIENT (SMILING): You will be happy to know that I didn't get drunk on Wednesday. That was the exception to the rule this week. Sorry doc!

CLINICIAN: Whether I am happy with your drinking is not important. If you are happy with your drinking as it is, it's your right to go on exactly as you are. But if you wish to make a change, we can talk about ways that we could work together towards that. So please tell me your decision: do you want your drinking this coming week to be like your drinking last week or not?

A patient from a different cultural background than the clinician

"I don't understand him at all," said the community psychiatric nurse who was reporting on a visit to her patient's home. "He's a Pakistani man who owns a fruit shop, aged about 60, very much the head of the family, with two grown-up sons who help in the business and take orders from their father. He and his wife have only a rather poor understanding of English. He has a bottle of whisky at the back of the shop, and he swigs at it steadily throughout the day. When I went round, I was treated with kindness, loaded with presents of fruit, and met with massive denial. He says that he uses a little whisky now and then for medicine."

The nurse had the openness to admit that she did not understand this patient's cultural position, and no doubt the shopkeeper was flummoxed as to the role, credentials, and purpose of this person whom his doctor had asked to call.

The cultural meaning of the drinking itself can be puzzling. What does "normal" drinking mean within a particular culture, and how are religious prohibitions in practice interpreted? What are the legitimate functions of alcohol? What are the culturally determined ideas that define "drinking too much?" Are men and women held to similar or different expectations for drinking behaviour? The questions that relate to difficulties in understanding the drinking itself constitute only a small part of the total cross-cultural puzzle. The essential background issues comprise family and family roles, religion, social class and status, and who has a right to say what to whom (Galvan & Caetano, 2003; Heim et al., 2004; Lee, Law, & Eunjoo, 2003; Rao, 2006). Different cultures will also carry different assumptions as to what constitutes "treatment," the primacy given to the prescription of medicines, or the degree of directiveness that is expected.

The case of the shopkeeper is one example of the many and varied cross-cultural problems in understanding that can be met whatever the country in which the clinician is practising. The presentation may be the recently immigrated family, the postgraduate student from abroad, the immigrant labourer, the refugee, or the patient of the clinician's own culture but with a different regional or social class identity. Alcohol treatment agencies and clinicians who are not alert to ethnic and cultural differences risk making clumsy, disrespectful, and even destructive interventions.

Every such case has to be seen as an exercise in building bridges. With the fruit-shop owner it may, for instance, be possible to find a second-generation member of the family who can be a broker in understanding. The patient's son may identify the key figures within the extended family network that have a right to advise and intervene. It may also be possible to find a professional within the local agencies or hospitals who speaks the patient's native language, understands the culture, and who can help with an assessment or perhaps take over the case.

The aggressive/violent patient

A subset of patients with drinking problems will present as chronically brimming with rage. They engage in explosive rants about friends, family, and co-workers and may also raise their voice in harsh criticism when encountering any frustrations with the clinician, administrative staff, or other patients in the waiting room. Such behaviour can be an established and comfortable interpersonal style, a failed struggle for emotional self-control, or a considered tactic adopted to bully others into submission.

Being a patient in need is not a licence to abuse other people, and this expectation should be clearly conveyed to all patients in a matter-of-fact fashion. When faced with a pattern of seething anger and verbal aggression, the clinician should assess both the patient's history (e.g., any record of assaults on staff or incarcerations for violent crimes) and the function of the aggressive behaviour for the patient. Aggressive patients with some capacity for insight can often be productively engaged in an analysis of what drives and reinforces their behaviour and also what adverse effects it has on other people and the patient as well.

Some problem drinkers move beyond threatening verbal behaviour to physical violence (see Chapter 4). Every now and then, a clinician will be faced by the worrying problem set by the patient who repeatedly turns up drunk and violent and demands to be seen. The safety of staff and other patients may be at risk, and an enormous amount of anxiety can be engendered. If an alcohol treatment service is coexisting closely with other facilities, it will acquire a bad name if disruption is allowed to get out of hand:

> A 40-year-old man, after a long drinking history, had been thrown out of his home and was now drifting around temporary accommodation or sleeping rough. Over a period of 6 months, he was twice admitted to a hospital but, on each occasion, he came back drunk onto the ward, assaulted the nurses, and smashed the furniture. A few days after his last discharge, he came up to the hospital late at night and got into a fight with an orderly. He then arrived at the outpatient clinic drunk and demanding admission, with threats of further violence if admission was not granted.

In such circumstances, two courses of action are anti-therapeutic and should not be followed. The first of these is to tolerate further violence or the threat of violence. The patient will not be helped, the morale of the treatment service will be torn apart, and staff may indeed be hurt. The second non-answer is to ban the patient from the hospital. Even if the banning is successful, it will only transfer the problem of violence onto someone else's doorstep, and things will not look too good if a week later the man is on an assault charge with the court told that a hospital had abrogated its responsibilities. The principle guiding the therapeutic response to this kind of patient is the realization that violence is often triggered by contextual cues that provoke that reaction (Graham et al., 1998).

Such a problem is dealt with more easily by a treatment service than by anyone working in isolation. A hospital, for instance, ought to be able to meet this type of problem, and the general practitioner and other local services will not be grateful if the hospital seeks to pass the buck. What is needed is a firm treatment policy drawn up for the individual, one that sets explicit limits but that, nonetheless, is a treatment rather than a mere containment policy (see Table 17.2). It must reward constructive behaviour and in no way reinforce unacceptable behaviour, and it must be communicated fairly and openly to the patient themselves, put at the front of the case notes (or prominently in the electronic record), and a copy given

Table 17.2. An example of an agreed treatment plan for a violent patient (Mr. Smith)

So that we can go on helping this patient within a treatment programme, the following guidelines have been agreed by the treatment team, and we would be grateful if everyone will give this plan support.

1. Mr Smith will only be seen by appointment, and if he comes up without an appointment he should be asked to leave.
2. He will then only be seen at the appointment if he is not intoxicated. If there is any suspicion of intoxication, he will be asked to leave without being seen further.
3. If Mr Smith refuses to leave when asked, or if he threatens or offers violence, help should be summoned through the hospital's usual emergency system and the police should be telephoned. The number is ... and the police station has been alerted. On no account should an individual staff member attempt to argue with this patient.
4. Mr Smith has been told that if he commits any chargeable offence on the hospital premises, the hospital will not hesitate to press charges.
5. These ground rules have been explained to Mr Smith personally, and they have been set up not only to protect the staff but also to make it possible for us to go on working with this patient within a constructive treatment plan.

to the patient and to all staff who may be involved. It is useful to hold a staff meeting for formulation of the care plan so that things go forward by agreement, with everyone fully in the picture. It may be wise to ensure that the treatment centre administrative staff are consulted and supported and a legal opinion obtained if necessary.

Contained within Table 17.2's seemingly flinty guidelines is a plan designed to enable the team to go on offering help to a man who would probably be rejected by many centres as unhelpable. In practice, this drawing of limits is reassuring to the patient himself. A disorganized and inconsistent response, which may even involve a sort of complicity with his violence, is likely to exacerbate anxiety and aggression, whereas a firm policy often results in the patient showing a capacity to go along with constructive expectations. They are able to come to appointments sober and make a new and positive therapeutic engagement. Things do not, however, always run smoothly, and if the patient does turn up drunk and tries to hit someone, a charge may have to be brought, for otherwise no learning can take place. To be able to use the police in support of the treatment plan requires careful liaison.

With the immediate threat of violence contained, it should be possible to get down to an individually planned and positive treatment programme. Violence is then no longer the central issue, and the patient's reputation should not be allowed to overshadow therapeutic dealings. There will be need to talk about the violence, and the patient has to come to terms with the full implications of the fact that alcohol increases his propensity for violence.

Another problem is how the stated rules are to be interpreted flexibly in certain difficult circumstances. For instance, if there is anxiety about the possibility of head injury, deterioration in the patient's physical condition, or concern as to whether underlying mental illness is now hidden within the picture, appropriate help should be obtained. Therefore, there has to be an understanding that individual clinical judgment allows a flexible response to an emergency, but the team should, whenever possible, be brought into the decision or promptly informed as to what has been done. There are some patients who pose extreme dangers of violence, and staff and public safety should then be the paramount consideration without prevarication or apology.

The "very important patient"

Frequently, and despite every supposed personal advantage, the man or woman with a large public reputation is the person whose alcohol problem is mishandled. Because of the aura of prestige, no-one quite dares make the diagnosis or take a firm line. Phone calls are made in the middle of the night, and a quick visit is demanded to a hotel room. Instead of a full history, there is a superficial and interrupted conversation, and everything is a whispering game. The clinician may need considerable confidence to stand their ground when dealing with the demands and expectations of the tycoon, the politician, the famous actress, the judge, or the distinguished surgeon. Matters become only more intimidating if the patient is eminent in the clinician's own ambit: a respected Professor at the same university, the director of a local hospital, or a senior official in the National Health Service. But unless the clinician is willing to hold to a therapeutic position, their patient will not be well served.

Paradoxically, the rich and famous may be as much at hazard of receiving inadequate treatment as the drinker on skid row. The fundamental risk to quality care is for the clinician to become dazzled by the patient and his or her lifestyle. Conversation becomes directed not to where it is maximally effective, but where it is the most fascinating for the clinician. Excuses for continued drinking (e.g., "You know what these Hollywood parties are like...")

are accepted that would never serve with the typical patient. Needed therapeutic confrontations are avoided because the clinician wants to be liked by such an eminent individual or because the clinician knows that the person is used to flattery and will react unusually aggressively or defensively to candid words. In some settings, there may also be institutional pressures on the clinician to coddle the patient (e.g., "Don't make him angry, his mother is a major philanthropic supporter of the hospital"). Clinicians may also be tempted to forget their ethical commitments and find subtle ways to let colleagues and friends suspect that they are the savior of a famous patient.

In a few respects, VIPs are indeed different, most particularly in that they have legitimately greater fear of wide public exposure if they, for example, have to walk into an alcohol treatment agency off a busy street or if they attend group therapy with other patients who might gossip. A dockworker in alcohol treatment is not fodder for the media, but a Member of Parliament is. That said, famous patients often underestimate the extent to which their drinking habits are already public knowledge and a known embarrassment to their colleagues. News that they are getting help can do more good than harm. The extent to which it is possible for someone in an important position to admit publicly that they have had to deal with a drinking problem varies from country to country and across professions but has clearly lessened in recent years due to the rise of the international "recovery movement" (White, 2007).

So much for a brief consideration of what may be "special." It must, however, be obvious that what has been instanced as "special" could be turned around and argued the other way. There is nothing unique about the fear of public exposure, and it may affect the driver of the company car as well as the company president, whereas stress and fear of failure are common themes whatever the stratum from which patients are drawn. Although it is necessary to be alert to the intensity and clustering of certain factors that affect the "special" patient, one is soon brought back to the need to hold onto the basics of the therapeutic approach. A full assessment must, for instance, be carried out, rather than the argument accepted that the patient is too busy for proper time to be given to this task. The formulation has to be discussed, the diagnosis agreed on, and goals appropriately set. And, as always, the quality of the relationship is fundamental. At one level, the encounter may be between public figure and psychiatrist or counsellor, but, more fundamentally, it is between a human being with a drinking problem and a person seeking, as best possible, to offer help.

The patient with a hidden agenda

A middle-aged man with a long-standing drinking problem presents for behavioural marital therapy with his wife. Both aver that they want to work together to end the drinking and thereby save the marriage. A month into treatment, after a therapeutic alliance has been formed, the wife shocks her husband (and the clinician) with this: "I've filed for divorce. I'm sick of trying, and I've been sick of it for years. I just wanted to get you with a doctor who could take care of you before I walked out because I know you need the help."

Patients enter alcohol treatment for myriad reasons, not all of which may be revealed at intake or even long after. Obtaining objective evidence of "doing something about the drinking" may be desired by the patient who is awaiting court trial for drink-driving (drunk-driving) or is in a divorce custody battle with an embittered ex-spouse. An actual desire to change drinking behaviour may or may not coexist with such ulterior motives. Other patients may pursue alcohol treatment in order to generate a record of real or manufactured ills (e.g., drinking, depression, suicidal impulses) that will prove useful in a lawsuit or disability claim.

A different type of patient may attempt to manipulate the clinician into providing regular absolution that removes internal pressure to change. Intellectually, they know what suffering they are causing to themselves and others, but they are able to divorce this insight from any deep feelings provided they are given repeated doses of forgiveness. They are, in fact, seeking the therapist's connivance as actor in a repetitive and unproductive play. Here is a case extract that illustrates one such presentation:

> The patient settled into a chair and said that he knew he was an "alcoholic," had been going to AA for years, and knew that all he now had to do was to get through one day without drink. His wife was threatening to leave him, and, after this last "slip" and all that she had been through, he entirely saw her point of view and did not blame her in the least. He was most dreadfully sorry and knew that he had behaved "like a swine." Furthermore, he had let the doctor down again and was thoroughly ashamed of himself. He had said exactly the same thing on many occasions with a similar show of contrition coupled with detachment from real feeling.

Things go wrong if the clinician falls into the position of aiding and abetting this cycle of behaviour. Such a story is not uncommon, and the patient may sometimes be a long-term AA attendee who has managed to get little out of AA. For the clinician to continue contact on this nontherapeutic or anti-therapeutic basis is useless. It is more helpful to redirect the responsibility back on the patient and refuse to be the confessor. An element of challenge and confrontation may produce new possibilities, but there is always the risk that the patient will instead go off and find another therapist who will at least temporarily provide the absolutions.

With all patients who have a hidden agenda, clinicians may find themselves feeling angry, duped, or even abused. These understandable reactions are entirely appropriate to disclose to supportive colleagues but should never be used to justify punitive conduct toward the patient. Even if the proper course is to terminate treatment, this should be implemented in a calm, professional manner free of recrimination.

A few words about medical negligence

We cannot close a chapter on clinical challenges without mentioning that it is not unknown for a doctor treating a drinking problem to find him- or herself facing an action for negligence. At the extreme, there may be risk of action for medical malpractice. This is a difficult area of practice, but that does not excuse practitioners from the inalienable responsibility to deliver high-quality care. As ever, the practitioner's best defence is to ensure that their treatment is of a kind and quality that would be seen as reasonable good practice by their peers. Scrupulous attention to note keeping and letter writing is important. When a patient poses the danger of self-harm or harm to others, in addition to the good medical practice of fully recording the consultation on file and discussing it with a colleague, it may also be good to seek a medico-legal opinion as well.

Here is a list of the kind of problems that good practice will in this arena seek most strenuously to avoid:

- Adverse outcomes of risky prescribing; for example, a heavy drinking patient overdosing after receiving a large supply of benzodiazepines and/or opioid pain medication is a not uncommon cause for legal action.

- Failure of an emergency room doctor to diagnose and immediately treat incipient Wernicke's encephalopathy may lead to brain damage for the patient and enormous legal damages against the hospital and doctor.
- Failure of a general hospital ward to deal adequately with withdrawal and to maintain a safe environment (see Chapter 11) may see staff held responsible for a tragedy.
- Careless prescribing of disulfiram can lead to dangerous interactions with alcohol.

None of these types of accident should ever be allowed to happen, but unfortunately these accidents still continue to occur, proof that, in every medical setting, enhanced alertness and better training on drinking problems are required.

Managing when setbacks are encountered

This chapter has reviewed some potentially intimidating and anxiety-provoking aspects of the treatment of drinking problems. But this should not reduce optimism about a disorder that has a far higher rate of recovery than most chronic health problems that come to the attention of clinicians. This is in part because many strategies exist for righting the course of treatment when it goes wrong (see Table 17.3)

Treating the person with a drinking problem is about moving that individual by every available strategy toward alliance with his or her own recovery. The richest arena for learning is the actuality of contact, the experience of things sometimes going wrong, and the discovery that, with patience, flexibility, and mutual effort, things often very happily come right.

Every individual and team should explore the question of how, within their practice circumstances, they are going to address problems positively and effectively to help the patient through and ensure that they themselves learn in the process. Younger and more experienced clinicians have needs in this regard, and male and female staff members may at times need different kinds of support. The sharing of problems rather than a drift to isolation is vital, and the availability for staff support of an experienced clinician from outside the team can be valuable. There should be an open and unashamed willingness to see oneself as having needs rather than yielding to the destructive belief that one can endlessly give without being given to.

Table 17.3. The positive therapeutic response to clinical setbacks

- Problems should be shared. Talk through the situation with a colleague.
- Problems can be two-way. Try to understand your own behaviour, attitudes, and expectations as well as those of the patient.
- Identify blocks – in particular the therapeutic approach losing its balance.
- Motivation is essential to change – does further work need to be done on readiness to change?
- Check back on the original assessment and formulation, review the case, and get a purposive plan in place – with the patient participating – to recover the therapeutic motivation.
- Remember, no-one is omnipotent, and clinicians have rightful needs.

References

Galvan, F. H., & Caetano, R. (2003). Alcohol use and related problems among ethnic minorities in the United States. *Alcohol Health and Research World*, **27**, 87–94.

Graham, K., Leonard, K. E., Room, R., et al. (1998). Current directions in research on understanding and preventing intoxicated aggression. *Addiction*, **93**, 659–676.

Heim, D., Hunter, S. C., Ross, A. J., Bakshi, N., Davies, J. B., Flatley, K. J., & Meer, N. (2004).

Alcohol consumption, perceptions of community responses and attitudes to service provision: results from a survey of Indian, Chinese and Pakistani young people in greater Glasgow. *Alcohol and Alcoholism*, **39**, 220–226.

Lee, M. Y., Law, P. F. M., & Eunjoo, E. (2003). Perception of substance use problems in Asian American communities by Chinese, Indian, Korean and Vietnamese populations. *Journal of Ethnicity in Substance Abuse*, **2**, 1–30.

Rao, R. (2006). Alcohol misuse and ethnicity. *British Medical Journal*, **332**, 682.

White, W. (2007). The new recovery advocacy movement in America. *Addiction*, **102**, 696–703.

Epilogue

Griffith Edwards began writing the first edition of this book almost a half-century ago, and the treatment of drinking problems has in some respects changed enormously since then. Treatment is much more commonly provided in the community rather than the hospital. The clinical focus on highly dependent, severely impaired alcoholics has been expanded to include problem drinkers with less severe but still significant problems. Female patients, once an uncommon sight in alcohol treatment, are now a significant portion of clinical caseloads. New medications and psychotherapies provide different options for clinicians engaged in face-to-face care with patients, and new Internet technologies provide treatment options that don't involve face-to-face care at all. These and other changes are reflected in the pages you have just read.

Yet certain essentials of the treatment enterprise have remained constant through the years and will do so in the future. The case for treatment remains a humanitarian one: the goal is to reduce the suffering of struggling human beings and those around them. And, regardless of which techniques described in this book are employed, the heart of treatment will always be an empathic, respectful human relationship that motivates and facilitates lasting change. The authors will be very pleased if their book helps those engaged in the treatment of drinking problems form such relationships with patients and apply the evidence-based therapeutic techniques that can restore health, promote public safety, and transform lives.

Index